PREVENTING MEDICATION ERRORS

Committee on Identifying and Preventing Medication Errors

Board on Health Care Services

Philip Aspden, Julie A. Wolcott, J. Lyle Bootman, Linda R. Cronenwett,
Editors

INSTITUTE OF MEDICINE
OF THE NATIONAL ACADEMIES

THE NATIONAL ACADEMIES PRESS
Washington, DC
www.nap.edu

THE NATIONAL ACADEMIES PRESS   500 Fifth Street, N.W.   Washington, DC 20001

NOTICE: The project that is the subject of this report was approved by the Governing Board of the National Research Council, whose members are drawn from the councils of the National Academy of Sciences, the National Academy of Engineering, and the Institute of Medicine. The members of the committee responsible for the report were chosen for their special competences and with regard for appropriate balance.

This study was supported by Contract No. HHSM-500-2004-00020C between the National Academy of Sciences and Department of Health and Human Services (Centers for Medicare and Medicaid Services). Any opinions, findings, conclusions, or recommendations expressed in this publication are those of the author(s) and do not necessarily reflect the view of the organizations or agencies that provided support for this project.

Library of Congress Cataloging-in-Publication Data

Preventing medication errors / Committee on Identifying and Preventing Medication Errors, Board on Health Care Services ; Philip Aspden ... [et al.], editors.
    p. ; cm. — (Quality chasm series)
  Includes bibliographical references and index.
  ISBN-13: 978-0-309-10147-9 (hardcover)
  ISBN-10: 0-309-10147-6 (hardcover)
  1. Medication errors—Prevention. I. Aspden, Philip. II. Institute of Medicine (U.S.). Committee on Identifying and Preventing Medication Errors. III. Series.
    [DNLM: 1. Medication Errors—prevention & control—United States. 2. Safety Management—United States. QZ 42 P9435 2006]
  RM146.P744 2006
  615'.6—dc22
                                        2006029215

Additional copies of this report are available from the National Academies Press, 500 Fifth Street, N.W., Lockbox 285, Washington, DC 20055; (800) 624-6242 or (202) 334-3313 (in the Washington metropolitan area); Internet, http://www.nap.edu.

For more information about the Institute of Medicine, visit the IOM home page at: **www.iom.edu.**

The serpent has been a symbol of long life, healing, and knowledge among almost all cultures and religions since the beginning of recorded history. The serpent adopted as a logotype by the Institute of Medicine is a relief carving from ancient Greece, now held by the Staatliche Museen in Berlin.

*"Knowing is not enough; we must apply.
Willing is not enough; we must do."*
—Goethe

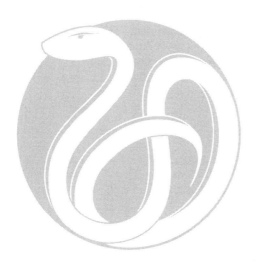

INSTITUTE OF MEDICINE
OF THE NATIONAL ACADEMIES

Advising the Nation. Improving Health.

THE NATIONAL ACADEMIES
Advisers to the Nation on Science, Engineering, and Medicine

The **National Academy of Sciences** is a private, nonprofit, self-perpetuating society of distinguished scholars engaged in scientific and engineering research, dedicated to the furtherance of science and technology and to their use for the general welfare. Upon the authority of the charter granted to it by the Congress in 1863, the Academy has a mandate that requires it to advise the federal government on scientific and technical matters. Dr. Ralph J. Cicerone is president of the National Academy of Sciences.

The **National Academy of Engineering** was established in 1964, under the charter of the National Academy of Sciences, as a parallel organization of outstanding engineers. It is autonomous in its administration and in the selection of its members, sharing with the National Academy of Sciences the responsibility for advising the federal government. The National Academy of Engineering also sponsors engineering programs aimed at meeting national needs, encourages education and research, and recognizes the superior achievements of engineers. Dr. Wm. A. Wulf is president of the National Academy of Engineering.

The **Institute of Medicine** was established in 1970 by the National Academy of Sciences to secure the services of eminent members of appropriate professions in the examination of policy matters pertaining to the health of the public. The Institute acts under the responsibility given to the National Academy of Sciences by its congressional charter to be an adviser to the federal government and, upon its own initiative, to identify issues of medical care, research, and education. Dr. Harvey V. Fineberg is president of the Institute of Medicine.

The **National Research Council** was organized by the National Academy of Sciences in 1916 to associate the broad community of science and technology with the Academy's purposes of furthering knowledge and advising the federal government. Functioning in accordance with general policies determined by the Academy, the Council has become the principal operating agency of both the National Academy of Sciences and the National Academy of Engineering in providing services to the government, the public, and the scientific and engineering communities. The Council is administered jointly by both Academies and the Institute of Medicine. Dr. Ralph J. Cicerone and Dr. Wm. A. Wulf are chair and vice chair, respectively, of the National Research Council.

www.national-academies.org

WILSON D. PACE, Professor of Family Medicine and Green-Edelman Chair for Practice-based Research, University of Colorado; Director, American Academy of Family Physicians National Research Network

KATHLEEN R. STEVENS, Professor and Director, Academic Center for Evidence-Based Practice, University of Texas Health Science Center, San Antonio

EDWARD WESTRICK, Vice President of Medical Management, University of Massachusetts Memorial Health Care

ALBERT W. WU, Professor of Health Policy and Management and Internal Medicine, The Johns Hopkins University

Health Care Services Board

CLYDE J. BEHNEY, Acting Director (June 2005 to December 2005 and from May 2006)

JOHN C. RING, Director (from December 2005 to May 2006)

JANET M. CORRIGAN, Director (September 2004 to May 2005)

ANTHONY BURTON, Administrative Assistant

Study Staff

PHILIP ASPDEN, Study Director

JULIE A. WOLCOTT, Program Officer (to April 2006)

ANDREA M. SCHULTZ, Research Associate (from June 2006)

RYAN L. PALUGOD, Research Assistant (from December 2005)

TASHARA BASTIEN, Senior Program Assistant (to January 2006)

WILLIAM B. MCLEOD, Senior Librarian

GARY J. WALKER, Senior Financial Officer (from December 2005)

TERESA REDD, Financial Advisor (to December 2005)

ELIZABETH E. LAFALCE, Intern (April to May, 2005)

Reviewers

This report has been reviewed in draft form by individuals chosen for their diverse perspectives and technical expertise, in accordance with procedures approved by the NRC's Report Review Committee. The purpose of this independent review is to provide candid and critical comments that will assist the institution in making its published report as sound as possible and to ensure that the report meets institutional standards for objectivity, evidence, and responsiveness to the study charge. The review comments and draft manuscript remain confidential to protect the integrity of the deliberative process. We wish to thank the following individuals for their review of this report:

LOWELL ANDERSON, Watauga Corporation
MARGE BOWMAN, University of Pennsylvania Health System
PATRICIA FLATLEY BRENNAN, School of Nursing and College of Engineering, University of Wisconsin-Madison
DAVID COUSINS, National Patient Safety Organization, London
DON E. DETMER, American Medical Informatics Association and The University of Virginia
WILLIAM EVANS, St. Jude Children's Research Hospital, Memphis
ANN HENDRICH, Ascension Health, St. Louis, MO
CRAIG HOESLEY, University Hospital, University of Alabama at Birmingham
WILLIAM J. KOOPMAN, Department of Medicine, University of Alabama at Birmingham
GERALD D. LAUBACH, Pfizer Inc., Past President

LUCIAN LEAPE, Department of Health Policy and Management, Harvard School of Public Health
ART LEVIN, Center for Medical Consumers, New York, NY
G. STEVE REBAGLIATI, Department of Emergency Medicine, Oregon Health and Sciences University
HUGH TILSON, School of Public Health, University of North Carolina

Although the reviewers listed above have provided many constructive comments and suggestions, they were not asked to endorse the conclusions or recommendations nor did they see the final draft of the report before its release. The review of this report was overseen by **Paul F. Griner,** University of Rochester, Professor Emeritus and **Charles E. Phelps,** University of Rochester. Appointed by the National Research Council and Institute of Medicine, they were responsible for making certain that an independent examination of this report was carried out in accordance with institutional procedures and that all review comments were carefully considered. Responsibility for the final content of this report rests entirely with the authoring committee and the institution.

Preface

In 2000, the Institute of Medicine (IOM) report *To Err Is Human: Building a Safer Health System* raised awareness about medical errors and accelerated existing efforts to prevent such errors. The present report makes clear that with regard to medication errors, we still have a long way to go. The current medication-use process, which encompasses prescribing, dispensing, administering, and monitoring, is characterized by many serious problems and issues that threaten both the safety and positive outcomes of the process. Each of the steps in the process needs improvement and further study.

At the beginning of the medication-use process, prescribers often lack sufficient knowledge about how the drugs they are prescribing will work in specific patient populations. If the balance of medication risks and benefits is not known (as is common, for example, with children and the elderly), it is impossible to say whether medication use is safe. Improving medication use and reducing errors, therefore, requires improving the quality of information generated by the pharmaceutical industry and other researchers regarding drug products and their use in clinical practice. We also need to better understand how to communicate such information to clinicians and patients via packaging, leaflets, and health information technology systems. Lastly, we need to understand how better to prevent medication errors in all care settings and in transitions between care settings. In this report, the IOM Committee on Identifying and Preventing Medication Errors proposes a research agenda for industry and government that can help meet these critical needs.

Despite the lack of data regarding many interventions that might improve the quality and safety of medication use, the committee offers recommendations for change that should be implemented and evaluated. People who use medications to meet their health care needs have a huge stake in that effort. The most powerful strategy for improving safety may be motivating providers and organizations to support the full engagement of patients and surrogates in improving the safety of medication use. In addition, providers and leaders of health care organizations must create the climate and infrastructure necessary to continuously learn about and improve the safety of all steps in the medication-use process. This report provides guidance on the types of error prevention strategies that should be implemented in each care setting. It also presents the committee's recommendations for the pharmaceutical industry, government, and regulatory, certification, and accreditation bodies, each of which has a role to play in improving the quality and safety of medication use.

This report represents the culmination of the dedicated efforts of three groups of people. We would like to thank our fellow committee members who have worked long and diligently on this challenging study, the many experts who provided formal testimony to the committee and informal advice throughout the study, and the staff of the Health Care Services Board who managed the study and coordinated the writing of the final report.

J. Lyle Bootman, Ph.D., Sc.D.
Linda R. Cronenwett, Ph.D., M.A., R.N.
Cochairs
July 2006

Acknowledgments

The Committee on Identifying and Preventing Medication Errors wishes to acknowledge the many people whose contributions and support made this report possible. The committee benefited from presentations made by a number of experts over the past 2 years. The following individuals shared their research, experience, and perspectives with the committee: Tom Abrams, Food and Drug Administration; Bruce Bagley, American Academy of Family Physicians; Robert Ball, Food and Drug Administration; Jim Battles, Agency for Healthcare Research and Quality; Karen Bell, Centers for Medicare and Medicaid Services; Douglas Bierer, Consumer Healthcare Products Association; David Bowen, Office of Senator Edward Kennedy; Bill Braithwaite, eHealth Initiative; Dan Budnitz, Centers for Disease Control and Prevention; Betsy Chrischilles, University of Iowa; John Clarke, ECRI; David Classen, First Consulting Group; Ilene Corina, Patients United Limiting Substandards and Errors in Healthcare; Diane Cousins, U.S. Pharmacopeial Convention; Loriann De Martini, California Department of Health Services; Noel Eldridge, Veterans Health Administration; Frank Federico, Institute for Healthcare Improvement; Susan Frampton, Planetree; David Gustafson, University of Wisconsin; Ed Hammond, Duke University; Mark Hayes, Office of Senator Chuck Grassley; Carol Holquist, Food and Drug Administration; David Hunt, Centers for Medicare and Medicaid Services; Gordon Hunt, Sutter Health; John Jenkins, Food and Drug Administration; Mike Kafrissen, Johnson & Johnson; Ken Kizer, National Quality Forum; Richard Moore, Massachusetts State Senator; Bill Munier, Agency for Healthcare Research and Quality; Dianne Murphy, Food and Drug Administration; Steve Northrop, Office of Senator Chuck Grassley; Jerry

Osheroff, Micromedex; Emily Patterson, Ohio State University; John Reiling, Synergy Health and St. Joseph's Hospital; Lisa Robin, Federation of State Medical Boards; William Rollow, Centers for Medicare and Medicaid Services; Jeffrey Rothschild, Brigham and Women's Hospital Partners Healthcare; Lee Rucker, American Association of Retired Persons; Luke Sato, Harvard Risk Management Foundation; Stephen Schondelmeyer, University of Minnesota; David Schulke, American Health Quality Association; Paul Schyve, Joint Commission on Accreditation of Healthcare Organizations; Paul Seligman, Food and Drug Administration; Vickie Sheets, National Council of State Boards of Nursing; Pat Sodomka, Medical College of Georgia; Scott Stanley, University Health System Consortium; Jonathan Teich, Health Vision; Anne Trontell, Food and Drug Administration; Tim Vanderveen, Alaris & Cardinal Health; and Ed Weisbart, Express Scripts.

The following individuals were important sources of information, generously giving their time and knowledge to further the committee's efforts: Michele Boisse, American Society for Clinical Pharmacology and Therapeutics; Anne Burns, American Pharmacists Association; Francis Dobscha, Advance Med; Melody Eble, Johnson & Johnson; Atheer Kaddis, Blue Cross and Blue Shield of Michigan; Lucinda Maine, American Association of Colleges of Pharmacy; Gary Merica, York Hospital; Joseph Morris, Health Care Improvement Foundation; Richard Park, *IVD Technology* magazine; Ken Reid, Washington Information Source Co.; Ed Staffa, National Association of Chain Drug Stores; Kasey Thompson, American Society of Health-system Pharmacists; Marissa Schlaifer, Academy of Managed Care Pharmacy; Junelle Speller, American Academy of Pediatrics; Sharon Wilson, Center for Nursing Practice; and Charles Young, Massachusetts Board of Registration in Pharmacy.

The committee commissioned eight papers that provided important background information for the report, and would like to thank all the authors for their dedicated work and helpful insights: Harvey J. Murff, Vanderbilt University; Ginette A. Pepper, University of Utah College of Nursing; Grace M. Kuo, Baylor College of Medicine; Marlene R. Miller, Karen A. Robinson, Lisa H. Lubomski, Michael L. Rinke, and Peter J Pronovost, The Johns Hopkins University; Benjamin C. Grasso, The Institute for Self-Directed Care; Albert I. Wertheimer and Thomas M. Santella, Temple University; Eta Berner, University of Alabama at Birmingham with assistance from Lorri Zipperer, Zipperer Project Management; Richard Maisiak, consultant; and Brent Petty, The Johns Hopkins University.

The committee also benefited from the work of other committees and staff of the Institute of Medicine that conducted studies relevant to this report, particularly the Committee on Quality of Health Care in America and the Committee on Identifying Priority Areas for Quality Improvement. The Committee on Quality of Health Care in America produced the 2000 report *To Err Is Human: Building a Safer Health System* and the 2001 report *Crossing the Quality Chasm: A New Health System for the 21st Century*. The committee on Identifying Priority Areas for Quality Improvement produced the 2003 report *Priority Areas for National Action: Transforming Health Care Quality.*

Finally, funding for this project was provided by the Centers for Medicare and Medicaid Services. The committee extends special thanks for that support.

Contents

xv

APPENDIXES

Summary

ABSTRACT

The use of medications is ubiquitous. In any given week, more than four of five U.S. adults take at least one medication (prescription or over-the-counter [OTC] drug, vitamin/mineral, or herbal supplement), and almost a third take at least five different medications.[1] Errors can occur with any of these products at any point in the medication-use process and in any care setting. The frequency of medication errors and preventable medication-related injuries represents a very serious cause for concern.

The Centers for Medicare and Medicaid Services sponsored this study by the Institute of Medicine (IOM) with the aim of developing a national agenda for reducing medication errors based on estimates of the incidence of such errors and evidence on the efficacy of various prevention strategies. The study focused on the safe, effective, and appropriate use of medications in the major components of the medication-use system, addressing the use of prescription drugs, OTC drugs, and complementary and alternative medications, in a wide range of care settings—hospital, long-term, and community.

The committee estimates that on average, a hospital patient is subject to at least one medication error per day, with considerable

---

[1]In this report, the terms *medication* and *drug* are used interchangeably.

1

variation in error rates across facilities. The few existing studies of the costs associated with medication errors are limited to the health care costs incurred by preventable injuries, and these are substantial.

At least a quarter of all medication-related injuries are preventable. Many efficacious error prevention strategies are available, especially for hospital care; examples are electronic prescribing and clinical decision-support systems that check dosages and monitor for harmful drug–drug interactions. This report provides guidance on how to implement error prevention strategies in hospitals, long-term care, and ambulatory care.

Establishing and maintaining a strong provider–patient partnership is a key approach for reducing medication errors. The report outlines how such a partnership can be achieved and what roles providers, patients, and third parties must play. For example, consumers should maintain careful records of their medications, providers should review a patient's list of medications at each encounter and at times of transition between care settings (e.g., hospital to outpatient care), and the federal government should seek ways to improve the quality of pharmacy leaflets and medication-related information on the Internet for consumers.

Health care providers in all settings should seek to create high-reliability organizations that constantly improve the safety and quality of medication use. To this end, they should implement active internal monitoring programs so that progress toward improved medication safety can be accurately demonstrated. The report offers guidance on appropriate monitoring systems for each major care setting.

In carrying out this study, the IOM committee identified enormous gaps in the knowledge base with regard to medication errors. Current methods for generating and communicating information about medications are inadequate and contribute to the incidence of errors. Likewise, incidence rates of medication errors in many care settings, the costs of such errors, and the efficacy of prevention strategies are not well understood. The report proposes a research agenda to address these and other knowledge gaps.

STUDY SCOPE

The Institute of Medicine (IOM) report *To Err Is Human: Building a Safer Health System* (IOM, 2000) accelerated existing efforts to prevent medication errors and improve the quality of health care, efforts that are just now gaining acceptance as a discipline requiring investment in individuals who specialize in error prevention and quality improvement. Against this background, at the urging of the Senate Finance Committee, the United States

---

BOX S-1
Scope of the Study

Congress, through the Medicare Modernization Act of 2003 (Section 107(c)), mandated the Centers for Medicare and Medicaid Services to sponsor the Institute of Medicine to carry out a study:

• To develop a fuller understanding of drug safety and quality issues through the conduct of an evidence-based review of the literature, case studies and analysis. This review will consider the nature and causes of medication errors; their impact on patients; and the differences in causation, impact and prevention across multiple dimensions of health care delivery including patient populations, care settings, clinicians, and institutional cultures.

• If possible, to develop estimates of the incidence, severity and costs of medication errors that can be useful in prioritizing resources for national quality improvement efforts and influencing national health care policy.

• To evaluate alternative approaches to reducing medication errors in terms of their efficacy, cost-effectiveness, appropriateness in different settings and circumstances, feasibility, institutional barriers to implementation, associated risk, and quality of evidence supporting the approach.

• To provide guidance to consumers, providers, payers, and other key stakeholders on high-priority strategies to achieve both short-term and long-term drug safety goals, to elucidate the goals and expected results of such initiatives and support the business case for them, and to identify critical success factors and key levers for achieving success.

• To assess opportunities and key impediments to broad nationwide implementation of medication error reductions, and to provide guidance to policymakers and government agencies in promoting a national agenda for medication error reduction.

• To develop an applied research agenda to evaluate the health and cost impacts of alternative interventions, and to assess collaborative public and private strategies for implementing the research agenda through the Agency for Healthcare Research and Quality and other government agencies.

Congress directed the Centers for Medicare and Medicaid Services (CMS) to contract with the IOM for a study to formulate a national agenda for reducing medication errors by developing estimates of the incidence of such errors and determining the efficacy of prevention strategies (see Box S-1).

THE LEVEL AND CONSEQUENCES OF MEDICATION ERRORS ARE UNACCEPTABLE

Rates of Errors and Preventable Harmful Events Are High

The frequency of medication errors and preventable adverse drug events (ADEs) (defined in Box S-2) is a very serious cause for concern. In

BOX S-2
Key Definitions

Error: The failure of a planned action to be completed as intended (error of execution) or the use of a wrong plan to achieve an aim (error of planning). An error may be an act of commission or an act of omission (IOM, 2004).

Medication error: Any error occurring in the medication-use process (Bates et al., 1995a). Examples include wrong dosage prescribed, wrong dosage administered for a prescribed medication, or failure to give (by the provider) or take (by the patient) a medication.

Adverse drug event: Any injury due to medication (Bates et al., 1995b). Examples include a wrong dosage leading to injury (e.g., rash, confusion, or loss of function) or an allergic reaction occurring in a patient not known to be allergic to a given medication.

hospitals, errors are common during all steps of the medication-use process—procuring the drug, prescribing, dispensing, administering, and monitoring the patient's response. In hospitals, they occur most frequently at the prescribing and administration stages.

Published error rates depend on the intensity and specifics of the error detection methods used. In particular, some methods are better suited to certain stages of the medication-use process. Detection methods addressing all stages but not including direct observation of administration found a rate of 0.1 prescribing errors per patient per day in a study of hospital pediatric units (Kaushal et al., 2001) and a rate of 0.3 prescribing errors per patient per day in a study of hospital medical units (Bates et al., 1995a). A major study using direct observation of administration (Barker et al., 2002) carried out at 36 different health care facilities found an administration error rate of 11 percent, excluding doses administered outside the scheduled time ("wrong-time" errors). Since a hospital patient receives on average at least ten medication doses per day, this figure suggests that on average, a hospital patient is subject to one administration error per day. Further, since prescribing and administration errors account for about three-fourths of medication errors (Leape et al., 1995), the committee conservatively estimates that on average, a hospital patient is subject to at least one medication error per day. Substantial variations in error rates are found, however. For the 36 facilities in the study mentioned above, the administration error rate (excluding wrong-time errors) ranged from 0 to 26 percent, with a median value of 8.3 percent (Barker et al., 2002).

A preventable ADE is a serious type of medication error. ADEs, defined as any injury due to medication (Bates et al., 1995b), are common in hospitals, nursing homes, and the outpatient setting. ADEs associated with a medication error are considered preventable. The committee estimates that at least 1.5 million preventable ADEs occur each year in the United States:

• Hospital care—Classen and colleagues (1997) projected 380,000 preventable ADEs occurring annually, and Bates and colleagues (1995b) 450,000. These are likely underestimates given the higher preventable ADE rate of another study using more comprehensive ADE identification methods (Jha et al., 1998).
• Long-term care—Gurwitz and colleagues (2005) projected 800,000 preventable ADEs, again likely an underestimate given the higher ADE rates of other studies.
• Ambulatory care—Among outpatient Medicare patients alone, Gurwitz and colleagues (2003) projected 530,000 preventable ADEs. Their approach was conservative, however, because it did not involve direct contact with patients, which yields much higher rates (Gandhi et al., 2003).

The above data exclude errors of omission—failure to prescribe medications for which there is an evidence base for the ability to reduce morbidity and mortality. With respect to such errors, the committee found well-documented evidence of inadequate treatments for acute coronary syndromes, heart failure, chronic coronary disease, and atrial fibrillation, as well as inadequate antibiotic and thrombosis prophylaxis in hospitals.

Morbidity Due to Medication Errors Is Costly

Current understanding of the costs of medication errors is highly incomplete. Most of what is known relates to additional health care costs associated with preventable ADEs, which represent the injuries caused by errors.

For hospital care, there is one estimate of the extra costs of inpatient care for a preventable ADE incurred while in the hospital—$5,857 (Bates et al., 1997). This figure excludes health care costs outside the hospital and was derived from 1993 cost data. Assuming conservatively an annual incidence of 400,000 in-hospital preventable ADEs, each incurring extra hospital costs of $5,857, yields an annual cost of $2.3 billion in 1993 dollars or $3.5 billion in 2006 dollars.

For long-term care, as noted earlier, Gurwitz and colleagues (2005) projected an annual incidence of 800,000 preventable ADEs. However, there is no estimate of the associated health care costs for this group of preventable ADEs.

For ambulatory care, the best estimate derives from a study (Field et al., 2005) that calculateed the annual cost of preventable ADEs for all Medicare enrollees aged 65 and older. The cost in 2000 per preventable ADE was estimated at $1,983, while national annual costs were estimated at $887 million.

In addition to the likelihood of underestimation, the above estimates are characterized by some important omissions. First, the costs of some highly common medication errors, such as drug use without a medically valid indication and failure to receive drugs that should have been pre-scribed, were excluded from the Medicare study of ambulatory ADEs (Field et al., 2005). Moreover, the costs of morbidity and mortality arising from the failure of patients to comply with prescribed medication regimens were not assessed. Second, all the studies omitted some important costs: lost earnings, costs of not being able to carry out household duties (lost house-hold production), and compensation for pain and suffering. Third, few data are available for any setting regarding the costs of medication errors that do not result in harm. While no injury is involved, these errors often create extra work, and the costs involved may be substantial.

Effective Error Prevention Strategies Are Available

According to most studies, at least a quarter of all harmful ADEs are preventable. Moreover, many efficacious error prevention strategies are available, especially for hospital care. In the hospital setting, there is good evidence for the effectiveness of computerized order entry with clinical decision-support systems (Bates et al., 1998), for clinical decision-support systems themselves (Evans et al., 1994), and for pharmacist participation on hospital rounds (Leape et al., 1999). Bar coding and smart intravenous (IV) pumps show promise for the hospital setting, but their efficacy has not yet been clearly demonstrated.

Interventions consisting of educational visits appear to hold promise for improving prescribing practices and patient outcomes in nursing homes. Involving pharmacists in the management of medications in nursing homes and ambulatory care also shows promise, but requires additional study. This intervention has been most successful to date in populations with certain conditions, such as diabetes.

IMPROVED PROVIDER–PATIENT COMMUNICATION IS VITAL

Achieving the patient-centered model of care envisioned in the IOM report *Crossing the Quality Chasm: A New Health System for the 21st Century* (IOM, 2001) will require a paradigm shift away from a paternalis-tic, provider-centric model of care. Consumers (and their surrogates) should be empowered as partners in their care, with appropriate communication, information, and resources in place to support them. For medication safety, consumers and providers (including physicians, nurses, and pharmacists) should know and act on patients' rights, providers should engage in meaningful communication about the safe and effective use of medications at multiple points in the medication-use process, and government and other participants should improve consumer-oriented written and electronic information resources.

Patient Rights

Patient rights are the foundation for the safe and ethical use of medications (see Box S-3). Ignoring these rights can have lethal consequences. Millions of Americans take prescription drugs each year without being fully informed by their providers about associated risks, contraindications, and side effects. When clinically significant medication errors do occur, they usually are not disclosed to patients or their surrogates unless injury or death results.

Many but not all patient rights relating to medical care have been established broadly in the U.S. Constitution (Amendments I and XIV) and articulated by the courts through common law. Certain states have instituted a patient bill of rights relating to particular providers or care settings. One important point not specifically addressed by these laws is the right for a patient to be told when an adverse event occurs. Establishing a comprehensive set of patient rights in one document would facilitate patient and

---

BOX S-3
Patient Rights

Patients have the right to:

• Be the source of control for all medication management decisions that affect them (that is, the right to self-determination).
• Accept or reject medication therapy on the basis of their personal values.
• Be adequately informed about their medication therapy and alternative treatments.
• Ask questions to better understand their medication regimen.
• Receive consultation about their medication regimen in all health settings and at all points along the medication-use process.
• Designate a surrogate to assist them with all aspects of their medication management.
• Expect providers to tell them when a clinically significant error has occurred, what the effects of the event on their health (short- and long-term) will be, and what care they will receive to restore their health.
• Ask their provider to report an adverse event and give them information about how they can report the event themselves.

provider understanding and exercise of these rights and improve the safety and quality of medication use.

Actions for Consumers

For sound medication management, providers and consumers[2] should maintain an up-to-date record of medications being administered, including prescription medications, over-the-counter (OTC) drugs, and dietary supplements, as well as all known drug and/or food allergies. Such records are especially important for patients who have chronic conditions, see multiple providers, or take multiple medications.

By becoming more informed and engaged, consumers (and their surrogates) may decrease the probability of experiencing a medication error (Cohen, 2000). Such actions can range from the simple and routine, such as double-checking their prescription when dropping it off and picking it up from the pharmacy, to the more involved, such as forming an active partnership with providers in managing their health care. When using OTC medications, herbal remedies, and dietary supplements, consumers should seek the information they need to make informed decisions. When obtaining medical care, consumers should ask questions and insist on answers from providers to guide their decision making based on their personal values and preferences. They should ensure that their provider explains their medication regimen clearly and speak up if they do not understand. In addition, they should ensure that providers give them written information about their medications, as well as tell them where to obtain information from other sources. Finally, consumers should communicate with their providers if they experience any unexpected changes in the way they feel after initiating a new medication. Some specific actions consumers can take are outlined in Box S-4.

Actions for Providers

Providers can take several specific actions to improve medication safety (see Box S-5). First, they can verify the patient's current medication list for appropriateness at each encounter, and they can ensure that this list is accurate at times of transition between care settings. They can educate their patients about the medication regimen, understanding that patients need different kinds of information at different times and for different purposes. Providers can also respect patients' wishes and inform them of

---

[2]In this report, the term *consumers* is often used in referring to patients to emphasize the active role individuals need to take in ensuring the quality of the health care services they are purchasing.

BOX S-4
Consumer Actions to Enhance Medication Safety

Personal/Home

- Maintain a list of the prescription drugs, nonprescription drugs, and other products, such as vitamins and minerals, you are taking.
- Take the list with you when you visit any medical practitioner, and have him or her review it.
- Be aware of where to find educational material in your local community and at reliable Internet sites.

Ambulatory Care/Outpatient Clinic

- Have the prescriber provide in writing the name of the drug (brand and generic names, if available), what it is for, its dosage, and how often to take it, or provide other written material with this information.
- Have the prescriber explain how to use the drug properly.
- Ask about the side effects of the drug and what to do if you experience a side effect.

Pharmacy

- Make sure the name of the drug (brand or generic) and the directions for use received at the pharmacy are the same as what is written down by the prescriber.
- Know that you can review your list of medications with the pharmacist for additional safety.
- Know that you have the right to counseling by the pharmacist if you have any questions; you can ask the pharmacist to explain how to take the drug properly, what side effects it has, and what to do if you experience them (just as you did with your prescriber).
- Ask for written literature about the drug.

Hospital Inpatient (Patient or Surrogate)

- Ask the doctor or nurse what drugs you are being given at the hospital.
- Do not take a drug without being told the reason for doing so.
- Exercise your right to have a surrogate present whenever you are receiving medication and are unable to monitor the medication-use process yourself.
- Prior to surgery, ask whether there are medications, especially prescription antibiotics, that you should take or any you should stop taking preoperatively.
- Prior to discharge, ask for a list of the medications you should be taking at home, have a provider review them with you, and be sure you understand how the medications should be taken.

BOX S-5
Issues for Discussion with Patients by Providers
(Physicians, Nurses, and Pharmacists)

- Review the patient's medication list routinely and during care transitions.
- Review different treatment options.
- Review the name and purpose of the selected medication.
- Discuss when and how to take the medication.
- Discuss important and likely side effects and what to do about them.
- Discuss drug–drug, drug–food, and drug–disease interactions.
- Review the patient's or surrogate's role in achieving appropriate medication use.
- Review the role of medications in the overall context of the patient's health.

---

their rights, including the right to have a surrogate present and involved in their medication management whenever they are unable to monitor their own medication use.

When communicating about medication errors that occur with the potential for or actual harm, providers can tell patients how the error may affect their health and what is being done to correct it. The vast majority of patients want and expect to be told about errors, particularly those that cause them harm.

Barriers Experienced by Consumers and Providers

In the current system, a number of barriers affect the ability of consumers to engage in safe and effective use of medications and the ability of providers to change their day-to-day practices to support new consumer-oriented activities (Cohen, 2000). These barriers include (1) knowledge deficits, such as patients lacking sufficient education about their medications and providers lacking the latest pharmacological knowledge about particular drugs; (2) practical barriers, such as patients being unable to pay for their medications and providers having to operate burdensome prescribing arrangements required by payers; and (3) attitudinal factors, such as patients and providers having different cultural norms and beliefs about the use of medications. These barriers often result in errors, such as taking the wrong dose, taking a medication at the wrong time, or taking someone else's medication. Many of these barriers can be overcome by improved consumer-oriented drug information, efforts on the part of providers to respond to the challenges faced by their patients, and actions by health care organizations to adopt a culture of safety and make more extensive use of information technology.

Recommendation 1: To improve the quality and safety of the medication-use process, specific measures should be instituted to strengthen patients' capacities for sound medication self-management. Specifically:

• Patients' rights regarding safety and quality in health care and medication use should be formalized at the state and/or federal levels and ensured at every point of care.

• Patients (or their surrogates) should maintain an active list of all prescription drugs, over-the-counter drugs, and dietary supplements they are taking; the reasons for taking them; and any known drug allergies. Every provider involved in the medication-use process for a patient should have access to this list.

• Providers should take definitive action to educate patients (or their surrogates) about the safe and effective use of medications. They should provide information about side effects, contraindications, and how to handle adverse reactions, as well as where to obtain additional objective, high-quality information.

• Consultation on their medications should be available to patients at key points in the medication-use process (during clinical decision making in ambulatory and inpatient care, at hospital discharge, and at the pharmacy).

Actions for Government and Other Stakeholders

Consumers should be able to obtain high-quality information about medications not only from their providers, but also from the pharmacy and Internet and community-based resources. However, these resources need significant improvement in two overarching areas.

First, current materials (e.g., pharmacy information sheets [leaflets], Internet-based information) are inadequately designed to facilitate consumers' ability to read, comprehend, and act on medication information. Pharmacy leaflets are the source of such information most relied upon by consumers. Yet a number of studies have revealed the inadequate quality of these leaflets, as well as their variable quality from one pharmacy to another and from one drug to another (Svarstad and Mount, 2001). Internet-based health information has proliferated over the last decade, providing consumers with immediate access to valuable resources such as medical journals and libraries, but most consumers are unfamiliar with how to access this information since it usually does not figure prominently during online searches. Rather, consumers are directed to a multitude of other sources of information with differing standards for the content provided.

The federal government should develop mechanisms for improving pharmacy leaflets and the quality of Internet information for consumers.

Second, there is a need for additional resources beyond pharmacy leaflets and Internet information that can be provided on a national scale. In particular, a national drug information telephone helpline and community-based health resource centers should be developed to promote consumer education. Further, communication networks already in place, such as those associated with the public health infrastructure (e.g., the Centers for Disease Control and Prevention's National Center for Health Marketing) and consumer networks should be used for broad dissemination of national medication safety initiatives.

> **Recommendation 2: Government agencies (i.e., the Agency for Healthcare Research and Quality [AHRQ], the Centers for Medicare and Medicaid Services [CMS], the Food and Drug Administration [FDA], and the National Library of Medicine [NLM]) should enhance the resource base for consumer-oriented drug information and medication self-management support. Such efforts require standardization of pharmacy medication information leaflets, improvement of online medication resources, establishment of a national drug information telephone helpline, the development of personal health records, and the formulation of a national plan for the dissemination of medication safety information.**
>
> • **Pharmacy medication information leaflets should be standardized to a format designed for readability, comprehensibility, and usefulness to consumers. The leaflets should be made available to consumers in a manner that accommodates their individual needs, such as those associated with variations in literacy, language, age, and visual acuity.**
> • **The NLM should be designated as the chief agency responsible for Internet health information resources for consumers. Drug information should be provided through a consumers' version of the DailyMed program, with links to the NLM's Medline Plus program for general health and additional drug information.**
> • **CMS, the FDA, and the NLM, working together, should undertake a full evaluation of various methods for building and funding a national network of drug information helplines.**
> • **CMS, the FDA, and the NLM should collaborate to confirm a minimum dataset for personal health records and develop requirements for vendor self-certification of compliance. Vendors should take the initiative to improve the use and functionality of personal health records by incorporating basic tools to support consumers' medication self-management.**

• A national plan should be developed for widespread distribution and promotion of medication safety information. Health care provider, community-based, consumer, and government organizations should serve as the foundation for such efforts.

ELECTRONIC PRESCRIBING AND MONITORING FOR ERRORS IN ALL CARE SETTINGS ARE ESSENTIAL

Safe medication use requires that clinicians synthesize several types of information, including knowledge of the medication itself, as well as understanding of how it may interact with coexisting illnesses and medications and how its use might be monitored. Several electronic supports can help providers absorb and apply the necessary information.

Access to Automated Point-of-Care Reference Information

The underlying knowledge base is constantly changing, creating a situation in which it is almost impossible for health care providers to have current knowledge of every medication they prescribe. Clinicians therefore need access to critical syntheses of the evidence base. The Cochrane Collaboration (CC, 2005) is one such resource. In addition, many software applications now being developed provide decision support for prescribing clinicians (Epocrates, 2005). Applications of this type are typically available via the Internet or on personal digital assistants (PDAs). All prescribers should use point-of-care reference information.

Electronic Prescribing

Paper-based prescribing is associated with high error rates (Kaushal et al., 2003). Having all pharmacies receive prescriptions electronically would result in fewer errors than occur with current paper or oral approaches (Bates, 2001). Electronic prescribing is safer (Bates et al., 1998) because it eliminates handwriting and ensures that the key fields (for example, drug name, dose, route, and frequency) include meaningful data. More important, as noted above, computerization enables the delivery of clinical decision support (Evans et al., 1998), including checks for allergies, drug–drug interactions, overly high doses, and clinical conditions, as well as suggestions for appropriate dosages given the patient's level of renal function and age. It should be noted that recent studies have identified implementation problems and the unintended occurrence of new types of errors with these computerized approaches (for example, pharmacy inventory displays of available drug doses being mistaken for the usual or minimally effective doses). Avoiding these problems requires addressing business and cultural issues before such strategies are implemented and aggressively solving technological problems during the implementation process. Regulatory issues must also be addressed for electronic transmission of prescriptions to be practical.

Effective Use of Well-Designed Technologies

To deliver safe drug care, health care organizations should make effective use of well-designed technologies, which will vary by setting. Although the evidence for this assertion is strongest in the inpatient setting (AHRQ, 2005), the use of technology will undoubtedly lead to major improvements in all settings. In acute care, technologies should target prescribing by including computerized provider order entry with clinical decision support. Administration is also a particularly vulnerable stage in the medication-use process, and several technologies are likely to be especially important in this stage. These include electronic medication administration records, which can improve documentation of what medications have been given and when, as well as machine-readable identification, such as bar coding, and smart IV infusion pumps. All these technologies should be linked electronically.

In nursing homes, computerized prescribing with decision support will likely be important, although there has been little research on its efficacy (Gurwitz et al., 2005). Moreover, implementation of computerized prescribing in this setting will be challenging since most nursing homes have very limited resources.

Some evidence suggests that computerized prescribing will be important in the outpatient setting as well (Gandhi et al., 2003), although it may not yield significant safety benefits without added decision support. Equally important are likely to be approaches that improve communication between patients and providers.

Communication of Patient-Specific Medication-Related Information

The delivery of care often involves moving the locus of care among sites and providers. These "handoffs" are fraught with errors. One strategy for reducing errors during these care transitions is to reconcile medication orders between transition points, especially between care settings such as hospital and outpatient, but also between points within organizations, such as the intensive care unit and a general care unit. This reconciliation involves comparing what a patient is taking in one setting with what is being provided in another to avoid errors of transcription and omission, duplication of therapy, and drug–drug and drug–disease interactions. This process typically reveals many discrepancies (Pronovost et al., 2003).

Reconciliation is facilitated when medication data are transmitted electronically among providers, with confirmation by the patient. Three important steps are required. First, a complete and accurate medication list must be compiled. Second, the data must be structured into components such as the medication name, dose, route, frequency, duration, start date, and so on. Third, these data must be formatted in a way that allows disparate computer systems to understand both their structure and content.

The power of interoperable health care data was demonstrated after the devastation of Hurricane Katrina. Pharmacy chains were able to make patients' medication lists available quickly to care providers, and states with immunizations registries were able to retrieve immunization records, enabling the enrollment of children in new schools.

Monitoring for Errors

All health care provider groups should seek to be high-reliability organizations preoccupied with the possibility of failure (Reason, 2000). They should implement active internal monitoring programs so that progress toward improved medication safety can be accurately demonstrated. Voluntary internal reporting systems have recognized limitations for evaluating the true frequency of medication errors and ADEs (Flynn et al., 2002). Error detection methods that complement such systems should be used in all care settings. These include computerized detection of ADEs, observation of medication passes in hospitals to assess administration errors, and audits of filled prescriptions in community pharmacies to monitor dispensing errors.

Many external programs exist to which patients and providers can report a medication error or hazardous situation (IOM, 2004). Voluntary practitioner reporting to an external program will continue to be important, as it is often the only way practitioners can effect change outside their organizations. Errors need to be reported and analyzed if improvements in care are to be achieved.

Adopting a Safety Culture

Patient safety can best be achieved through the adoption of a culture of safety—an organizational commitment to continually seeking to improve safety. To achieve a safety culture, senior management of health care organizations must devote sufficient attention to safety, as well as make sufficient resources available for quality improvement and safety teams (IOM, 2004). Senior management must also authorize the investment of resources in technologies that have been demonstrated to be effective but are not yet widely implemented in most organizations, such as computerized provider order entry systems and electronic health records. It has become increasingly clear that the introduction of any of these technologies requires close attention to business processes and ongoing maintenance. As noted above, studies have shown that these tools can have unintended and adverse consequences, and that avoiding these consequences requires addressing both business and cultural issues.

> Recommendation 3: All health care organizations should immediately make complete patient-information and decision-support tools available to clinicians and patients. Health care systems should capture information on medication safety and use this information to improve the safety of their care delivery systems. Health care organizations should implement the appropriate systems to enable providers to:
>
> • Have access to comprehensive reference information concerning medications and related health data.
> • Communicate patient-specific medication-related information in an interoperable format.
> • Assess the safety of medication use through active monitoring and use these monitoring data to inform the implementation of prevention strategies.
> • Write prescriptions electronically by 2010. Also by 2010, all pharmacies should be able to receive prescriptions electronically. By 2008, all prescribers should have plans in place to implement electronic prescribing.
> • Subject prescriptions to evidence-based, current clinical decision support.
> • Have the appropriate competencies for each step of the medication-use process.
> • Make effective use of well-designed technologies, which will vary by setting.

ENORMOUS KNOWLEDGE DEFICITS MUST BE ADDRESSED

Current methods for generating and communicating information about medications are inadequate and contribute to a growing rate of medication errors. Likewise, error incidence rates, costs to the health system, and prevention strategies are not well understood. As a result, there are enormous gaps in the knowledge required to implement a safe medication-use system.

Risk/Benefit Information for Prescription Drugs

Being able to determine whether a medication error has been made depends on knowing the correct dose of the drug for that patient at that time and whether the indication for that drug is correct in comparison with alternative approaches to treatment. Over the past several decades, however, drug evaluations have not been sufficiently comprehensive. As a result, the balance of risk and benefit for a drug frequently is not known for a given population. Such gaps in therapeutic knowledge often result in devastating effects on clinical practice and patient health, as exemplified by adverse events involving hormone replacement therapy, cyclooxygenase-2 (COX-2) inhibitors, and nonsteroidal anti-inflammatory drugs that resulted in increased morbidity and mortality.

These issues are magnified in specific patient populations. For example, the majority of prescriptions written for children are off label—not based on empirical demonstration of safety and efficacy. Among those over age 80, the fastest-growing segment of the population, almost nothing is known about the balance of risks and benefits. Patients with renal dysfunction are another large and growing group for whom more comprehensive studies are needed. And patients with multiple comorbidities are typically excluded from premarketing clinical trials, yet many of the major problems with drug toxicity have occurred in those taking multiple medications because of multiple diseases. Thus the numbers and types of patients for whom clinical outcomes are measured must be greatly increased to elucidate the proper dosing of drugs in individuals and within subgroups.

Of critical concern is the need for transparency through the publication of clinical studies in a national repository to advance medication safety, error prevention, and public knowledge. Such a repository should include postmarket studies. The goal of such studies is to generate new data about a drug's effects in the population; often, however, these studies place insufficient emphasis on safety information. There is a need for comprehensive redesign and expansion of the mechanisms for undertaking clinical studies to improve understanding of the risks and benefits of drug therapies, prevent errors and ADEs, and meet the health needs of the population.

Communication of Drug Information

How information about a drug is communicated to providers and consumers can directly affect the frequency of medication errors and ADEs (see Box S-6). Drug information is communicated through labeling and packaging, marketing practices, and advertisements. Poorly designed materials and inadequate representation of the risks and benefits to providers and consumers have led to many errors, including inappropriate prescribing;

BOX S-6
Drug Naming, Labeling, and Packaging Problems

- Brand names and generic names that look or sound alike
- Different formulations of the same brand or generic drug
- Multiple abbreviations to represent the same concept
- Confusing word derivatives, abbreviations, and symbols
- Unclear dose concentration/strength designations
- Cluttered labeling—small fonts, poor typefaces, no background contrast, overemphasis on company logos
- Inadequate prominence of warnings and reminders
- Lack of standardized terminology

---

confusion among products, affecting dispensing and administration; and compromised ability to monitor the effects of drugs adequately.

In particular, drug names that look or sound alike increase the risk of medication errors. Abbreviations, acronyms, certain dose designations, and other symbols used for labeling also have caused errors. Even the layout and presentation of drug information on the drug container or package label can be visually confusing, particularly if it is designed for marketing rather than clinical purposes.

Unit-of-use packaging—containers that provide enough medication for a particular period, such as blister packs containing 30 individually wrapped doses—is not widely employed in the United States but is used extensively elsewhere. This form of packaging brings important safety and usage benefits. The committee believes the expanded implementation of unit-of-use packaging in this country warrants further investigation.

Another issue related to medication safety is the common practice of providers offering free samples of prescription drugs to patients to start them on their medications quickly, to adjust prescribed doses before the full prescription is filled, and to offset medication costs for indigent and underinsured patients. However, there has been growing unease about the way free samples are distributed. In particular, concern exists about the resulting lack of documentation of medication use and the bypassing of standard prescribing and dispensing services, which incorporate drug-interaction checking and pharmacy counseling services. There is a need for resrach on the impact of differing sample distribution methods on medication safety.

Recommendation 4: Enhancing the safety and quality of the medication-use process and reducing errors requires improved methods for labeling drug products and communicating medication information to providers and consumers. For such improve-

ments to occur, materials should be designed according to designated standards to meet the needs of the end user. Industry, AHRQ, the FDA, and others as appropriate (e.g., U.S. Pharmacopeia, Institute for Safe Medication Practices) should work together to undertake the following actions to address labeling, packaging, and the distribution of free samples:

- The FDA should develop two guidance documents for industry: one for drug naming and another for labeling and packaging. The FDA and industry should collaborate to develop (1) a common drug nomenclature that standardizes abbreviations, acronyms, and terms to the extent possible, and (2) methods of applying failure modes and effects analysis to labeling and packaging.
- Additional study of optimum designs for all drug labeling and information sheets to reflect human and cognitive factors should be undertaken. Methods for testing and measuring the effects of these materials on providers and consumers should also be established, including methods for field testing of the materials. The FDA, the NLM, and industry should work with consumer and patient safety organizations to improve the nomenclature used in consumer materials.
- The FDA, the pharmaceutical industry, and other stakeholders should collaborate to develop a strategy for expanding unit-of-use packaging for consumers to new therapeutic areas. Studies should be undertaken to evaluate different unit-of-use packaging and design approaches that will best support various consumer groups in their medication self-management.
- AHRQ should fund studies to evaluate the impact of free samples on overall patient safety, provider prescribing practices, and consumer behavior (e.g., adherence to the medication regimen), as well as alternative methods of distribution that can improve safety, quality, and effectiveness.

Health Information Technology

Realization of the full benefits of many health information technologies (such as decision-support systems, smart IV pumps, bar code administration systems, and pharmacy database systems) is hampered by the lack of common data standards for system integration and well-designed interfaces for end users.

Problems with data standards for drug information are threefold. First, there is no complete, standardized set of terms, concepts, and codes to represent drug information. Second, there is no standardized method for presenting safety alerts according to severity and/or clinical importance. Instead, providers are sometimes inundated with too many alerts, which can result in "alert fatigue." Third, many systems lack intelligent mechanisms for relating patient-specific data to allowable overrides, such as those associated with a particular patient and drug allergy alert or duplicate therapy request.

The ability of clinicians to use health information technologies successfully depends on how well the technologies have been designed at the level of human-machine interaction (i.e., the user interface). Displaying information in a cluttered, illogical, or confusing manner leads to decreased user performance and satisfaction. Moreover, a poorly designed user interface can contribute to medication errors. Addressing user interface issues requires greater attention to the cognitive and social factors influencing clinicians in their daily workflow and interaction with technologies (van Bemmel and Musen, 1997).

> **Recommendation 5: Industry and government should collaborate to establish standards affecting drug-related health information technologies. Specifically:**
>
> • The NLM should take the lead in developing a common drug nomenclature for use in all clinical information technology systems, based on standards for the national health information infrastructure.
>
> • AHRQ should take the lead in organizing mechanisms for safety alerts according to severity, frequency, and clinical importance to improve clinical value and acceptance.
>
> • AHRQ should take the lead in developing intelligent prompting mechanisms specific to a patient's unique characteristics and needs; provider prescribing, ordering, and error patterns; and evidence-based best-practice guidelines.
>
> • AHRQ should take the lead in developing user interface designs based on the principles of cognitive and human factors and the context of the clinical environment.
>
> • AHRQ should support additional research to determine specifications for alert mechanisms and intelligent prompting, as well as optimum designs for user interfaces.

Research on Medication Errors:
Incidence Rates, Costs, and Prevention Strategies

In reviewing the research literature, the committee concluded that large gaps exist in our understanding of medication error incidence rates, costs, and prevention strategies. The committee believes the nation should invest about \$100 million annually in the research proposed below.

The primary focus of research on medication errors in the next decade should be prevention strategies, recognizing that to plan an error prevention study, it is essential to be able to measure the baseline rate of errors. Evidence on the efficacy of prevention strategies for improving medication safety is badly needed in a number of settings, including care transitions, ambulatory care (particularly home care, self-care, and medication use in schools), pediatric care, psychiatric care, and the use of OTC and complementary and alternative medications. For hospitals, key areas are further investigation of some prevention strategies (particularly bar coding and smart IV pumps) and how to integrate electronic health records with computerized provider order entry, clinical decision support, bar coding, and smart IV pumps.

Overall, most data on medication error incidence rates come from the inpatient setting, but the magnitude of the problem is likely to be greater outside the hospital. Areas of priority for research on medication error and ADE incidence rates are care transitions, specialty ambulatory clinics, psychiatric care, the administering of medications in schools, and the use of OTC and complementary and alternative medications. Much more research is needed as well on the patient's role in the prevention of errors, specifically, what systems provide the most cost-effective support for safe and effective medication self-management or for surrogate participation in medication use when a patient is unable to self-manage.

Most studies of the costs of medication errors relate to hospitals, and some report data more than 10 years old (Bates et al., 1997). A better understanding of the costs and consequences of medication errors in all care settings is needed to help inform decisions about investing in medication error prevention strategies.

> **Recommendation 6: AHRQ should take the lead, working with other government agencies such as CMS, the FDA, and the NLM, in coordinating a broad research agenda on the safe and appropriate use of medications across all care settings, and Congress should allocate the funds necessary to carry out this agenda. This agenda should encompass research methodologies, incidence rates by type and severity, costs of medication errors, reporting systems, and in particular, further testing of error prevention strategies.**

OVERSIGHT, REGULATION, AND PAYMENT

Improving medication safety will require key changes in oversight, regulation, and payment. Accordingly, the following recommendation is addressed to the stakeholders that shape the environment in which care is delivered, including legislators, regulators, accreditors, payers, and patient safety organizations.[3]

> Recommendation 7: Oversight and regulatory organizations and payers should use legislation, regulation, accreditation, and payment mechanisms and the media to motivate the adoption of practices and technologies that can reduce medication errors, as well as to ensure that professionals have the competencies required to deliver medications safely.

> • Payers and purchasers should continue to motivate improvement in the medication-use process through explicit financial incentives.
> • CMS should evaluate a variety of strategies for delivering medication therapy management.
> • Regulators, accreditors, and legislators should set minimum functionality standards for error prevention technologies.
> • States should enact legislation consistent with and complementary to the Medicare Modernization Act's electronic prescribing provisions and remove existing barriers to such prescribing.
> • All state boards of pharmacy should undertake quality improvement initiatives related to community pharmacy practice.
> • Medication error reporting should be promoted more aggressively by all stakeholders (with a single national taxonomy used for data storage and analysis).
> • Accreditation bodies responsible for the oversight of professional education should require more training in improving medication management practices and clinical pharmacology.

MOVING FORWARD

The American people expect safe medication care. In this report, the committee proposes an ambitious agenda for making the use of medications safer. This agenda requires that all stakeholders—patients, care providers, payers, industry, and government, working together—commit to preventing medication errors. Given that a large proportion of injurious drug events are preventable, this proposed agenda should deliver early and measurable benefits.

---

[3]Patient safety organizations are regulated through the Patient Safety and Quality Improvement Act of 2005 (P.L. 109-41). Broadly, they are organizations separate from health care providers that collect, manage, and analyze patient safety data, and advocate safety improvements on the basis of analysis of the patient safety data they receive.

REFERENCES

AHRQ (Agency for Healthcare Research and Quality). 2005. *Advances in Patient Safety: From Research to Implementation*. Vols. 1–4. Rockville, MD: AHRQ.

Barker KN, Flynn EA, Pepper GA, Bates DW, Mikeal RL. 2002. Medication errors observed in 36 health care facilities. *Archives of Internal Medicine* 162(16):1897–1903.

Bates DW. 2001. A 40-year-old woman who noticed a medication error. *Journal of the American Medical Association* 285(24):3134–3140.

Bates DW, Boyle DL, Vander Vliet MB, Schneider J, Leape L. 1995a. Relationship between medication errors and adverse drug events. *Journal of General Internal Medicine* 10(4): 100–205.

Bates DW, Cullen DJ, Laird N, Petersen LA, Small SD, Servi D, Laffel G, Sweitzer BJ, Shea BF, Hallisey R, Vander Vliet M, Nemeskal R, Leape LL. 1995b. Incidence of adverse drug events and potential adverse drug events. Implications for prevention. ADE Prevention Study Group. *Journal of the American Medical Association* 274:29–34.

Bates DW, Spell N, Cullen DJ, Burdick E, Laird N, Petersen LA, Small SD, Sweitzer BJ, Leape L. 1997. The costs of adverse drug events in hospitalized patients. Adverse Drug Events Prevention Study Group. *Journal of the American Medical Association* 277(4):307–311.

Bates DW, Leape LL, Cullen DJ, Laird N, Petersen LA, Teich JM, Burdick E, Hickey M, Kleefield S, Shea B, Vander Vliet M. 1998. Effect of computerized physician order entry and a team intervention on prevention of serious medication errors. *Journal of the American Medical Association* 280(15):1311–1316.

CC (Cochrane Collaboration). 2005. *What Is the Cochrane Collaboration?* [Online]. Available: http://www.cochrane.org/docs/descrip.htm [accessed October 6, 2005].

Classen DC, Pestotnik SL, Evans RS, Lloyd JF, Burke JP. 1997. Adverse drug events in hospitalized patients. Excess length of stay, extra costs, and attributable mortality. *Journal of the American Medical Association* 277(4):301–306.

Cohen MR. 2000. *Medication Errors: Causes, Prevention, and Risk Management*. Sudbury, MA: Jones and Bartlett Publishers.

Epocrates. 2005. *All-One-Guide to Drugs, Diseases and Diagnostics*. [Online]. Available: http://www2.epocrates.com [accessed October 6, 2005].

Evans RS, Classen DC, Pestotnik SL, Lundsgaarde HP, Burke JP. 1994. Improving empiric antibiotic selection using computer decision support. *Archives of Internal Medicine* 154(8):878–884.

Evans RS, Pestotnik SL, Classen DC, Clemmer TP, Weaver LK, Orme JF, Lloyd JF, Burke JP. 1998. A computer-assisted management program for antibiotics and other antiinfective agents. *New England Journal of Medicine* 338(4):232–238.

Field TS, Gilman BH, Subramanian S, Fuller JC, Bates DW, Gurwitz JH. 2005. The costs associated with adverse drug events among older adults in the ambulatory setting. *Medical Care* 43(12):1171–1176.

Flynn EA, Barker KN, Pepper GA, Bates DW, Mikeal RL. 2002. Comparison of methods for detecting medication errors in 36 hospitals and skilled-nursing facilities. *American Journal of Health-System Pharmacy* 59(5):436–446.

Gandhi TK, Weingart SN, Borus J, Seger AC, Peterson J, Burdick E, Seger DL, Shu K, Federico F, Leape LL, Bates DW. 2003. Adverse drug events in ambulatory care. *New England Journal of Medicine* 348(16):1556–1564.

Gurwitz JH, Field TS, Harrold LR, Rothschild J, Debellis K, Seger AC, Cadoret C, Garber L, Fish LS, Kelleher M, Bates DW. 2003. Incidence and preventability of adverse drug events among older person in the ambulatory setting. *Journal of the American Medical Association* 289(94):1107–1116.

Gurwitz JH, Field TS, Judge J, Rochon P, Harrold LR, Cadoret C, Lee M, White K, LaPrino J, Mainard JF, DeFlorio M, Gavendo L, Auger J, Bates DW. 2005. The incidence of adverse drug events in two large academic long-term care facilities. *American Journal of Medicine* 118(3):251–258.

IOM (Institute of Medicine). 2000. *To Err Is Human: Building a Safer Health System.* Washington, DC: National Academy Press.

IOM. 2001. *Crossing the Quality Chasm: A New Health System for the 21st Century.* Washington, DC: National Academy Press.

IOM. 2004. *Patient Safety: Achieving a New Standard for Care.* Washington, DC: The National Academies Press.

Jha AK, Kuperman GJ, Teich JM, Leape L, Shea B, Rittenberg E, Burdick E, Seger DL, Vander Vliet M, Bates DW. 1998. Identifying adverse drug events: Development of a computer-based monitor and comparison with chart review and stimulated voluntary report. *Journal of the American Medical Informatics Association* 5(3):305–314.

Kaushal R, Bates DW, Landrigan C, McKenna KJ, Clapp MD, Federico F, Goldmann DA. 2001. Medication errors and adverse drug events in pediatric inpatients. *Journal of the American Medical Association* 285(16):2114–2120.

Kaushal R, Shojania KG, Bates DW. 2003. Effects of computerized physician order entry and clinical decision support systems on medication safety: A systematic review. *Archives of Internal Medicine* 163(12):1409–1416.

Leape LL, Bates DW, Cullen DJ, Cooper J, Demonaco HJ, Gallivan T, Hallisey R, Ives J, Laird N, Laffel G, Nemeskal R, Petersen L, Porter K, Servi D, Shea B, Small S, Weitzer B, Thompson B, Vander Vleit M. 1995. Systems analysis of adverse drug events. *Journal of the American Medical Association* 274(1):35–43.

Leape LL, Cullen DJ, Clapp MD, Burdick E, Demonaco HJ, Erickson JI, Bates DW. 1999. Pharmacists participation on physician rounds and adverse drug events in the intensive care unit. *Journal of the American Medical Association* 282(3):267–270.

Pronovost P, Weast B, Schwarz M, Wyskiel RM, Prow D, Milanovich SN, Berenholtz S, Dorman T, Lipsett P. 2003. Medication reconciliation: A practical tool to reduce the risk of medication errors. *American Journal of Critical Care* 18(4):201–205.

Reason J. 2000. Human error: Models of management. *British Medical Journal* 320(7237): 768–770.

Svarstad BL, Mount JK. 2001. *Evaluation of Written Prescription Information Provided in Community Pharmacies, 2001.* Rockville, MD: U.S. FDA.

van Bemmel JH, Musen MA. 1997. *Handbook of Medical Informatics.* Heidelberg, Germany: Springer-Verlag.

1

Introduction

The Institute of Medicine (IOM) report *To Err Is Human: Building a Safer Health System* (IOM, 2000) identified medication errors as the most common type of error in health care and attributed several thousand deaths to medication-related events. The report had an immediate impact. In response, Congress apportioned $50 million in fiscal year 2001 for a major federal initiative to improve patient safety research and directed the Agency for Healthcare Research and Quality (AHRQ) to establish a Center for Quality Improvement and Patient Safety. The American people also took notice: 51 percent of respondents to a national survey conducted in late 1999 reported closely following the media coverage on the report (Kaiser Family Foundation, 1999).[1] The report's impact has continued. Five years after its release, two members of the committee that produced the report (Leape and Berwick, 2005) reflected that it had led to:

- Broader acceptance within the health care community that preventable medical errors are a serious problem.
- A number of important stakeholders (for example, the federal government, the Veterans Health Administration, and the Joint Commission on Accreditation of Healthcare Organizations [JCAHO]) taking up the challenge to improve patient safety.
- Accelerated implementation of safe health care practices. For example, JCAHO in 2003 required hospitals to implement a number of evidenced-based safe-care practices, and the Institute for Healthcare Im-

---

[1]The IOM report was released in 1999, prior to the survey, and formally published in 2000.

provement undertook its 100,000 Lives Campaign, aimed at fostering the use of safe practices.

Likewise, an article in *Health Affairs* reviewing the impact of *To Err Is Human* (Wachter, 2004) noted that the report had led to improved patient safety processes through stronger regulation (for example, expanded patient safety regulation by JCAHO). The article also pointed to the accelerated implementation of clinical information systems that can help reduce medication errors. In addition, progress had been made on workforce issues, particularly in hospitals through the emergence of hospitalists—physicians who coordinate the care of hospitalized patients. Overall, however, the review suggested that much more needed to be done. Examples cited were the limited impact of error reporting systems and scant progress in improving accountability.

The key messages of *To Err Is Human* were that there are serious problems with the quality of health care delivery; that these problems stem primarily from poor health care delivery systems, not incompetent individuals; and that solving these problems will require fundamental changes in the way care is delivered. A subsequent IOM report, *Crossing the Quality Chasm: A New Health System for the 21st Century* (IOM, 2001), took up the challenge of suggesting how the health care delivery system should be redesigned. It identified six aims for quality improvement: health care should be safe, effective, patient-centered, timely, efficient, and equitable (IOM, 2001).

The *Quality Chasm* report and the later IOM report, *Patient Safety: Achieving a New Standard for Care* (IOM, 2004), also emphasized the need for an information infrastructure to support the delivery of quality health care. The latter report called specifically for a national health information infrastructure to provide real-time access to complete patient information and decision-support tools for clinicians and their patients, to capture patient safety information as a by-product of care, and to make it possible to use this information to design even safer delivery systems (IOM, 2004).

To Err Is Human focused on injuries arising as a direct consequence of treatment, that is, errors of commission, such as prescribing a medication that has harmful interactions with another medication the patient is taking. *Patient Safety* focused not only on those errors, but also errors of omission, such as failing to prescribe a medication from which the patient would likely have benefited. Box 1-1 portrays in stark terms an example of the failure of the care delivery system to catch and mitigate a medication error and the tragic outcome that resulted.

MEDICATION ERRORS: THE MAGNITUDE OF THE CHALLENGE

Regardless of whether one considers errors of commission or omission, error rates for various steps in the medication-use process, adverse drug

BOX 1-1
The Betsy Lehman Case

Betsy Lehman, a 39-year-old wife and mother of two and health reporter for the *Boston Globe*, was diagnosed with breast cancer in September 1993. She was admitted to the Dana-Farber Cancer Institute in Boston on November 14, 1994, for her third round of cyclophosphamide, a toxic chemotherapy agent. Betsy was participating in a dose-escalating phase 1 clinical trial in which higher-than-normal doses of the drug were being administered to wipe out cancer cells. She was undergoing a bone marrow transplant to restore immune and blood-forming cells.

Betsy received the wrong dose of cyclophosphamide. The correct dose was 1,000 milligrams (mg) per square meter (m^2) of body surface area, given each day for a total of 4 days (or, for her height and weight, a total of 4,000 mg/m^2 or 6,520 mg infused over the 4-day course of therapy). But after reading the trial protocol, a physician fellow wrote the order as "4,000 mg/m^2 × 4 days." The erroneous dosing went unrecognized, and Betsy died as a result of the overdose on December 3, 1993. The error was not discovered until 10 weeks later, when her treatment data were entered into the computer for the clinical trial (Bohmer, 2003; Bohmer and Winslow, 1999).

Experts at the hospital, as well as outside consultants, recognized that many factors contributed to this tragedy (Conway and Weingart, 2005). System issues included minimal double-checks, orders written by fellows without attending MD signoff, and unclear protocols that were not current and not easily available to RNs and pharmacists. Some dosages were written in total dose and some in daily dose formats, often in the same protocol. Maximum dose checking was not a feature of the pharmacy computer system. Both the patient and her family had felt that Betsy was not being listened to and mechanisms for reporting issues were not clear. When reporting did occur, it did not move up the organization in a timely fashion.

Today, the hospital has a strong culture of safety and engages interdisciplinary groups of front-line clinicians in the design and implementation of chemotherapy protocols. There is an understanding that safe cancer care requires an extraordinarily high level of communication, coordination, and vigilance, with a strong focus on being aware of and acting on the incidence of errors (Gandhi et al., 2005). Authority to prescribe cancer chemotherapy is reserved for attending staff, and dosages must be expressed only in terms of daily dose. Computer system warnings prevent physicians from placing drug orders that exceed the safe maximum, and the computerized provider order entry system is extensively supported by online protocols and templates. Alerts such as a red "WARNING: HIGH CHEMOTHERAPY DOSE" appear on the screen. To override the computer and exceed current guidelines, doctors must show the pharmacist new scientific results that prove a higher dose may be safe and effective. Much has been done to encourage independent checks of prescribed doses by nurses and pharmacists, and staff have been explicitly authorized to question openly any presumed dosing error. The organization describes the key lessons learned in the 10 years since Betsy's overdose as the importance of the engagement of governance and leadership, vigilance by all every day, support for victims of errors, system support for safe practice, interdisciplinary practice, and patient- and family-centered care (Conway and Weingart, 2005; Conway et al., 2006).

event rates in various care settings, or estimates of the economic impact of drug-related morbidity and mortality, it is clear that medication safety represents a serious cause of concern for both health care providers and patients. Data from a variety of settings demonstrate that medication errors are common, although the frequency reported depends on the identification technique used and the definition of error employed.

A 1999 study in 36 hospitals and skilled nursing facilities found a 10 percent medication administration error rate (excluding wrong-time errors) (Barker et al., 2002). In observational studies of hospital outpatient pharmacies, prescription dispensing error rates of 0.2 to 10 percent have been found (Flynn et al., 2003). And in a national observational study of the accuracy of prescription dispensing in community pharmacies, the error rate was 1.7 percent—equivalent to about 50 million errors during the filling of 3 billion prescriptions each year in the United States (Flynn et al., 2003).

The mortality projections documented in *To Err Is Human* were derived from adverse event data collected in a New York State study (Brennan et al., 1991; Leape et al., 1991) and a Colorado/Utah study (Thomas et al., 2000). In these two studies, medication-related adverse events were found to be the most common type of adverse event—representing 19 percent of all such events. In a variety of studies, moreover, researchers have found even higher rates of inpatient adverse drug events than were observed in the New York State and Colorado/Utah studies (Classen et al., 1991; Bates et al., 1995b) using less restrictive definitions of adverse drug events and more rigorous detection methods. More recently, major studies have shown that many adverse drug events occur in the period after discharge from the hospital (Forster et al., 2003), in nursing homes (Gurwitz et al., 2000, 2005), and in ambulatory care settings (Gandhi et al., 2003; Gurwitz et al., 2003).

In a major recent study, moreover, researchers found high levels of errors of omission in the U.S. health care system across a wide range of measures. The chance of receiving high-quality care was only about 55 percent (McGlynn et al., 2003).

Nearly 10 years ago, researchers estimated that the annual cost of drug-related illness and death in the ambulatory care setting in the United States was approximately $76.6 billion (Johnson and Bootman, 1997). Using the same approach, this cost was estimated to be $177.4 billion in 2000 (Ernst and Grizzle, 2001).

MEASURES TO IMPROVE MEDICATION SAFETY

Efforts to improve medication safety are made at all levels of the health care system: by helping the patient avoid medication errors; by organizing health care units so that care is delivered safely; by creating health care organizations (collections of health care delivery units) that foster safe care, for example, through training for health care workers; and by encouraging health care organizations to deliver safe care by such means as regulatory and fiscal measures. Many of these efforts are long-standing and predate *To Err Is Human*. Key examples of such efforts are described below.

Helping the Patient Avoid Medication Errors

Since the early 1980s, the People's Medical Society has developed guidelines to help consumers avoid medication errors in hospitals and at community and mail-order pharmacies (Personal communication, Charles Inlander, March 25, 2005). Medication errors can also take place in the home, and in June 2004, the National Consumers League, jointly with the Food and Drug Administration (FDA), launched Take with Care, a public education campaign addressing the need to be careful when taking over-the-counter (OTC) pain relievers (National Consumers League, 2004).

Organizing Health Care Units to Deliver Care Safely

For more than a decade, many organizations have provided guidance on safe medication practices for health care delivery units. Since 1994 the Institute for Safe Medication Practices has provided guidance on eliminating medication errors through newsletters, journal articles, and communications with health care professionals and regulatory authorities. In 1996 the National Coordinating Council for Medication Error Reduction and Prevention began publishing a series of recommendations on strategies for reducing medication errors (NCCMERP, 2005). Professional organizations have also offered guidance on medication safety. For example, the American Society of Health-System Pharmacists has provided guidance on safe pharmacy practices in hospitals and integrated health systems. Recently, the American Academy of Pediatrics published guidelines on the prevention of medication errors in the pediatric inpatient setting (Stucky et al., 2003).

Following the publication of *To Err Is Human*, AHRQ funded studies to evaluate best practices. The agency commissioned the Evidence-Based Practice Center of the University of California, San Francisco–Stanford University to evaluate the evidence supporting a long list of proposed safe practices, including many related to medication (Shojania et al., 2001).

In 2003, the National Quality Forum (NQF) identified 30 practices that should be adopted in applicable care settings, including implementing a computerized prescriber order entry system (safe practice 12) (NQF, 2003). In addition, JCAHO has been active in fostering patient safety for many years. In 1995 it implemented a Sentinel Event Policy that encourages the voluntary reporting of serious adverse events and requires the performance of root-cause analyses for such events. Beginning in 1998, JCAHO disseminated patient safety solutions via Sentinel Event Alerts, based on analyses of reported sentinel events. Since 2003, JCAHO has set annual National Patient Safety Goals (JCAHO, 2006). Many of these goals relate to medications; an example is goal 13: Encourage the active involvement of patients and their families in the patients' care as a patient safety strategy.

In parallel with the development of guidance on the delivery of safe care, emerging technologies have been developed to improve safety. These include electronic prescribing that automates the medication ordering process; clinical decision-support systems (usually combined with electronic prescribing systems), which may include suggestions or default values for drug doses and checks for drug allergies, drug laboratory values, and drug–drug interactions; automated dispensing systems that dispense medications electronically in a controlled fashion and track medication use; bar coding for positive identification of patients, prescriptions, and medications; and computerized adverse drug event monitors that search patient databases for data that may indicate the occurrence of such an event.

Creating Health Care Organizations That Foster Safe Care

The full benefits of technologies for preventing medication errors will not be achieved unless a culture of safety is created within health care organizations that are adequately staffed with professionals whose knowledge, skills, and ethics make them capable of overseeing the medication management of patients who are vulnerable and unable to manage their medications knowledgeably themselves (IOM, 2004). Indeed, the first safe practice in the NQF report *Safe Practices for Better Healthcare* is the creation of a culture of safety (NQF, 2003). The IOM's (2004) *Patient Safety* report outlined the elements of a culture of safety: a shared understanding that health care is a high-risk undertaking, recruitment and training with patient safety in mind, an organizational commitment to detecting and analyzing patient injuries and near misses, open communication regarding patient injury results, and the establishment of a just culture seeking to balance the need to learn from mistakes and the need to take disciplinary action (IOM, 2004).

Two of NQF's safe practices relate to the need for adequate resources. Safe practice 3 calls for use of an explicit protocol to ensure an adequate level of nursing based on the institution's usual patient mix and the experience and training of its nursing staff. Safe practice 5 calls for pharmacists to participate actively in the medication-use process, including, at a minimum, being available for consultation with prescribers on medication ordering, interpretation and review of medication orders, preparation of medications, dispensing of medications, and administration and monitoring of medications.

Establishing an Environment That Enables Health Care Organizations to Deliver Safe Care

Many important systems, including accreditation, information technology, education, and knowledge generation, foster safe medication use. Important developments have occurred in each of these areas since the release of *To Err Is Human*. The medication-related National Patient Safety Goals and associated requirements established by JCAHO are an example in the area of accreditation. With regard to information technology, several IOM reports have stressed the need for an information infrastructure to support the delivery of quality health care. A key element of this infrastructure is the development and implementation of national health care data standards. In May 2004, Secretary of Health and Human Services Thompson announced 15 health care data standards for use across the federal health care sector, building on an initial set of 5 standards adopted in March 2003 (DHHS, 2004). In 2003 the Accreditation Council on Graduate Medical Education promulgated new residency training work-hour limitations (ACGME, 2003), drawing on published research on the relationship between fatigue and errors. And in response to *To Err Is Human*, Congress apportioned $50 million to support patient safety research; in early 2005, AHRQ published the results of this research (AHRQ, 2005).

STUDY CONTEXT[2]

Attempts to improve medication safety must be considered against the background of a number of important contextual issues. First, it is essential to recognize the ubiquitous nature of the use of prescription and OTC drugs and of complementary and alternative medications in the United States. In the 2004 Slone Survey (Slone, 2005), 82 percent of adults reported taking at least one medication (prescription or OTC drug, vitamin/mineral, or herbal supplement) during the week preceding the interview, and 30 percent reported taking at least five medications. The three most commonly used drugs were all OTC—acetaminophen (used by 20 percent of the adult population in the week prior to the interview), aspirin, and ibuprofen. In 2003, 3.4 billion prescriptions were purchased in the United States; on average there were 11.8 prescriptions per person (Kaiser Family Foundation, 2004). Fifty-

---

[2]The discussion here, as well as elsewhere in the report, draws on a paper commissioned by the committee: "Trends in Medication Use: Implications for Medication Errors," by Brent Petty, MD, The Johns Hopkins Hospital.

five percent of the adults interviewed in the 2004 Slone Survey reported taking at least one prescription drug in the week prior to the interview, and 11 percent reported taking five or more such drugs (Slone, 2005). In the same survey, 42 percent of the adults surveyed reported taking vitamins and 19 percent herbal or other natural supplements.

Another key contextual issue is ongoing cost containment efforts. In recent years, these efforts have failed to limit increases in health care costs to the general inflation rate or less. National health spending in 2003 was $1.679 trillion, an increase of 7.7 percent over the previous year (Smith et al., 2005). This growth rate is not much below that for the previous year; in 2002 national health spending increased 9.3 percent over that in 2001 (Levit et al., 2004). U.S. prescription drug sales have been rising more rapidly yet. IMS Health Inc., a leading provider of information and consulting services to the pharmaceutical and health care industries, reported that prescription drug sales in the United States grew 8.3 percent to $235 billion in 2004, compared with $217 billion the previous year (IMS, 2005). This increase followed an 11.5 percent growth in 2003 over 2002 and an 11.8 percent growth in 2002 over 2001 (IMS, 2003, 2004). One critical implication of these figures relevant to this study is that efforts to control health care costs at the federal and state levels and within health care organizations mean that any new investments, including investments in medication safety, will need to be thoroughly justified.

Efforts to contain health care costs have had limited success because of a number of important cost drivers (IFoM, 2003). Innovative new pharmaceuticals are displacing older agents, which are usually cheaper because they are off patent. An aging population is leading to higher consumption of health care in general and pharmaceuticals in particular. A more demanding patient population is less accepting of restrictions on health care use for cost containment reasons. And a broader definition of treatable disease is increasing the demand for health care. Implementation of the Medicare prescription drug benefit is also likely to increase the demand for pharmaceuticals. The Administration's Financial Year Budget projected that the net federal cost of the Medicare prescription drug benefit would be $37.4 billion in 2006, rising to $109.2 billion in 2015 (Kaiser Family Foundation, 2005).

The FDA is a key player in ensuring the safety of medications, both prescription and nonprescription. The FDA approves a drug for sale in the United States after determining that its clinical benefits outweigh its potential risks. After a drug has been approved, the FDA continues to assess its benefits and risks, primarily on the basis of reports made to the agency on the effects of its use. In 2004, withdrawal of the drug rofecoxib (Vioxx) by Merck & Co. Inc. for safety reasons increased public concern about the procedures used for assessing drug safety. In response to this concern, the

FDA requested that the IOM convene an ad hoc committee of experts (the IOM Committee on Assessment of the U.S. Drug Safety System) to conduct an independent assessment of the current system for evaluating and ensuring drug safety postmarketing.

Implementation of the Medication Modernization Act of 2003 (P.L. 108-173) will make the Centers for Medicare and Medicaid Services (CMS) the largest purchaser of prescription drugs in the United States and a major player in the way prescription medications are used. The next few years will be a pivotal period as CMS decides how it will administer the prescription drug benefit. There will be opportunities for introducing into the drug benefit rules safety guidelines for both prescribing and dispensing, and to use pay-for-performance incentives to enhance adoption of whatever guidelines are proposed. Further, there will be opportunities for medication safety research arising from the data CMS will collect as part of the drug benefit (CMS, 2005).

CMS will also become an important driver of electronic prescribing standards, whose development and implementation are called for by the Medication Modernization Act. The Medicare Prescription Drug Benefit final rule (42 Code of Federal Regulations Parts 400, 403, 411, 417 and 423) requires that Part D sponsors (e.g., participating Prescription Drug Plans and Medicare Advantage Organizations) support and comply with such standards once they are in effect. The final rule does not require providers to write prescriptions electronically; if prescribers send prescription information electronically, however, they will have to use the standards.

STUDY CHARGE AND APPROACH

In this context, at the urging of the Senate Finance Committee, the United States Congress, through the Medicare Modernization Act of 2003 (Section 107(c)), mandated that CMS sponsor a study by the IOM to address the problem of medication errors. The IOM convened the Committee on Identifying and Preventing Medication Errors to conduct this study, with the following charge:

• To develop a fuller understanding of drug safety and quality issues through the conduct of an evidence-based review of the literature, case studies and analysis. This review will consider the nature and causes of medication errors; their impact on patients; and the differences in causation, impact and prevention across multiple dimensions of health care delivery including patient populations, care settings, clinicians, and institutional cultures.

• If possible, to develop estimates of the incidence, severity and costs of medication errors that can be useful in prioritizing resources for national quality improvement efforts and influencing national health care policy.

- To evaluate alternative approaches to reducing medication errors in terms of their efficacy, cost-effectiveness, appropriateness in different settings and circumstances, feasiblity, institutional barriers to implementation, associated risk, and quality of evidence supporting the approach.
- To provide guidance to consumers, providers, payers, and other key stakeholders on high-priority strategies to achieve both short-term and long-term drug safety goals, to elucidate the goals and expected results of such initiatives and support the business case for them, and to identify critical success factors and key levers for achieving success.
- To assess opportunities and key impediments to broad nationwide implementation of medication error reductions, and to provide guidance to policy-makers and government agencies in promoting a national agenda for medication error reduction.
- To develop an applied research agenda to evaluate the health and cost impacts of alternative interventions, and to assess collaborative public and private strategies for implementing the research agenda through AHRQ and other government agencies.

The committee comprised 17 members representing a range of expertise related to the scope of the study, as described below (see Appendix A for biographical sketches of the committee members). The committee addressed its charge by reviewing the salient research literature, government reports and data, empirical evidence, and additional materials provided by government officials and others. In addition, a workshop was held to augment the committee's knowledge and expertise through more focused discussion of specific issues of concern, and to obtain input from a wide range of researchers, providers of health care services, and interested members of the public. The committee also commissioned several background papers to avail itself of expert, detailed, and independent analyses of some of the key issues beyond the time and resources of its members.

SCOPE OF THE STUDY

CMS determined that this study should focus on issues related to the safe, effective, appropriate, and efficient *use of medications*. As mentioned above, a parallel IOM committee, the Drug Safety Committee, was tasked with assessing the *postmarketing surveillance system for medications*. There is some overlap between the present study and the work of that committee. The two committees and their staffs have worked together closely to define common areas in the two studies and develop consistent sets of recommendations.

Definitions

Drugs and Dietary Supplements

This study addressed the quality of the five steps in the medication-use process: selecting and procuring by the pharmacy, selecting and prescribing for the patient, preparing and dispensing, administering, and monitoring effects on the patient. The study examined medication use in a wide range of care settings—hospital, long-term, and community. The term *medication* encompasses three broad categories of products—prescription and nonprescription drugs and dietary supplements—all regulated by the FDA (see Chapter 2).

According to the FDA (2004), a *drug* is defined as a substance that is recognized by an official pharmacopeia or formulary; intended for use in the diagnosis, cure, mitigation, treatment, or prevention of disease; intended to affect the structure or any function of the body (excluding food); and intended for use as a component of a medicine, but not a device or a component, part, or accessory of a device.

Biologic products (including vaccines, blood, and blood products) are a subset of drug products. Biologics are distinguished from other drugs by their manufacturing process—biological as opposed to chemical. Some biologics, principally vaccines (excluding their long-term effects), are within the scope of this study; blood and blood products and tissues for transplantation are excluded.

Drugs include both those that require a prescription and those that do not. Nonprescription drugs are usually termed *over-the-counter* (OTC). The characteristics of OTC drugs are such that the potential for misuse and abuse is low, consumers are able to use them successfully for self-diagnosable conditions, they can be adequately labeled for ease and accuracy of use, and oversight by health practitioners is not needed to ensure safe and effective use (FDA, 2005).

Dietary supplements, often called *complementary and alternative medications*, are another group of products often used for medicinal or general health purposes. The Dietary Supplement Health and Education Act of 1994 (P.L. 103-147) defined a dietary supplement as a product (other than tobacco) intended to supplement the diet that bears or contains one or more of the following dietary ingredients: a vitamin; a mineral; an herb or other botanical; an amino acid; a dietary substance for use by man to supplement the diet by increasing the dietary intake; or a concentrate, metabolite, constituent, extract, or combination of any ingredient cited above. While the primary emphasis of the study was on prescription and OTC drugs, attention was given to dietary supplements as well, and the discussion of drugs often applies also to the latter products.

Medication Error, Adverse Drug Event, and Adverse Drug Reaction

The terms *medication error, adverse drug event,* and *adverse drug reaction* denote related concepts (see Figure 1-1) and are often used incorrectly. *To Err Is Human* (IOM, 2000, p. 28) defined *error* and *adverse event* as follows:

> An error is defined as the failure of a planned action to be completed as intended (i.e., error of execution), or the use of a wrong plan to achieve an aim (i.e., error of planning).

> An adverse event is an injury caused by medical management rather than the underlying condition of the patient.

The Committee on Data Standards for Patient Safety was concerned that the phrase *medical management* did not embrace *acts of omission.* The committee gave considerable thought to expanding on these two definitions and produced the following (IOM, 2004, p. 30, 32):

> An error is defined as the failure of a planned action to be completed as intended (i.e., error of execution), or the use of a wrong plan to achieve an aim (i.e., error of planning). An error may be an act of commission or an act of omission.

> An adverse event results in unintended harm to the patient by an act of commission or omission rather than by the underlying disease or condition of the patient.

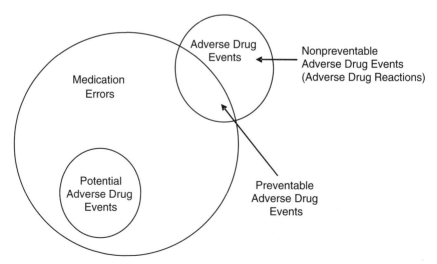

FIGURE 1-1 Relationship among medication errors, adverse drug events, and potential adverse drug events.
SOURCE: Gandhi et al., 2000.

The Committee on Data Standards for Patient Safety wanted to make clear that the potentially avoidable results of an underlying disease or condition—for example, a recurrent myocardial infarction in a patient without a contraindication who was not given a beta-blocker (an error of omission)—should be considered an adverse event (IOM, 2004). The Committee on Identifying and Preventing Medication Errors discussed the *adverse event* definition given in the *Patient Safety* report and decided to adopt this definition. Further attempts to operationalize the definition of adverse event may well lead eventually to additional modifications of the definition.

Consistent with the above definitions:

A medication error is defined as any error occurring in the medication use process (Bates et al., 1995a).

An adverse drug event is defined as any injury due to medication (Bates et al., 1995b).

An injury includes physical harm (for example, rash), mental harm (for example, confusion), or loss of function (for example, inability to drive a car).

Medication errors and adverse drug events have multiple sources. They may be related to professional practice; health care products, procedures, and systems, including prescribing; order communication; product labeling, packaging, and nomenclature; compounding; dispensing; distribution; administration; education of the patient or health care professional; and monitoring of use.

Implicit in the definition of medication errors is that they are preventable. However, most medication errors do not cause harm. Some do cause harm and are either potential adverse drug events or preventable adverse drug events (see Figure 1-1), depending on whether an injury occurred (Gandhi et al., 2000). Potential adverse drug events are events in which an error occurred but did not cause injury (for example, the error was detected before the patient was affected, or the patient received a wrong dose but experienced no harm) (Gandhi et al., 2000).

Adverse drug events can be preventable (for example, a wrong dose leads to injury) or nonpreventable (for example, an allergic reaction occurs in a patient not known to be allergic) (see Figure 1-1). Nonpreventable adverse drug events are also often termed adverse drug reactions[3] (Gandhi et al., 2000).

---

[3]The field of pharmacoepidemiology defines the terms *adverse drug event* and *adverse drug reaction* differently (Strom, 2005). An adverse drug event (or adverse drug experience) is an untoward outcome that occurs during or following clinical use of a drug, whether preventable or not. An adverse drug reaction is an adverse drug event that is judged to be caused by the drug.

The World Health Organization has defined an adverse drug reaction as a response to a drug that is noxious and unintended and occurs at doses normally used in man for prophylaxis, diagnosis, or therapy of disease or modification of physiological function (WHO, 1975). This definition excludes injuries due to drugs that are caused by errors, which are of obvious interest. As a result, drug safety researchers coined the term *adverse drug event* to include both adverse drug reactions (which are nonpreventable), and preventable adverse drug events (Bates et al., 1995b). From the safety perspective, preventable adverse drug events are most important because they are known to be preventable today; adverse drug reactions are also important, however, since it may become possible to prevent them in the future by using new approaches, such as pharmacogenomic profiling.

Audiences for the Report

The committee sought to assess the roles of and make recommendations for all of the major stakeholders involved in the safe use of medications:

- First and foremost, the consumer[4] or patient who uses a medication, as well as family members, friends, and neighbors who may be involved in assisting the patient.
- Individual health care providers—physicians, nurses, and pharmacists.
- The organizations responsible for delivering care, for example, hospitals, nursing homes, ambulatory clinics, pharmacies, and pharmacy benefit managers.
- Those responsible for salient policy (Congress and state legislators), payment (CMS and commercial insurers), regulation (for example, the FDA and state regulatory bodies), accreditation (for example, JCAHO), and professional education (for example, schools of nursing).
- Manufacturers of medications and the systems used in medication delivery (for example, intravenous pumps and health information technology systems) and providers of value-added services (for example, tools that indicate harmful drug–drug interactions).

In carrying out the study, the committee took the view that the goal of all these stakeholders with regard to medication use should be to optimize the relationship between the patient and the health care provider(s) so as to meet the six aims set forth in the *Quality Chasm* report (care should be safe, effective, timely, patient-centered, equitable, and efficient) (IOM, 2001). In

---

[4]In this report, the term *consumers* is often used in referring to patients to emphasize the active role individuals need to take in ensuring the quality of the health care services they are purchasing.

general, the health care system should enable the flow of all information needed to choose medications that optimize health to the extent possible in accordance with the preferences of the patient. In addition, all health care stakeholders should attempt to produce information on and inform patients and providers about the balance between effectiveness and safety, rather than addressing either in isolation. Effectiveness (tangible benefits— those that can be felt by the patient—in the actual setting in which the medication is used) rather than efficacy (benefit based on ideal circumstances of use) is the appropriate measure for the purpose of informing patients and providers. Further, all stakeholders should strive to produce a system in which the transactions that ensue following a decision about using a medication at a particular dose and time are free of errors.

REPORT OVERVIEW

Part I of this report addresses the causes, incidence, and costs of medication errors. By way of background, it begins with a case study illustrating how medication errors can arise through a combination of organizational and individual failures. Chapter 2 provides an overview of the system for drug development, regulation, distribution, and use, identifying the many points at which errors can occur. Chapter 3 summarizes the peer-reviewed literature on the incidence and costs of medication errors.

Part II of the report outlines the steps needed to establish a patient-centered, integrated medication-use system. It provides action agendas for achieving both short- and long-term improvements in medication safety for patients/consumers to support provider–consumer partnerships (Chapter 4), for health care organizations (Chapter 5), and for the industry that provides medications and medication-related products and services (Chapter 6). In Chapter 7, the committee outlines an applied research agenda designed to foster safe medication use. Finally, Chapter 8 proposes action agendas for those who set the environment in which care is delivered (for example, legislators, payers, and regulators). Appendix B provides a glossary and acronym list for the report, while Appendices C and D present detailed discussion of medication incidence rates and prevention strategies, respectively.

REFERENCES

ACGME (Accreditation Council for Graduate Medical Education). 2003. *For Insertion into the Common Program Requirements for All Core and Subspecialty Programs by July 1, 2003: V.F. Resident Duty Hours and the Working Environment.* [Online]. Available: http://www.acgme.org/acWebsite/dutyHours/dh_Lang703.pdf [accessed May 26, 2005].
AHRQ (Agency for Healthcare Research and Quality). 2005. *Advances in Patient Safety: From Research to Implementation.* Vols. 1–4. Rockville, MD: AHRQ.

Barker KN, Flynn EA, Pepper GA, Bates DW, Mikeal RL. 2002. Medication errors observed in 36 health care facilities. *Archives of Internal Medicine* 162(16):1897–1903.
Bates DW, Boyle DL, Vander Vliet MB, Schneider J, Leape L. 1995a. Relationship between medication errors and adverse drug events. *Journal of General Internal Medicine* 10(4): 100–205.
Bates DW, Cullen DJ, Laird N, Petersen LA, Small SD, Servi D, Laffel G, Sweitzer BJ, Shea BF, Hallisey R, Vander Vliet M, Nemeskal R, Leape LL. 1995b. Incidence of adverse drug events and potential adverse drug events. Implications for prevention. ADE Prevention Study Group. *Journal of the American Medical Association* 274:29–34.
Bohmer R, Winslow A. 1999. *The Dana-Farber Cancer Institute. HBS Case #699-025*. Boston, MA: Harvard Business School Publishing.
Bohmer RMJ. 2003. *Dana-Farber Cancer Institute, The (TN). Harvard Business School Teaching Note 603-092*. Boston, MA: Harvard Business School Publishing.
Brennan TA, Leape LL, Laird NM, Hebert L, Localio AR, Lawthers AG, Newhouse JP, Weiler PC, Hiatt HH. 1991. Incidence of adverse events and negligence in hospitalized patients. Results of the Harvard Medical Practice Study I. *New England Journal of Medicine* 324(6):370–376.
Classen DC, Pestotnik SL, Evans RS, Burke JP. 1991. Computerized surveillance of adverse drug events in hospital patients. *Journal of the American Medical Association* 266:2847–2851.
CMS (Centers for Medicare and Medicaid Services). 2005. *Speech by Administrator Mark B. McClellan, M.D., Ph.D., PCMA Drug Use Safety Symposium, May 11, 2005*. [Online]. Available: http://www.pcmanet.org/events/presentation/McClellan%20Drug%20Data%20speech.pdf [accessed May 26, 2005].
Conway JB, Weingart SN. 2005. *Organizational Change in the Face of Highly Public Errors: The Dana-Farber Cancer Institute Experience*. [Online]. Available: http://www.webmm.ahrq.gov/perspective.aspx?perspectiveID=3 [accessed January 25, 2006].
Conway JB, Nathan DG, Benz EJ. 2006. *Key Learning from the Dana-Farber Cancer Institute's 10-Year Patient Safety Journey. American Society of Clinical Oncology: 2006 Education Book*. Alexandria, VA: American Society of Clinical Oncology. Pp. 615–619.
DHHS (U.S. Department of Health and Human Services). 2004. *Secretary Thompson, Seeking Fastest Possible Results, Names First Health Information Technology Coordinator: HHS Also Announces Milestones in Developing Health IT*. [Online]. Available: http://www.hhs.gov/news/press/2004pres/20040506.html [accessed May 26, 2005].
Ernst FR, Grizzle AJ. 2001. Drug-related morbidity and mortality: Updating the cost-of-illness model. *Journal of the American Pharmacists Association* 41:192–199.
FDA (U.S. Food and Drug Administration). 2004. *Drugs @ FDA: Glossary of Terms*. [Online]. Available: http://www.fda.gov/cder/drugsatfda/glossary.htm [accessed June 7, 2005].
FDA. 2005. *Office of Nonprescription Drugs*. [Online]. Available: http://www.fda.gov/cder/offices/otc/default.htm [accessed June 7, 2005].
Flynn EA, Barker KN, Carnahan BJ. 2003. National observational study of prescription dispensing accuracy and safety in 50 pharmacies. *Journal of the American Pharmacists Association* 43(2):191–200.
Forster AJ, Murff HJ, Peterson JF, Gandhi TK, Bates DW. 2003. The incidence and severity of adverse events affecting patients after discharge from the hospital. *Annals of Internal Medicine* 138(3):161–167.
Gandhi TK, Seger DL, Bates DW. 2000. Identifying drug safety issues: From research to practice. *International Journal for Quality in Health Care* 12(1):69–76.
Gandhi TK, Weingart SN, Borus J, Seger AC, Peterson J, Burdick E, Seger DL, Shu K, Federico F, Leape LL, Bates DW. 2003. Adverse drug events in ambulatory care. *New England Journal of Medicine* 348(16):1556–1564.

Gandhi TK, Bartel SB, Shulman LN, Verrier D, Burdick E, Cleary A, Rothschild JM, Leape LL, Bates DW. 2005. Medication safety in the ambulatory chemotherapy setting. *Cancer* 104(11):2477–2483.

Gurwitz JH, Field TS, Avorn J, McCormick D, Jain S, Eckler M, Benser M, Edmondson AC, Bates DW. 2000. Incidence and preventability of adverse drug events in nursing homes. *American Journal of Medicine* 109(2):87–94.

Gurwitz JH, Field TS, Harrold LR, Rothschild J, Debellis K, Seger AC, Cadoret C, Fish LS, Garber L, Kelleher M, Bates DW. 2003. Incidence and preventability of adverse drug events among older persons in the ambulatory setting. *Journal of the American Medical Association* 289(9):1107–1116.

Gurwitz JH, Field TS, Judge J, Rochon P, Harrold LR, Cadoret C, Lee M, White K, LaPrino J, Mainard JF, DeFlorio M, Gavendo L, Auger J, Bates DW. 2005. The incidence of adverse drug events in two large academic long-term care facilities. *American Journal of Medicine* 118(3):251–258.

IFoM (International Forum on Medicine). 2003. *Presentation of the Forum and Current Agenda Areas*. The Hague, The Netherlands: International Pharmaceutical Federation.

IMS (Intercontinental Marketing Services). 2003. *IMS Reports 11.5% Dollar Growth in 2002 U.S. Prescription Sales*. [Online]. Available: http://imshealth.com/ims/portal/front/articleC/0,2777,6372_3665_41276589,00.html [accessed October 27, 2005].

IMS. 2004. *IMS Reports 11.5 Percent Dollar Growth in '03 U.S. Prescription Sales*. [Online]. Available: http://www.imshealth.com/ims/portal/front/articleC/0,2777,6599_40183881_44771558,00.html [accessed October 27, 2005].

IMS. 2005. *IMS Reports 8.3 Percent Dollar Growth in 2004 U.S. Prescription Sales*. [Online]. Available: http://ir.imshealth.com/phoenix.zhtml?c=67124&p=irol-newsArticle&ID=674505&highlight= [accessed October 27, 2005].

IOM (Institute of Medicine). 2000. *To Err Is Human: Building a Safer Health System*. Washington, DC: National Academy Press.

IOM. 2001. *Crossing the Quality Chasm: A New Health System for the 21st Century*. Washington, DC: National Academy Press.

IOM. 2004. *Patient Safety: Achieving a New Standard for Care*. Washington, DC: The National Academies Press.

JCAHO (Joint Commision on Accreditation of Healthcare Organizations). 2006. *Facts About the 2006 National Patient Safety Goals*.[Online]. Available: http://www.jcipatientsafety. org/show.asp?durki=9726 [accessed August 16, 2006].

Johnson JA, Bootman JL. 1997. Drug-related morbidity and mortality and the economic impact of pharmaceutical care. *American Journal of Health-System Pharmacy* 54: 554–558.

Kaiser Family Foundation. 1999. *Kaiser/Harvard Health News Index: November-December 1999*. [Online]. Available: http://www.kff.org/kaiserpolls/upload/13350_1.pdf [accessed May 25, 2005].

Kaiser Family Foundation. 2004. *Prescription Drug Trends—October 2004*. [Online]. Available: http://www.kff.org/rxdrugs/3057-03.cfm [accessed October 26, 2005].

Kaiser Family Foundation. 2005. *Medicare Fact Sheet: March 2005*. [Online]. Available: http://www.kff.org/medicare/loader.cfm?url=/commonspot/security/getfile.cfm& PageID=33325 [accessed May 25, 2005].

Leape LL, Berwick DM. 2005. Five years after To Err Is Human: What have we learned? *Journal of the American Medical Association* 293(19):2384–2390.

Leape LL, Brennan TA, Laird N, Lawthers AG, Localio AR, Barnes BA, Hebert L, Newhouse JP, Weiler PC, Hiatt H. 1991. The nature of adverse events in hospitalized patients. Results of the Harvard Medical Practice Study II. *New England Journal of Medicine* 324(6):377–384.

Levit K, Smith C, Cowan C, Sensenig A, Catlin A, Health Accounts Team. 2004. Health spending rebound continues in 2002. *Health Affairs (Millwood)* 23(1):147–159.

McGlynn EA, Asch SM, Adams J, Keesey J, Hicks J, DeCristofaro A, Kerr EA. 2003. The quality of health care delivered to adults in the United States. *New England Journal of Medicine* 348(26):2635–2645.

National Consumers League. 2004. *New Campaign Focuses on Preventing Common Medication Errors in the Home.* [Online]. Available: http://www.nclnet.org/news/2004/take_with_care.htm [accessed May 25, 2005].

NCCMERP (National Coordinating Council on Medical Error Reduction and Prevention). 2005. *National Coordinating Council on Medical Error Reduction and Prevention: Council Recommendations.* [Online]. Available: http://www.nccmerp.org/councilRecs.html [accessed May 25, 2005].

NQF (National Quality Forum). 2003. *Safe Practices for Better Healthcare: A Consensus Report.* Washington, DC: NQF.

Shojania K, Duncan B, McDonald K, Wachter RM. 2001. *Making Health Care Safer: A Critical Analysis of Patient Safety Practices.* Rockville, MD: AHRQ.

Slone. 2005. *Patterns of Medication Use in the United States 2004.* Boston, MA: Slone Epidemiology Center at Boston University.

Smith C, Cowan C, Sensenig A, Catlin A, Health Accounts Team. 2005. Health spending growth slows in 2003. *Health Affairs (Millwood)* 24(1):185–194.

Strom BL (editor). 2005. *Pharmacoepidemiology, 4th edition.* Chichester, England: Wiley.

Stucky ER, American Academy of Pediatrics Committee on Drugs, American Academy of Pediatrics Committee on Hospital Care. 2003. Prevention of medication errors in the pediatric inpatient setting. *Pediatrics* 112(2):431–436.

Thomas EJ, Studdert DM, Burstin HR, Orav EJ, Zeena T, Williams EJ, Howard KM, Weiler PC, Brennan TA. 2000. Incidence and types of adverse events and negligent care in Utah and Colorado. *Medical Care* 38(3):261–271.

Wachter RM. 2004. The end of the beginning: Patient safety five years after "To Err Is Human." *Health Affairs (Millwood)* (Suppl. Web Exclusives:W4):534–545.

WHO (World Health Organization). 1975. *Requirements for Adverse Drug Reporting.* Geneva, Switzerland: WHO.

Part I

Understanding the Causes and
Costs of Medication Errors

Numerous factors in the health care system contribute to medication safety and errors. Some of these factors can be attributed directly to provider organizations, while others can be attributed to the medication-use system itself. In many cases, multiple factors are involved. The following case study, discussed in *Hospital Pharmacy* (Smetzer and Cohen, 1998), illustrates the complexity of the health care system and the medication-use process and the interrelatedness of the factors involved in medication safety and quality.

In 1996, a Denver hospital acknowledged that a medication error had led to the death of a day-old infant, born to a mother with a prior history of syphilis. Because the infant's parents spoke only Spanish, communication was difficult, and treatment of the disease could not be verified easily. Despite incomplete information about the mother's past treatment for syphilis and the current status of both mother and child, a decision was made to treat the infant for congenital syphilis. After telephone consultation with infectious disease specialists and the health department, an order was written for one dose of "Benzathine penicillin G 150,000U IM."

The hospital physicians, nurses, and pharmacists, unfamiliar with the treatment of congenital syphilis, had limited knowledge about this drug. The pharmacist filling the order consulted both the infant's progress notes (where a nurse practitioner had documented a recommendation from the health department) and a drug reference book to determine the usual dose of penicillin G benzathine for an infant. However, the pharmacist misread the dose in both sources as 500,000 units/kilogram (kg), a typical adult dose, instead of 50,000 units/kg. Consequently, she misread the order as 1,500,000 units, especially since the "U" for units appeared to add a zero to the dose. She prepared the order accordingly—a 10-fold overdose. Because there was no consistent pharmacy procedure for independent double-checking, the error was not detected. A pharmacy label on the bag that was dispensed indicated that 2.5 milliliters (ml) of medication was to be administered IM (intramuscularly) to equal a dose of 1,500,000 units.

After glancing at the medication sent from the pharmacy, one of the nurses expressed concern to her colleagues about the number of injections required to give the infant the medication. Normally, because a baby's muscles are so tiny, a maximum of 0.5 ml per injection is allowed in infants. The labeled dose would require five injections. Wishing to prevent any unnecessary pain to the infant, two of the nurses decided to investigate the possibility of administering the medication IV (intravenously) instead of IM. They checked with a popular medication reference book to determine whether penicillin G benzathine could be administered IV. However, the reference did not mention penicillin G benzathine specifically; instead, it referred to aqueous crystalline penicillin G IV slow push or penicillin G procaine IM. Nowhere in the two-page text in the reference book was penicillin G benzathine mentioned, nor were there any specific warnings regarding "IM use only" for penicillin G procaine and penicillin G benzathine.

Unfamiliar with the various forms of penicillin G, the nurse practitioner believed that "benzathine" was a brand name for penicillin G. This misconception was reinforced by the fact that the physician had written the order with benzathine capitalized and placed on a line above "penicillin G" rather than after it on the same line. In addition, many texts use ambiguous synonyms when referring to various forms of penicillin. For example, penicillin G benzathine is frequently associated with the terms "crystalline penicillin" and "aqueous suspension" in texts. Believing that aqueous crystalline penicillin G and penicillin G benzathine were the same drug, the nurse practitioner concluded that the drug could be safely administered IV. The nurses knew that, while having been taught that only clear liquids can be injected IV, certain milky-looking substances, such as lipid-based drug products, can be given IV. Therefore, they did not recognize the problem with giving penicillin G benzathine, a milky-white substance, IV.

While hospital policies and practices gave prescribing authority to nurse practitioners, they did not clearly define such authority in terms of the ability to change prescription orders. However, the neonatal nurse practitioner assumed that she was operating under a national protocol that allows neonatal nurse practitioners to plan, direct, implement, and change drug therapy. Consequently, the nurse practitioner, not wanting to cause pain to the infant with the large IM injection dose, made the decision to administer the drug IV.

While preparing for drug administration, neither of the nurses noticed the 10-fold overdose or the manufacturer's label on the syringe "IM use only." They had no idea that IV administration would be lethal because the drug is insoluble and obstructs blood flow in the lungs required for the transfer of oxygen from the baby's airways. The manufacturer's warning is very difficult to see because it is not prominently placed; it can be viewed only if the syringe is rotated 180 degrees away from the drug name. The nurses began to administer the first syringe of Permapen slow IV push. After about 1.8 ml had been administered, the infant became unresponsive, and resuscitation efforts were unsuccessful. Later, upon autopsy, it was confirmed that the baby had not had congenital syphilis, and therefore never needed treatment.

The three nurses involved in this medication error were later indicted by a grand jury for negligent homicide. Two of the nurses agreed to legal sanctions before the trial, but a third pled not guilty, and a trial ensued. Expert testimony presented during the trial served as convincing evidence that, while the nurse and her colleagues had played a part in the tragedy, more than 50 latent[1] and active failures had occurred throughout the medication-use process (see Table I-1), most of which, such as the poor syringe labeling, the pharmacist's mistake, and the confusing drug information, had not been under the control of the nurses. It was these failures that had set the stage for the nurses' tragic mistakes. The experts advised against the tendency to focus on the errors of the providers. Had even one of these failures not occurred, either the accident would not have happened, or the error would have been detected and corrected before reaching the infant. Since most of what people do is governed by the system within which they act, the causes of errors belong to the system and often lie outside the control of individuals, despite their best efforts. This case illustrates that medication errors are almost never the fault of a single practitioner or caused by the failure of a single element. The analysis presented during the trial had a powerful influence on the jury, which acquitted the nurse in the one case that was tried. The lesson learned from this case study is that we must look beyond blaming individuals and focus on the multiple underlying system failures that shape individual behavior and create the conditions under which medication errors occur.

---

[1]Weaknesses in the structure of an organization, such as faulty information management, ineffective personnel training, or faulty drug labeling. By themselves, latent failures are often subtle and may cause no problems. Their consequences are hidden, becoming apparent only when they occur in proper sequence and combine with active failures of individuals to penetrate or bypass the system's safety nets (Reason, 1990). Providing an optimal level of medication safety requires that we recognize and correct the latent failures in the system.

TABLE I-1 Latent and Active Failures Associated with Key Elements of the Medication-Use System, Denver Case Study

Key Element	Latent Failures	Active Failures
1. Prescribing Phase		
Patient Information	• Incomplete clinical information on prior treatment and current status of mother for syphilis. • Incomplete clinical information on current status of infant for congenital syphilis. • Lack of systematic method of communicating mother's prenatal care to infant's physicians.	• Decision made to treat infant for congenital syphilis.
Patient Education	• Inefficient education of parents regarding the possibility of congenital syphilis in the infant and their treatment options.	• Decision made to treat the infant prior to discharge from the hospital without informing the mother, who later said she would have refused therapy because she had been treated previously and had two other children at home without congenital syphilis.
Communication Dynamics	• Lack of efficient means of communicating with parents when a language barrier was present. • Incomplete communication of drug information. • Nonstandard method of communicating drug order.	• Health department recommendation documented in progress notes only as "penicillin G," not "penicillin G benzathine;" route of administration not documented. • Failure to question a seemingly excessive number of IM injections.
Drug Information	• Insufficient drug information (rarely used in practice, nonformulary drug).	• Order for the drug written with "Benzathine" capitalized and placed above "penicillin G;" "IM" written over "IV." "U" used to denote units, making it look like added zero or 1,500,000 instead of 150,000.

TABLE I-1 continued

Key Element	Latent Failures	Active Failures
2. Ordering Phase		
Drug Information	• Insufficient drug information (rarely used in practice, nonformulary drug).	• Misread both health department recommendation and drug resource in determining units/kg dose for infant; consequently misread order, resulting in a 10-fold overdose.
Staff Education and Staffing Patterns	• Lack of specialized training/education in neonatal/pediatric pharmacy. • Failure to staff pharmacy with neonatal/pediatric pharmacist in a hospital providing these services.	
Quality Control	• Lack of maximum-dose warning system on pharmacy computer.	• Ten-fold overdose not detected.
3. Drug Dispensing Phase		
Quality Control	• Inconsistent pharmacy procedure for independent double-check of doses prior to dispensing.	• Ten-fold overdose prepared and dispensed.
Labeling, Packaging, and Nomenclature of Drug	• Lack of unit dose system for dispensing medications in neonatal unit. • Communication of dose in the millions numerically instead of phonically.	• Dispensed two full syringes of drug labeled "1,200,000 units" and "1,500,000 units" (instead of "1.2 million units" and "1.5 million units"), with "note dosage strength" stickers on plungers. • Pharmacy label and syringes did not carry an auxiliary warning of "for IM use only."
Staff Education	• No procedure for educating staff prior to dispensing a nonformulary drug.	• Nonformulary drug dispensed without briefing of staff responsible for administering it.

continued

TABLE I-1 continued

Key Element	Latent Failures	Active Failures
Drug Information	• Insufficient information on volume of medication that can be safely administered IM to neonates (maximum of 0.5 ml per injection). • Insufficient drug information regarding significant serious effects of IM injection of the drug in neonates.	• Dispensed medication with directions to administer 2.5 ml of drug IM to neonate, requiring five IM injections.

4. Drug Administration Phase

Drug Information	• Insufficient drug information about various forms of penicillin G (never used penicillin G benzathine in practice, nonformulary drug). • Inadequate drug references: penicillin G benzathine is frequently referred to in texts with the ambiguous synonyms "crystalline penicillin" and "aqueous suspension." • Inadequate drug reference: *Neofax'95* does not mention penicillin G benzathine in monograph, but notes aqueous crystalline penicillin G IV push is used to treat congenital syphilis; no specific warnings that penicillin G benzathine (or procaine) can be administered IM only. • Inadequate drug reference: *NICU Medication Administration* does not mention penicillin G benzathine in monograph on penicillin G. • Inadequate resource text: 1994 *Red Book* does not	• Misunderstood benzathine to be brand name for aqueous penicillin G. • Incorrectly thought that aqueous crystalline penicillin G and penicillin G benzathine were the same drug; consequently, problem with IV administration went unrecognized. • Made decision to administer the drug IV to avoid pain from multiple IM injections.

TABLE I-1 continued

Key Element	Latent Failures	Active Failures
	warn that drug can be administered IM only. • Conflicting information about IV use of milky-white substances. • Lack of FDA requirement for "black box" or other vivid warning regarding IV administration of penicillin G benzathine in drug monographs.	
Competency	• Hospital had an unclear definition of prescriptive authority for nonphysicians.	• Nurse practitioner assumed authority to change route of administration based on national protocol and current practice in hospital.
Labeling, Packing, and Nomenclature	• Manufacturer's warning for "IM use only" not prominently placed on syringe: syringe had to be rotated 180 degrees away from drug name to view the warning; plunger obscured the view after syringe prepared; "1,200,000" used instead of "1.2 million" units (errors occur when comma is misread).	• Warning on syringe for "IM use only" not seen. • Ten-fold overdose not recognized. • Penicillin G benzathine administered intravenously.

SOURCE: Smetzer and Cohen, 1998.

REFERENCES

Reason, J. 1990. The contribution of latent human failures to the breakdown of complex systems. *Philosophical Transactions of the Royal Society of London, Series* B 327, 475–484.

Smetzer JL, Cohen MR. 1998. Lessons from the Denver medication error/criminal negligence case: Look beyond blaming individuals. *Hospital Pharmacy* 33(6):640–657.

2

Overview of the Drug Development, Regulation, Distribution, and Use System

CHAPTER SUMMARY

The drug system encompasses four main stages—research and development; regulatory review; medication manufacturing, distribution, and marketing; and medication use—that each contain multiple critical control points at which quality, safety, and efficacy can be addressed, and at which breakdowns can occur. This chapter provides an overview of the major components of the drug system and the points that might lead directly or indirectly to errors as well as opportunities for learning, recovery, and improvement.

As noted in two previous Institute of Medicine (IOM) reports—*To Err Is Human: Building a Safer Health System* (IOM, 2000) and *Crossing the Quality Chasm: A New Health System for the 21st Century* (IOM, 2001), redesigning health care to improve quality and safety requires definitive action by all stakeholder groups interacting with the health system. Applied to this report, stakeholders of the drug system associated with research, innovation, regulation, clinical practice, payment, education, legislation, and reporting should be assessed according to how well quality and safety are (or can be) achieved, among other factors. Advancing this concept requires that the disciplines of human factors engineering, organizational psychology, sociology, and informatics must become the basic sciences of quality just as molecular biology, pharmacology, and genetics are the basic sciences of medicine (Brennan et al., 2005). Quality and safety in medication use depends directly on the extent to which the principles of these sciences are built into the overall drug system (Califf et al., 2002). Integrating the sciences of quality with the biomedical and health sciences will ultimately facilitate the translation of safety and quality in medication use from theory to clinical practice.

As a first order of business, the points at which safety and quality can be compromised must be identified. Currently, the potential for harm is present throughout the system. Harm can be due to any number of factors, many of which are now in the national spotlight, including undisclosed harmful side effects of a drug for specific patient populations; lax follow-through on regulatory responsibility after product approval; human error in prescribing, dispensing, administering, and monitoring effects in patients; and inadequate patient activation and education. This chapter identifies the key issues of the overall drug system that affect safety and quality in medication use. Subsequent chapters in this report provide recommendations for improvement, many of which incorporate the "sciences of quality" mentioned above.

STRUCTURE OF THE OVERALL DRUG SYSTEM

Currently more than 10,000 prescription drugs and biologics (FDA, 1999) and more than 300,000 over-the-counter (OTC) products are on the market in the United States (RSW, 2001). In 2004, 215 prescription and 71 OTC drugs were recalled because of manufacturing and distribution problems or serious adverse reactions (FDA, 2004a).

The regulatory element of the drug system evolved over the past century from being focused on regulating interstate transport and misbranded products to being built on an infrastructure with the goal of reliable standards, processes, and laws to ensure some degree of safety and efficacy in medicinal agents. The result is a sophisticated, comprehensive drug system encompassing four stages that interact with, support, and reinforce each other to varying degrees (see Figure 2-1): (1) *research and development (R&D)*, where ideas for new drugs are conceived and candidates are clinically tested; (2) *regulatory review* by the Food and Drug Administration (FDA) to validate or counter the research findings and ensure proper labeling; (3) *manufacture, distribution, and marketing* of products that have received regulatory approval; and (4) *use of medications* available either through a prescription or OTC. Prescription drugs, biologics, and some OTCs follow this model. The product development and regulatory review stages are abbreviated for other OTCs and for generics.

Each element of the drug system is governed by its own set of standards and methods for scientific analysis to advance the safety, quality, and efficacy of products and their use. As the chief protector of the public health, the FDA has responsibility for developing and enforcing the standards in all

52

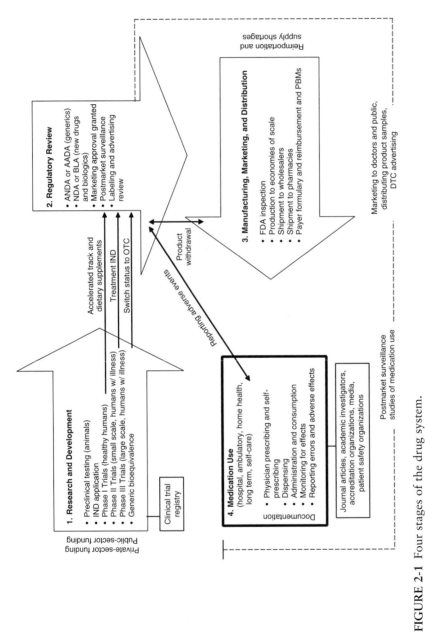

FIGURE 2-1 Four stages of the drug system.

NOTE: AADA = Abbreviated Antibiotic Drug Application; ANDA = Abbreviated New Drug Application; BLA = Biologic Licensing Application; DTC = direct to consumer; FDA = U.S. Food and Drug Administration; IND = Investigational New Drug Application; NDA = New Drug Application; OTC = over-the-counter; PBM = Pharmacy Benefits Manager.

areas except clinical practice, which is governed by state boards of medicine, nursing, and pharmacy; professional societies; and accreditation organizations.[1] Compliance with FDA regulatory standards is the responsibility of the manufacturers who promote their products in the marketplace. Safe and effective use of medications is the responsibility of providers who prescribe the medications and patients who take them.

Standards[2] for each component of the drug system act as links in a chain of events that have an important bearing on the competence and effectiveness of drug therapies in medical care. The key points at which important interventions can be implemented are identified in Figure 2-1. Building safety and quality into the system starts with rational ideas for new drug products, followed by sound scientific research; reliable clinical testing; rigorous regulatory reviews; appropriate labeling; use of good manufacturing processes; proper distribution techniques; adequate supplies; ethical marketing practices; competent prescribing, dispensing, and administration of medications; and finally suitable monitoring of the patient, reporting of errors, and measurement of outcomes (Martin, 1978). If standards do not exist, are inadequate, have not been met, or are not enforced at any point along this chain, patient safety and quality of care can be compromised. For example, restriction on the publication of a drug's side effects can affect a prescriber's ability to choose the best drug for a patient or to identify and respond to an adverse reaction in a timely manner; lax enforcement of regulatory requirements for drug labeling can result in product confusion in a high-stress, fast-paced clinical setting; formulary restrictions can force a switch to a medication that may be less appropriate for a patient than the one initially prescribed; or the failure to document all of the medications a patient is taking (including OTCs and dietary supplements) can cause a drug–drug interaction that could have been prevented.

In the first three of these examples, problems in the drug development, regulation, and distribution systems contribute to medication-use errors that should be corrected. Yet most links or components of the drug system operate in a quasi-silo state with less-than-ideal means of sharing important

---

[1]The Center for Drug Evaluation and Research (CDER) regulates prescription (including therapeutic biologics), generic, and nonprescription drugs; the Center for Biologics Evaluation and Research (CBER) regulates the remaining biologics and blood products; and the Center for Devices and Radiological Health regulates medical devices, including those used to administer medications. The FDA's authority, established by the Federal Food, Drug, and Cosmetic Act of 1938, has evolved steadily over the past 60 years through a series of legislative and regulatory actions to foster safety and efficacy through all stages of the drug system.

[2]A set of characteristics or quantities that describes features of a product, process, service, interface, or material. The description can take many forms, such as the definition of terms; specification of design and construction; detailing of procedures; or performance criteria against which a product, process, and other factors can be measured (NRC, 1995).

information or responding to safety-related problems. In the last example, the problem results from an error within the medication-use system itself (e.g., insufficient information). Most often this is the case: medication errors are the result of a problem incurred during the prescribing, dispensing, administration, or monitoring phases of the medication-use system.

Nevertheless, both aspects of causation—how the drug is prepared (developed, regulated, distributed) and how it is used in clinical practice or self-care—must be addressed if errors in the medication-use system are to be reduced and prevented. The remainder of this section addresses the former (research and development; regulatory review; and manufacture, distribution, and marketing). The second section of the chapter addresses medication use.

Research and Development

The R&D process involves more than the development of new products; it encompasses the overall generation and disclosure of high-quality data that can be used with confidence by providers and patients in medical care, by providers and technology vendors to populate knowledge bases and clinical decision-support systems, by regulators in assessing benefit/risk balances for protection of the public health, and by researchers for continued innovation and advancement of science and medicine (Califf, 2004). Issues related to study design, data quality, and disclosure can have direct bearing on the development of the medication knowledge base needed to support clinicians and pharmacists in clinical decision making and prescribing; preparation and administration of appropriate dosages; and monitoring of patient response (positive and negative) to a medication, particularly the ability to discern symptoms of disease from effects of the drug. Public availability of information from trials also is necessary to support consumers in their self-care, disease management, and medication self-management. Data quality can be compromised by poor clinical study designs, less-than-optimal methods of data analysis, and/or conflicts of interest that affect the objectivity of investigators (Califf and DeMets, 2002a,b; Strom, 2004; March et al., 2005). The failure to disclose negative study results (e.g., serious adverse side effects) can have fatal effects on patients (Bodenheimer, 2000; Moore et al., 1998).

Current State of R&D

Pharmaceutical R&D for new drugs and biologics aims to meet a medical need in a specified patient population by creating medications with characteristics of high activity, low toxicity, and relatively few side effects. Fundamentally, approval for marketing a drug is based on an assessment of the balance of the benefit and risk of using the drug in the specified population. The ability to separate toxic and side effects from therapeutic effects on the basis of preclinical evaluation is an ongoing challenge. Sizable amounts of time and effort are spent on trying to increase this margin, but ultimately the balance of benefit and risk cannot be defined until clinical trials have been conducted in relevant populations (Martin, 1978; Califf, 2004). Trends in drug development over the past few decades have led to significant improvements in study designs, reducing the incidence of incorrect conclusions concerning dosage, efficacy, and safety while deepening understanding of how the molecular structures of potential new drugs interact with specific human cellular structures. More recent scientific discoveries in the areas of genomics, biotechnology, and informatics are expected to increase significantly the number of new molecular targets and the ability to develop medicines with greater specificity and fewer side effects (NRC, 2004), although this promise has not been realized, and the time frame for pragmatic advances remains unclear (Califf, 2004).

Clinical Study Design

Traditionally, the R&D process has been performed in sequential stages. After *discovery* of potential compounds for new medicines and *preclinical testing* in the laboratory and in animals for safety and biological activity against the targeted disease, the manufacturer (i.e., sponsor) submits an *Investigational New Drug Application* (IND) to the FDA or other international regulatory authority for review.[3] The IND contains plans for clinical studies in humans (Phases I, II, and III), all data from preclinical testing, and complete structural and manufacturing information. At any time after the IND has been submitted, the sponsor may request an accelerated development and approval track ("fast track") for drugs that promise substantial benefit over existing therapies for serious or life-threatening illnesses. Granting of fast track status is based on the case that the drug would fulfill a critical unmet health need, early evidence of the drug's effects on a surrogate end point,[4] commitments to undertake postmarket studies, and/or agreement to restrict distribution and use after approval (FDA, 1999).

Most *Phase I* studies use healthy volunteers to test the drug's actions, both metabolic (pharmacokinetics [PK]) and pharmacologic (pharmacody-

---

[3]The FDA performs clinical, chemistry, toxicology, and safety reviews of the IND and, if it is accepted, makes adjustments to clinical trial parameters as needed. The IND sets the stage for the FDA's interaction with the sponsor during clinical studies.

[4]A surrogate end point is a laboratory finding or physical sign that may not, in itself, be a direct measurement of how a patient feels, functions, or survives, but nevertheless is considered likely to predict therapeutic benefit (FDA, 1999).

namics [PD]);[5] side effects associated with increasing doses; and if possible, early evidence of efficacy (FDA, 1998). *Phase II* studies use a small group of patients with the condition in well-controlled circumstances to evaluate the dose that optimally affects the chosen biological target, the method of delivery (e.g., oral, intravenous), the dosing interval, and short-term side effects, and to extend the preliminary evidence of safety from Phase I (Walters, 1992; Leonard, 1994; FDA, 1998). A substantial number of drug trials are discontinued after both Phases I and II because of ineffectiveness, safety problems, or intolerable side effects. If the Phase I and II trials are successful, the sponsor may apply for *Treatment IND* status to provide promising drugs to patients with a life-threatening disease (e.g., AIDS) if no comparable therapy exists or the patients cannot participate in clinical studies.

Phase III trials are the most critical in the determination of a drug's approval for labeling by the FDA and international regulatory authorities. Typically, Phase III trials are structured as randomized controlled trials involving enough patients carefully selected, often across multiple sites, to obtain data on the drug's overall benefit/risk relationship so that regulators, often guided by expert panels, can be comfortable that the balance is favorable for the defined population (Nies, 2001). While such studies typically can last from 1 to 4 years and commonly include from 1,000 to 10,000 patients, generally only a few hundred patients are treated for more than 3 to 6 months with the drug, regardless of the duration of treatment required in clinical practice. As a result, only the most profound and overt risks and side effects that occur immediately after taking a drug can be detected if the occurrence rate is 1 in 100 administrations. Risks that are medically important but delayed, less frequent than 1 in 1,000 administrations, or not evenly distributed across the population may not be revealed prior to marketing (Nies, 2001). In particular, serious adverse effects for a specific patient population (e.g., pediatric, geriatric, those with renal dysfunction or multiple comorbidities) usually will not be known, as those groups are not well represented in the trials (Lee et al., 2001; Klein et al., 2002). Accordingly, postmarket surveillance and evaluation studies (*Phase IV*) are often requested for further evaluation of safety issues (e.g., adverse effects) after approval.

During a January 2005 meeting on drug development science sponsored by the FDA and the Association of American Medical Colleges (AAMC), participants from academia, industry, and government identified

---

[5]*Pharmacodynamics* denotes the biochemical and physiological effects of a drug and the relationship between drug concentration and effect. *Pharmacokinetics* is the activity or fate of drugs in the body over a period of time, including the processes of absorption, distribution, localization in tissues, biotransformation, and excretion.

crucial problems with the current model and opportunities for improvement (AAMC, 2005). The participants found that study designs often are not tailored to the pharmacology of potential new drugs and the patient populations that will use them, and frequently are not structured to allow adequate evaluation of a broad range of doses.

Each of the above factors can contribute to issues of patient safety and quality of care in the medication-use process. For example, drugs can produce very different effects in elderly patients and younger adults. The elderly are more likely to have impaired kidney and renal function, to be taking other medications, or to have other medical conditions. Few clinical studies include substantial numbers of elderly patients, however, even though the elderly are a growing proportion of the general population (FDA, 1999; Noah and Brushwood, 2000; Boyd et al., 2005).

Data Quality

While randomized controlled trials are considered the gold standard for assessing efficacy, they rarely provide all the information needed in clinical practice (Teutsch et al., 2005). Drugs are usually compared with a placebo, and studies frequently use surrogate or intermediate measures of efficacy, such as blood pressure, low-density lipoprotein cholesterol, or tumor shrinkage, rather than tangible patient outcomes, such as mortality, morbidity, and quality of life. Placebo-based comparisons serve regulatory requirements, leaving long-term studies comparing treatments to post-approval. Without data on health outcomes, extrapolation from the carefully selected patient populations used in clinical trials to patient populations seen in typical practice settings and from the patient population used in a trial to another patient population introduces uncertainty (Teutsch et al., 2005).

A variety of leaders have voiced concern about the threat posed to scientific integrity by conflicts of interest among industry and academic researchers, private-sector investigators, and regulators (Bodenheimer, 2000; Chopra, 2003; Fontanarosa et al., 2004; Psaty et al., 2004). There is evidence that research has tended to overemphasize drug benefits while downplaying risks (Rochon et al., 1994; Rothman and Michels, 1994; Bero and Rennie, 1996; Bekelman et al., 2003).

Disclosure of Results

Currently, public disclosure of results through registration is required only for clinical gene-transfer trials registered with the National Institutes of Health (NIH) and studies conducted under INDs (FDA, 2004b). Nondisclosure (failure to register) of all clinical trials from start to completion and

---

BOX 2-1
Summary of Key Problems with the Research and
Development Process Affecting Safety and Quality
in the Medication-Use System

- Study designs are insufficient to generate data for the full range of knowledge needs (for example, to evaluate metabolic and pharmacologic effects and clinical outcomes in specific populations).
- Studies are short-term, but medication use can be long-term; thus long-term effects are unknown.
- Public disclosure of clinical trial results may be selective.

---

failure to report results (both positive and negative) in a public database have left sizable gaps in the knowledge base that can affect decision making by regulators and clinicians, as well as the work of researchers and editors of medical journals (Steinbrook, 2004; IOM, 2006). (See Box 2-1 for a summary of key problems with the research and development process.)

Regulatory Review

Prior to marketing in the United States, all new prescription drugs (including generics), OTC drugs, and biologics are subjected to formal regulatory review and approval by the FDA's Center for Drug Evaluation and Research (CDER). The primary objectives of the regulatory review are to evaluate a drug's safety and effectiveness and to determine whether its benefits outweigh its risks. Regulatory review also verifies that industry has taken the appropriate measures to prepare the products properly for the market.

The balance of benefit and risk is influenced significantly by intended use, and varies from drug to drug and from one patient group to another (FDA, 1999; University of Utah, 2006). For example, greater risk may be tolerated for a drug designed to treat a life-threatening illness than for one designed to treat the common cold. Likewise, lower risk may be required for drugs intended for geriatric patients, who are more likely to have renal or hepatic impairment and multiple conditions (FDA, 1994). As genomics and proteomics enable drug development to become increasingly individualized, it will be possible to establish more specific benefit and risk assessments for particular patient populations with certain clinical or genetic characteristics. This capability will necessitate reexamination of the current benefit/risk model used for regulatory approval (Califf, 2004).

Review of Clinical Data for New Drugs and Biologics

Assessment of new drugs (i.e., new molecular entities [NMEs]) is based on the New Drug Application (NDA) or the Biologic Licensing Application (BLA)—dossiers submitted by the drug sponsor that include all data from preclinical and clinical studies on safety and efficacy, proposed labeling, and manufacturing details. A team from CDER's Office of New Drugs reviews the dossiers; communication with the sponsor occurs throughout the process to address scientific, medical, and procedural issues. The FDA uses advisory committees of external scientific experts for advice and opinions to broaden its basis for decision making on an NDA/BLA or regulatory issue.

For a drug to win approval, the FDA does not require that it be better than products already available, only that it be effective (better than nothing [i.e., placebo]) and fairly safe (Deyo, 2004). A drug is determined to be effective if it achieves a "surrogate outcome" (e.g., lowers cholesterol) without its effects on life expectancy being known. The FDA does not approve every use for which a drug may be prescribed by a clinician, only the use evaluated during its clinical trial.

Postmarket Surveillance of New Drugs

Some of the risks associated with a new drug are not known at the time of regulatory review because the data from clinical trials are limited in terms of patient population, study size, and/or duration. Consequently, drugs must continue to be evaluated as they are used in clinical settings to detect less frequent but significant adverse side effects, long-term effects, or effects in different patient populations. Two mechanisms are available for this purpose: (1) postmarket surveillance studies, and (2) the FDA's adverse event reporting systems (see later in the chapter). Both approaches rely on manufacturers to collect, evaluate, and report data on their own products (Fontanarosa et al., 2004).

Postmarket studies can be designed to observe a drug's effects in a larger, more heterogeneous population over 3–4 years (Berndt et al., 2005). The FDA requires postmarket studies as a condition for approval in only two product categories—drugs granted fast track status and drugs for which the manufacturer desires a pediatric indication (Fontanarosa et al., 2004). Such studies are optional for other product categories, although strongly encouraged. Manufacturers complete fewer than half of the postmarket studies they commit to undertaking as a condition for approval (FR, 2004a; Fontanarosa et al., 2004). At the request of the FDA, the IOM Committee on Assessment of the U.S. Drug Safety System is evaluating the agency's postmarketing surveillance. More detail on surveillance systems is given in the section on adverse event reporting and surveillance systems later in the chapter.

Review of Clinical Data for Generics and OTCs

The FDA uses a process similar to that for NMEs to review new generic drugs and OTCs. Sponsors of generics file an Abbreviated New Drug Application (ANDA) or Abbreviated Antibiotic Drug Application (AADA) that provides information supporting equivalence to an FDA-approved brand-name drug in terms of active ingredients, dosage, safety, strength, administration, quality, performance, and intended use. Generic manufacturers are not required to replicate the extensive clinical trials of the original drug, but must demonstrate bioequivalence; this can be done by measuring bioavailability (e.g., rate and extent of absorption) of the generic in 24 to 36 healthy subjects (FDA, 1999).

For OTCs the FDA has established drug monographs for each OTC product class, covering acceptable ingredients, doses, and formulations (FDA, 1998). An FDA team assesses a product's conformance to the monograph, as well as to OTC labeling guidelines.

Product Labeling

After deciding to approve a drug for a specific indication, the FDA evaluates the product labeling. Labeling is a broad term that encompasses a number of materials developed by pharmaceutical companies, including the professional product label (also known as the package insert); medication guides (for drugs posing a serious public health concern); patient package inserts (with content often used in media advertisements); product packaging (which pertains to the external package labeling of the drug); and any written, printed, or graphic material used for marketing (Kenny, 2001).

Professional product labels (package inserts) are developed by companies on the basis of Phase III data. They are evaluated by the FDA for compliance with federal regulations, rather than for usefulness[6] to health care professionals and consumers. Medication guides and patient package inserts are written for consumers in a more user-friendly language. However, problems with the design and content of all labeling materials affect their readability, comprehensibility, and usefulness (FR, 2006; Hubal and Day, 2006). The FDA's recently published new rule on drug labeling is an

---

[6]The Code of Federal Regulations requires that labels describe the drug's ingredients, structural formula, and clinical pharmacology; its indications, contraindications, warnings, and precautions; its associated adverse reactions and potential for abuse; the signs and symptoms of overdose; guidelines for proper use; and how the drug is supplied.

improvement (FR, 2006), but additional work is still needed on better incorporating the principles of cognitive and human factors engineering to address remaining issues concerning information presentation and nomenclature (http://www.fda.gov/cder/regulatory/physLabel/default.htm).

FDA Risk and Safety Communication

As a drug is used in clinical practice, new information and precautions for safety may be needed. The FDA can require the manufacturer to revise some of the information in the product labeling materials, although it can take close to 2 years to reach agreement with the manufacturer and incorporate labeling changes. Changes may include the addition of a "black box warning"—the strongest warning on a label, highlighting serious adverse reactions or special problems that could lead to injury or death (Wagner et al., 2006). Black box warnings are not easy for consumers to access as they are applied to the label (i.e., package insert and external package); most consumers do not read the insert and do not receive their prescriptions in the manufacturers' packaging (Szefler et al., 2006). Furthermore, companies tend to resist adding such a warning to a drug's label (Weatherby et al., 2002; Wagner et al., 2006). Of note, there are virtually no black box warnings on OTC products even though serious errors in administration occur with these products, and such warnings could greatly benefit consumers, particularly parents who must administer OTC medications to infants and children (Presecky, 2006). The FDA also distributes "dear doctor letters" to communicate new risk information directly to providers, yet these communications are relatively ineffective in changing prescribing behavior unless they are widely publicized (Smalley et al., 2000; Weatherby et al., 2001, 2002).

Recently, the FDA began developing and posting on its website supplemental emerging safety information derived from its reporting system (the MedWatch program; see later in the chapter) in an effort to improve the quality of postmarket information about prescription drugs for health care providers and consumers. Also, there is renewed interest in earlier efforts to improve the design and content of consumer drug information distributed through the pharmacy (i.e., pharmacy leaflets) (see Chapter 4).

Review of Product Packaging

Poor labeling on product packaging has contributed to serious medication errors (see Chapter 6) (Cohen, 2000). For example, packaging-related problems can make it easy for busy clinicians to misread poorly presented drug dosing units (e.g., concentration and strength) or to confuse drugs with names that sound similar (e.g., Lamictal, for seizure disorders, and

Lamisil, an antifungal) (Cohen, 2005). For all drugs, inserts and packaging that lack highly visible, easy-to-read instructions, warnings, and contra-indications presented in layman's terms (versus complex medical jargon) can lead to incorrect perceptions and poor retention by prescribers and patients alike.

To address labeling or packaging errors that occur after approval, the FDA sends a request for changes to the manufacturer. If the manufacturer has failed to respond to requests for labeling changes and patient harm recurs as a result of related errors, the FDA seeks to bring about the required changes through negotiation. Labeling for a generic must be identical to that for the reference drug. And recent requirements for the labeling of OTC drugs have created more consumer-friendly labels. The uniform labeling requirements standardized the presentation of "Drug Facts" on the outside of the OTC package in an easy-to-follow format using simpler language and clear visual markings. The FDA recommends, but does not require, manufacturers to include a phone number if more information is needed or if an adverse reaction occurs.

Monitoring of Marketing Materials

Labeling for marketing and advertising purposes is reviewed by CDER's Division of Drug Marketing, Advertising and Communications to ensure that product claims are truthful and not misleading. Promotional materials (i.e., advertisements) are submitted for review at the time of their initial use, but the FDA does not evaluate these materials before they are used by companies in the marketplace. (See section on marketing practices later in this chapter.) (See Box 2-2 for a summary of key problems with the regulatory review process.)

BOX 2-2
Summary of Key Problems with the Regulatory Review Process Affecting Safety and Quality in the Medication-Use System

- Confusing presentation of important drug information in naming, labeling, and packaging can contribute to medication errors.
- Procedures to address product labeling and packaging problems are cumbersome.
- Many companies fail to complete postmarket study commitments, so knowledge about important drug benefits/risks is not obtained.

Manufacture, Distribution, and Marketing

Plans for the manufacture, distribution, and marketing of drugs are developed by manufacturers and evaluated by the FDA. Although by this time products have passed the regulatory approval process, including validation of the data from clinical trials, issues affecting the medication-use system can arise during these processes as well. For example, drug shortages or discontinuations in certain dosages force patients to switch their prescription to another drug that may not be as appropriate for them or to resort to potentially unsafe practices, such as manipulating doses manually (e.g., tablet cutting) or purchasing from unknown Internet vendors. Restrictive formularies or lack of drug coverage for prescribed medications can lead to prescription sharing among family and friends. Marketing practices and campaigns that overemphasize the benefits of a drug to providers and consumers without appropriate disclosure of its risks can lead to inappropriate prescribing and adverse drug effects.

Manufacturing Controls

During the last stages of regulatory review for new drugs and generics, the FDA evaluates the adequacy of the sponsor's plans/controls for manufacturing to ensure the product's identity, strength, quality, and purity. The agency may even inspect a sample of clinical trial locations to verify the accuracy of the data in the NDA, as well as to inspect manufacturing and repackaging facilities to confirm compliance with international standards known as Current Good Manufacturing Practices (CGMP) (FDA, 2003). Inspections are a significant step in the review process, aimed at minimizing consumers' exposure to adulterated drug products. The inspections demonstrate a company's ability to manufacture a drug within tight parameters from batch to batch, day to day, year to year, and to prove that the same controls that received regulatory approval are being applied in the actual manufacture of the product (FDA, 1999).

Distribution to Pharmacies and Consumers

Once products have been produced to standards, they are ready to enter the distribution system that transfers drug products from manufacturers to pharmacies or retail outlets. Traditionally, wholesalers have functioned as the key intermediaries, providing services for storage and delivery to pharmacies. However, the rising cost of health care and prescription drugs, as well as other factors, has prompted the use of other methods to bring drug products to pharmacies, consumers, and patients. Some pharmacies, both provider- and community-based, now receive drug supplies directly from the manufacturer, delivered through the company's own services. A growing method of bringing drugs to consumers is through mail order pharmacies (such as those established by pharmacy benefits managers [PBMs]), Internet pharmacies, and pharmacies of general (usually large) retail outlets (e.g., Walmart, Target).

Mail Order and Internet Pharmacies

As the demand for and cost of prescription medications have increased, so, too, has the demand for more cost-efficient models for distributing drugs to consumers through mail order systems. Such systems include both the businesses of PBMs and the Internet. PBMs are third-party entities that evolved from claims administration and mail order pharmacies into organizations that also provide a range of drug benefit and clinical-based services (HPA, 2003).

Use of PBMs has grown considerably over the past decade with the expansion of their services to utilization management, disease management, and, more recently, medication safety for individuals with chronic diseases and associated polypharmacy-related issues. PBMs generally make pharmacists available to assist consumers with questions about their medications. Nonetheless, a substantial portion of consumers continue to prefer the convenience of their local pharmacy and personal contact with the community pharmacist.

The Internet has emerged as a growing marketplace for the purchase of drugs (GAO, 2004). It offers consumers the benefit of being able to shop from home at any time, and the ability to compare prices of multiple vendors and purchase from a wide range of drug categories (GAO, 2004). Although the Internet pharmacy market is subject to the same laws that govern traditional pharmacies, it is global and difficult to regulate. A recent report by the Government Accountability Office (GAO, 2004) notes that many Internet pharmacies do not comply with state pharmacy laws; for example, they sell drugs that are improperly packaged, counterfeit, or unapproved. Most important from a consumer safety standpoint, in some instances, prescription drugs can be purchased without a prescription.

Marketing to Consumers, Providers, and Payers

Most stakeholders in the drug system are introduced to drug products for the first time through marketing and advertising campaigns. The FDA's Division of Drug Marketing, Advertising and Communication estimates that industry spends $25 billion annually to promote drug products in the marketplace (Abrams, 2005). Marketing can take the form of visits by company representatives to physicians' offices to discuss new drugs in person and provide sample packs and gifts[7]; rebates to health plans and PBMs for preferential formulary placement; industry-sponsored continuing medical education (CME) programs focused on new drugs; funding of disease management programs; direct payment of travel expenses to attend medical association conferences; and direct-to-consumer advertising that promotes new drugs to the public at large in print, broadcast, and electronic media (Chung et al., 2003; Blumenthal, 2004).

A body of evidence confirms that these strategies have an influence on physicians' objectivity and behaviors, especially prescribing practices, formulary choices, and assessment of medical information (Levy, 1994; Wilkes et al., 2000; Carney et al., 2001; Goodman, 2001; NIHCMREF, 2002; Blumenthal, 2004; Chimonas and Rothman, 2005). Wazana's (2000) extensive literature review on physician–pharmaceutical industry interactions revealed that some positive outcomes were identified (for example, an improved ability to identify the treatment for complicated illnesses), but most studies found negative outcomes, although no study evaluated the impact on patient outcomes. The impact of physician–pharmaceutical industry interactions is particularly concerning since these strategies are employed even for new drugs that may have little or no discernable advantage over existing drugs or other treatment options (Avorn, 2004), and for which there may be only limited data from short-term clinical trials that may not have uncovered serious adverse effects (Califf and DeMets 2002a,b). In some cases, drugs attain preferential placement in formularies because of company financial incentives (e.g., discounts, rebates) rather than quality and evidence-based decision making (Chung et al., 2003). Thus many groups within the medical community are calling for changes in the way the industry interacts with the medical community (Katz et al., 2003; Blumenthal, 2004; Studdert et al., 2004; Brennan et al., 2006).

Distribution of Free Samples

The primary promotional tool for new drugs is the distribution of free samples to providers. In 2003, companies distributed about $16 billion worth of free samples (although this figure represents retail value, only 20–30 percent of which is the actual value) (IMS Health, 2004). While making samples broadly available to patients, particularly those with lower incomes, may be well intentioned, there is growing evidence that the provision of free samples directly affects physician's patterns in selecting and prescribing medications and in addressing issues of medication safety (Chew et al., 2000; Maguire, 2001; Petersen, 2000). Free samples are frequently taken by patients without a prescription and without documentation in

---

[7]Gift giving has been deterred by professional societies, government regulators, and industry itself (Coyle, 2002; Loucks, 2003; Moynihan, 2003; Angell, 2004).

BOX 2-3
Summary of Key Problems with the Manufacturing,
Distribution, and Marketing Processes
Affecting Safety and Quality in the Medication-Use System

- Many Internet pharmacies are inappropriately dispensing medications.
- The current system for distributing free samples leads to a lack of documentation that represents a threat to patient safety.
- Restrictive formularies and switching between formularies may lead to medication errors.

---

health records, thus bypassing the safety check on drug–drug interactions that may otherwise flag a potential error (Chew et al., 2000; Groves et al., 2003; Taira et al., 2003). Furthermore, free samples are most often the newest, least well tested drugs, and patients are thus being encouraged to take these drugs when others might, in fact, be safer for them (Avorn, 2004). (See the discussion in Chapter 6.)

Formularies

Companies also interact with insurance payers and PBMs to secure listing and reimbursement pricing in drug formularies. A formulary is a payer's list of covered drugs, designed to restrict the listing of drugs and/or the level of coverage in each therapeutic class for cost-saving purposes (Husakamp et al., 2003). Unlike other nations that use formularies to determine access, payers in the United States maintain an open system to accommodate the broadest population and its potential medication needs; formularies for prescription drugs are used solely to determine tiered copayment and reimbursement structures, not access. For example, the Veteran Health Administration (VHA), private-sector health maintenance organizations (HMOs), private-sector payers, and now the Centers for Medicare and Medicaid (CMS) with the new prescription drug benefit use open formularies, although coverage is tiered (also called incentive based) (Thomas, 2003; Landon et al., 2004; Shrank et al., 2005). HMOs tend to have more restrictive formularies (prohibiting payment for certain drugs), but many have also moved to tiered structures (Shrank et al., 2005). (See Box 2-3 for a summary of key problems with the manufacturing, distribution, and marketing process.)

STRUCTURE AND FUNCTION OF THE
MEDICATION-USE SYSTEM

The steps described above provide the basic foundation for safety in producing and distributing medications that meet consumers' medical and health needs. The medication-use system that is built on that foundation encompasses the continuum of (1) prescribing by the clinician (or self-prescribing), followed by transcribing; (2) preparing and dispensing by the pharmacist; (3) administering by the provider or consumer (self-care); and (4) monitoring for therapeutic and adverse effects (by nurse, surrogate, or self). Each of these steps includes critical control points at which decisions and actions can contribute to safety or errors. Figures 2-2, 2-3, and 2-4 outline these critical control points for the different health care settings.

The primary stakeholders involved in the medication-use system are patients/consumers and their families, providers, payers, regulators, employers, manufacturers, distributors, and policy makers. Secondary stakeholders include accrediting, patient safety, and quality improvement organizations; medical journal editors; and the general media. The dynamics of the system for medication delivery are shown, along with relevant stakeholders, in Figure 2-5.

Achieving safe and effective use of medications requires coordinated efforts by all stakeholders, with mutual recognition that each has unique perspectives on what constitutes appropriate or rational medication use (Knowlton and Penna, 2003). Patients/consumers and their families have an interest in maintaining their personal health and safety at a reasonable cost, as do their employers. Health care providers (physicians, nurse practitioners, physician assistants, nurses, pharmacists) have an interest in addressing patient problems effectively and achieving therapeutic objectives. Regulators have an interest in ensuring the safety of the general public and taking disciplinary action when necessary. Pharmaceutical manufacturers have an interest in developing and marketing new drugs in the service of society and their stockholders. Payers have an interest in providing their enrollees with insurance coverage at a reasonable cost (Knowlton and Penna, 2003). Community pharmacies and PBMs have an interest in providing patients and consumers with useful information about their medications and averting potential errors. Accrediting organizations have an interest in assessing health care providers' compliance with medical safety standards and best practices. Patient safety reporting organizations have an interest in collecting data on events and developing protocols to improve safety. Medical journal editors have an interest in publishing comprehensive and accurate information about medications and their use. And the general media have an interest in writing newsworthy stories about health care and exposing any problems.

Unfortunately, the complex and diverse interests of the primary stakeholders have resulted in a medication-use system that is disjointed and inefficient in terms of manpower and resource consumption. Errors in medication delivery are the largest single category of medical errors in health care (IOM, 2000). Errors occur with all types of medications (e.g., pre-

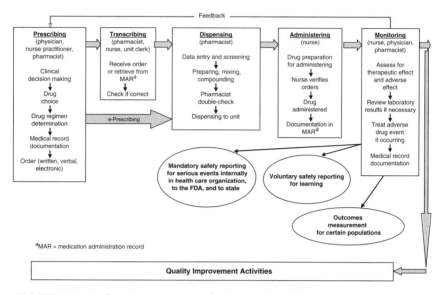

FIGURE 2-2 Medication-use process for hospital and long-term care.

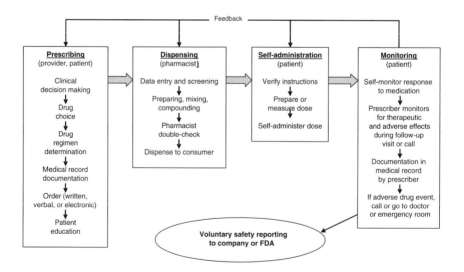

FIGURE 2-3 Medication-use process in community care.

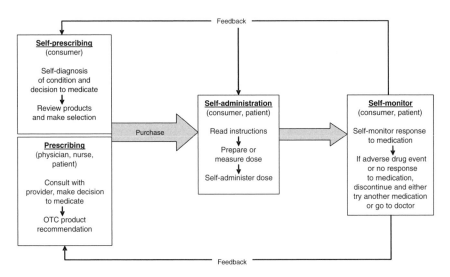

FIGURE 2-4 Medication-use process for over-the-counter drugs.

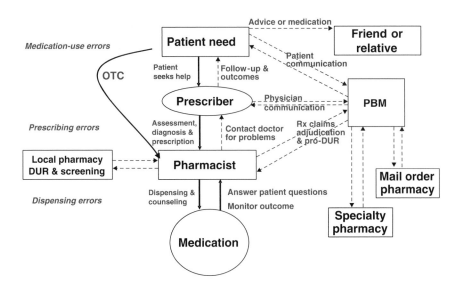

FIGURE 2-5 Dynamics of the medication-delivery system.
NOTE: DUR = drug utilization review; PBM = pharmacy benefits manager.
SOURCE: Adapted from Schondelmeyer, 2005.

scription, generic, OTC) and in all health care settings (e.g., hospital care, ambulatory care, nursing home care, and home self-care). Errors can be those of commission (e.g., prescribing the wrong dosage) or omission (e.g., failing to prescribe a medication that would likely benefit a patient). Errors can occur at any point along the medication-use continuum as a result of multiple factors in the health system, including those associated with the patient, the provider (e.g., experience, expertise, and overall human factors such as fatigue and stress), the care team (e.g., lack of communication between clinicians, shifts, and settings), the work environment (e.g., lack of clinical decision support, product labeling), and the department/institution (e.g., absence of a culture of safety) (Vincent, 2001). This section provides an overview of the points along the continuum of the medication-use system in community and inpatient care settings at which medication errors can occur: prescribing and ordering, self-prescribing, transcribing, preparing and dispensing, administering and consuming, self-administering, monitoring for effects, and self-monitoring.

Prescribing and Ordering

The prescribing domain in community, hospital, and long-term care settings involves clinical decision making, selection of a drug and drug regimen, medical record documentation, and ordering. The clinician has the responsibility to engage the patient in discussion about the appropriateness of a prescription drug as part of the treatment plan and about how to design the regimen to meet the patient's needs. Although the patient should participate in the decision making on whether to use medication therapy, the clinician retains responsibility for ensuring medically appropriate prescribing and accuracy in medical record documentation and prescription ordering.

Quality and safety in the medication-use system require good clinical decision making about patient care and therapeutic options. As stated in the *Quality Chasm* report (IOM, 2001), the best care results from the conscious, explicit, and judicious use of current best evidence and knowledge of patient values by well-trained, experienced clinicians. Thus, effective clinicians rely on best practices as appropriate for a given patient, yet they maintain the freedom to make choices that science cannot guide, such as those based on relationships and observation. These clinicians understand and respect the patient's special circumstances, preferences, and values, knowing they are vital to patient-centered care. They also are attuned to the patient's economic circumstances (e.g., uninsured, underinsured) and formulary restrictions as they may affect drug selection, especially if the patient must pay for the medications out of pocket.

Good decision making need not always be based on the results of randomized controlled trials for two reasons: (1) such results are not always available, and (2) other forms of knowledge may be definitive. For example, few drug products used for neonatal and pediatric patients have been tested in randomized controlled trials in these populations. When a drug exists that has been tested in the adult population, pediatricians must use their medical expertise and overall knowledge of therapeutics to make decisions regarding the "off-label" use of the drug to meet the needs of their patients (see Box 2-4).

Moreover, all illnesses do not require drug therapy. The need for a drug should be evaluated and weighed against alternative treatments to avoid overuse or inappropriate uses of medications (IOM, 2001). For instance, antibiotics are contraindicated for treating the common cold or a viral infection but are often requested and prescribed nonetheless, thus contributing to problems of antibiotic resistance. As another example, certain drugs, particularly antidepressants, analgesics, and muscle relaxants, are commonly and inappropriately prescribed for elderly patients, contributing to adverse drug events that necessitate health care services, physician contact, hospitalization, and emergency department visits (Golden et al., 1999; Hanlon et al., 2000a,b; Fick et al., 2004; Fialova et al., 2005).

When the decision is made to select a medication, care is necessary to screen the drug regimen for potential drug–drug and drug–food interactions; age- or gender-related metabolic or pharmacologic considerations; incidence and severity of side effects; tolerance effects over time; relationship to placebo effects; and comparability to other, nonmedication-related treatments (Nies, 2001). Poor decision making can result in prescribing that fails to help the patient or causes harm. Even if the correct decisions are made in determining the medication regimen, poor communication of prescription orders in any format (written, oral, electronic) can lead to serious adverse drug events (Cohen, 2000; USP, 2004).

A number of studies have cited prescribing as a principal source of overall medication errors, estimating incidence rates of 18.9 to 58.4 percent (Bates et al., 1995; Lesar et al., 1997; Gurwitz et al., 2000; USP, 2004). The numerous types of prescribing errors identified in the literature include the following (Lesar et al., 1990):

• Failure to alter drug therapy in patients with impaired renal or hepatic function.

• Failure to notice a patient's history of allergy to the prescribed drug class or missing critical information about a patient's known drug allergies.

• Use of the wrong drug name (e.g., sound-alike or look-alike names), wrong dosage form (e.g., intramuscular versus intravenous injection), or

BOX 2-4
Off-Label Use of Medications

Unlicensed use of medications is common when a health care need for a patient or patient population is not met by currently available therapies. A licensed medication (i.e., one that has received regulatory approval) is used off-label when prescribed by clinicians in a manner that they deem medically appropriate, but that is outside the agreed-upon statement of the medication's efficacy (Dick et al., 2003). Examples include administration by a different route, use outside a defined age range, use of a higher or more frequent dose, and prescription for a different indication. Unlicensed use includes modifications to a licensed medication, such as dispensing in a different formulation (e.g., crushing tablets to prepare a suspension); new medications available under a special manufacturing license; use of chemicals as medications (e.g., chemotherapy agents); medications used before a license is granted (e.g., those under an IND); and imported unlicensed medications (Dick et al., 2003). Although the FDA does not regulate off-label use, it can regulate the promotion of such uses (Loder and Biondi, 2004). Federal law and state insurance commissioners have attempted to define acceptable off-label use to prevent insurers from refusing to pay for such treatment. In 1990, the Omnibus Budget Reconciliation Act (OBRA) confirmed that "medically accepted indication" includes off-label use and should be supported by one of the following:

• American Hospital Formulary Service drug information
• American Medical Association drug evaluations
• United States Pharmacopeia drug information
• Scientific studies published in the peer-reviewed literature

Estimates of off-label medication use range from 20 to 60 percent, depending on the drug and patient population (Dick et al., 2003; NCI, 2004; Murphy, 2005). Off-label prescribing occurs most frequently with pediatric, oncology, obstetric, and

wrong abbreviation (e.g., "qd" [every day] instead of "qid" [4 times per day]).

• Incorrect dosage calculations, including wrongly placed decimal point and wrong rate, frequency, unit of measure, or route of administration.

• Wrong patient (i.e., faulty patient identification checking).

• Failure to prescribe when there is an indication (e.g., omission of beta-blockers post–acute myocardial infarction) or prescribing without an indication (e.g., use of antibiotics to treat the common cold).

• Other factors, such as failure to assess drug–drug or drug–food interactions or duplicative therapies (Lesar et al., 1997; Dean et al., 2002; Bobb et al., 2004; USP, 2004).

Prescribing errors are attributed chiefly to the provider's insufficient knowledge about the medication and its correct use or about the patient

AIDS patients, although it is by no means limited to these populations. The highest rate of such uses is with pediatric patients (Murphy, 2005). Up to 90 percent of these patients (especially neonates) are prescribed at least one drug off-label (Jong et al., 2001; Lifshitz et al., 2001) based on the modification of adult formulations, dosage strengths, and dosage levels (Jong et al., 2001). Published information from pediatric trials of other drugs and the clinical experiences of other physicians also are relied upon for decision making. While necessary, such methods can underscore the important differences between adults and children in development and the metabolism and excretion of a particular drug, increasing the risk of an adverse drug event (Christensen et al., 1999; Jong et al., 2001). Some drugs are now tested in pediatric populations, but significant ethical concerns about such testing mean that off-label use of drugs will continue to be necessary to meet the needs of these patients.

The second-largest rate of off-label use occurs with oncology patients (Poole and Dooley, 2004; Kos, 2005). A survey of oncologists found that 60 percent of these clinicians prescribe off-label for cancer patients who may require drugs approved for a different type of cancer or a different disease, or at different dosages, frequencies, or duration from those approved (NCI, 2004). One study found that about one-third of oncology prescriptions were off-label, and more than 50 percent of oncology patients received at least one drug off-label (NCI, 2004). Off-label use is common in oncology because cancer drugs rarely receive generalized approval, but are approved for a specific biological target or a particular type of tumor. Once the drug is on the market, however, further research and off-label use may demonstrate its action on different targets present in other types of cancer (NCI, 2004). Conversely, the side effects of cancer drugs can vary depending on the type of cancer being treated, such that the risk of an adverse event or reaction can increase when the side effects of an off-label use are unknown.

Because medical needs of certain patient populations cannot be met with approved uses of many medications, off-label prescribing will continue to be an important part of clinical practice.

(e.g., incomplete medical history), miscommunication among providers (e.g., illegible handwriting on written orders, misunderstanding of verbal orders, mistakes using electronic ordering), lapses in provider performance (e.g., nonadherence to policies and procedures, slips or memory lapses), and lapses in documentation (e.g., incomplete charting) (Cohen, 2000; IOM, 2000, 2004c; Phillips et al., 2001; USP, 2004). More specifically:

- Errors related to medication knowledge may be the result of gaps in timely access to drug information at the point of care, in understanding of the complexities of the use of specific drugs, and in access to comprehensive knowledge bases needed to build expertise in drug therapy (Lesar et al., 1997). Also, in some cases information that would be useful in preventing errors (e.g., the correct dose of aspirin to prevent coronary heart disease) does not exist.

• Incomplete medical histories contribute to prescribing errors. Many patients fail to list all the medications they are taking (e.g., OTCs, dietary supplements), or the provider may forget to ask about known drug allergies or to review laboratory data that would further improve prescribing for the patient (Lesar et al., 1997; Smith et al., 2005).

• Poorly handwritten prescription orders are the chief culprit in miscommunications among prescribing clinicians, nurses, and pharmacists, and have often resulted in serious injury or death due to incorrect understanding of the drug or its dosage, route, or frequency (Cohen, 2000).

• Although widespread use of computerized provider order entry or electronic prescribing systems has the potential to reduce errors associated with poorly handwritten prescriptions, errors can still occur in the interaction between the clinician and the technology as a result of issues in such areas as usability, readability, training, and suboptimal system safeguards (Horsky et al., 2005). Indeed, one study found that computerized provider order entry systems facilitated 22 different types of errors[8] (Koppel et al., 2005).

• Oral orders (e.g., those given over the phone to a pharmacy or between clinicians involved in emergency care) can result in an error if, for example, product names sound alike; dosages are unclear (e.g., "two 50 milligrams," which can be interpreted as 250 milligrams instead of 100 milligrams); or concentrations are not specified (Cohen, 2000).

• Performance lapses, or slips, can occur when a provider sets out to do one thing and actually does something else. Such lapses can be due to a lack of focus on the task at hand, distracting conversations (e.g., talking and listening to others talk about things unrelated to the task), interruptions, a poor working environment (e.g., high noise levels, low lighting), poor workflow (e.g., workflow that is not logical), and uneven workload (e.g., too little or too much) (Davis, 1996).

Self-Prescribing

During self-care with OTC products and dietary supplements, the consumer (or a family member) is responsible for prescribing based on his or her own (or the family member's) assessment and diagnosis of the condition. Determining which medication or supplement to take can be based on a review of labels and comparison of products deemed appropriate; the

---

[8]Examples include fragmented displays that prevent a coherent view of the patient's medications, pharmacy inventory displays mistaken for dosage guidelines, ignored antibiotic renewal notices placed on paper charts rather than in the computerized system, separation of functions that facilitate double dosing and incompatible orders, and inflexible ordering formats generating wrong orders (Koppel et al., 2005).

suggestion or experience of a family member, friend, community pharmacist, or community provider; and/or advertisements. Primary sources of information for selecting OTCs and dietary supplements vary according to the population group. A 2001 survey by the Consumers Healthcare Products Association, the industry trade group, found that consumers seek advice in treating minor ailments from family and friends first (27 percent), followed by physicians (20 percent), medical reference books (10 percent), pharmacists (7 percent), and the Internet (7 percent) (RSW, 2001). Generally, older Americans are much more likely than their younger counterparts to rely on their health care provider, regardless of the seriousness of their health condition (RSW, 2001). Individuals with lower incomes are more likely to rely on providers for recommendations, while those with higher incomes are more likely to turn to the Internet. Likewise, individuals who use dietary supplements (and alternative medicines) for minor ailments are significantly more likely than those who do not use dietary supplements to seek information from family and friends (25 percent), medical reference books (13 percent), and newspapers/magazines (8 percent) (RSW, 2001). Although pharmacists did not rank as the first choice for health-related information, an overwhelming majority of Americans (84 percent) agree that they are a good source of information for treatment of minor ailments.

A debatable issue concerns the ability of consumers to understand and use product labels when deciding to take an OTC or dietary supplement. The pharmaceutical industry asserts that an overwhelming majority of consumers take the necessary precautions, such as reading directions before using a product for first time use (95 percent), examining labels to help choose medications (89 percent), and reviewing possible side effects and interactions (91 percent) (RSW, 2001). This is an improvement over figures cited in an earlier poll by Harris Interactive (NPSF, 1997) that found only 20 percent of consumers read the label for side effects before making an OTC purchase, and 77 percent do not read the dosage instructions at all (Cropper, 2005). Language and literacy barriers exacerbate problems with consumers' understanding and use of drug labels (IOM, 2004a).

Transcribing

Once the drug regimen has been determined, orders from the prescribing clinician are sent to the pharmacy and, in the hospital setting, the nurses' station for processing. *Transcription* is the official term used to describe the complex set of tasks involved in interpreting and processing orders. Many medication errors are associated with the transcription process, particularly if a drug name looks or sounds like that of another drug or is illegible. In the order, the clinician must provide complete details on the drug regimen (patient name, drug name, dosage, formulation, route, frequency, units, flow rates, duration, reconstitution information) (Manasse and Thompson, 2005). Prior to processing, both the pharmacist and assigned nurse must communicate directly with the ordering clinician if there is even the slightest question concerning any aspect of the drug regimen or its clinical appropriateness (Cohen, 2000).

Because health care institutions and pharmacies vary widely in the extent to which they have implemented information technology, varying different methods are used to send medication orders to the pharmacy in the inpatient setting. Some pharmacies receive orders in written or typed form via fax, scanned image, a vacuum tube system, or carbon copies of the original; others may receive orders through a state-of-the-art computerized provider order entry system (Manasse and Thompson, 2005). Community pharmacies generally receive orders via fax or handwritten prescription or orally over the phone. Oral orders warrant greater caution given the ease with which miscommunication can occur, and should be read back, with spelling of the drug name and dosage, to the clinician (Cohen, 2000; Allinson et al., 2005). All health care organizations and pharmacies should have guidelines (e.g., readback of all verbal orders) in place to reduce the possibility of errors occurring in the transcription process (Cohen, 2000). While computerized provider order entry systems have been promoted as the primary method for reducing errors in transcription because they eliminate handwritten prescriptions, other factors, such as improved processes for drug naming to minimize look-alike, sound-alike names, also could improve the transcription process (see Chapter 6).

Preparing and Dispensing

Following transcription, the pharmacist begins the preparation and dispensing process. Entry of orders into the pharmacy database system allows for automated screening of orders for therapeutic duplications, drug interactions, allergies, or doses that are not within an acceptable range; if therapeutically appropriate, screening the order against the patient's laboratory test results can avert potential adverse events (Manasse and Thompson, 2005). About 91 percent of hospital or health system pharmacies have a computerized database system, and 87 percent have access to patient admission, discharge, and transfer data through links in the database (Ringold et al., 1999). If changes need to be made for therapeutic reasons or in response to a supply shortage, the pharmacist may do so only with the approval of the prescriber, and all of the initial steps in processing must be repeated. If pharmacists do not know all the drug-related products (i.e., prescription, OTC, dietary supplements) a consumer is taking, however, their ability to perform drug interaction checking is inhibited in both the inpatient and community setting. Interaction checking can be particularly difficult when consumers use multiple pharmacies to fill their prescriptions and fail to communicate this to each pharmacy.

Depending on the specific order and patient, preparation of the medication may require counting, measuring, or compounding (mixing of ingredients); repackaging (e.g., unit doses); and labeling. Activities associated with preparation present the greatest opportunity for error within the pharmacy (Manasse and Thompson, 2005). Most inpatient errors involve selection/dispensing of an incorrect drug (e.g., because of sound-alike, look-alike names or packaging), dosage strength (e.g., incorrect dilution), formulation (e.g., tablet versus intravenous), or dosage calculation (e.g., incorrect calculation of flow rate for intravenous medication) (Cohen, 2000; Phillips et al., 2001). Outpatient errors tend to center on incorrect drug labeling information (e.g., use or administration of the drug) (Buchanan et al., 1991; Flynn et al., 2003).

During preparation, a large percentage of oral and injectable medications used in the inpatient setting require further manipulation (compounding and/or repackaging) prior to administration, increasing the risk of error. Most drugs are licensed for adult use; reformulation and compounding are most often necessary to treat neonates or pediatric patients who cannot swallow tablets or capsules and require dosage concentrations and formulations tailored to their age, body weight, and body surface area (Nunn, 2003). Adult patients with a rare condition for which an orphan drug[9] is no longer manufactured may require the pharmacist's expertise to compound and formulate a medication from chemicals and ingredients available only in bulk (Kastango, 2003). Also, repackaging is common for inpatient facilities so as to provide medications in unit doses and thereby minimize dose manipulation and errors at the bedside. Currently, 79 to 99 percent of hospital pharmacists repackage oral medications, and 29 percent repackage injectables (Cohen, 2000; Pedersen et al., 2003). However, new federal regulations to go into effect in 2007 require manufacturers (or third-party repackagers) to provide all products to hospitals in unit dose form with bar codes (FR, 2004b). In a further effort to decrease errors, some hospitals also use decentralized automated dispensing systems (e.g., ward-based cabinets) for storing certain medications that are in unit dose form (e.g., narcotics, as-needed drugs, limited floor stock) (Cohen, 2000). These systems can be accessed by nurses with "swipe cards" or personal identification numbers. Finally, a growing number of community-based and most mail order pharmacies are using automated dispensing systems, including centralized systems that can produce unit doses (e.g., via strip or envelope packag-

---

[9]An *orphan drug* is a product that is used in the diagnosis or treatment of diseases or conditions considered rare in the United States.

ing),[10] or that use bottle-filling machines; others are experimenting with decentralized systems that rely on prefilled bottles and manufacturer-packaged items (Cohen, 2000).

Patient counseling in a pharmacy provides an opportunity for the pharmacist to inform the patient about his/her medications, encourage medication adherence, and answer any questions the patient may have. In the OBRA of 1990 (P.L. 101-508), Congress required that pharmacists counsel Medicaid patients. Since then, boards of pharmacy in most states have come to require some type of counseling for all patients (NABP, 2004). For many reasons (e.g., low patient demand, lack of cost-effectiveness data, time constraints, lack of reimbursement), however, pharmacies often offer counseling only as requested by a consumer. A study of 100 prescription orders dispensed in 1994 in community pharmacies in New Jersey, New York, and Florida found that oral counseling had been provided to 64 patients, covering on average 3 of the 14 categories[11] (i.e., dosage, frequency of administration, drug or food interactions) of drug information required by OBRA 1990 (Allan et al., 1995). Similar results were observed in a more recent, larger eight-state study. In this study, about two-thirds of consumers had been given oral information—on average 2.3 items from a 5-item list (Svarstad et al., 2004). The study also found that higher levels of pharmacist counseling were associated with younger pharmacists, less busy pharmacies, and more demanding state regulations. In terms of mail order pharmacies, counseling is generally available as requested by telephone.

Dispensing errors account for an estimated 6–12 percent of all medication errors (Buchanan et al., 1991; Allan et al., 1995; Flynn et al., 2003). Research suggests that the main causes of such errors are issues concerning workload and staffing, distractions during processing, suboptimal packaging and labeling, poorly designed work areas, and outdated or incorrect drug reference information (Cohen, 2000; Phillips et al., 2001). A review of the literature reveals that:

- Failure to double-check orders, medication, and labels is a common cause of dispensing errors.

---

[10]With strip and envelope packaging, instead of a 30-day bottled prescription containing 30 tablets (1 per day), a 30-pack "compliance strip" contains 1 pill per pack. Each pack contains the patient's name, the drug and its dose, and the date and time it is to be administered.

[11]The 14 categories for pharmacy counseling established by the Omnibus Budget Reconciliation Act of 1990 are drug name; use of medication; dosage (how much); route of administration; frequency of administration; duration of therapy; special directions, procedures for administration; side effects; drug or food interactions; disease state effects; storage; refills; directions if dose missed; and self-monitoring techniques (Allan et al., 1995).

- High workload/low staffing is the primary contributing factor to medication errors associated with preparing and dispensing medications in both community and institutional settings (Davis and Cohen, 1994; Roberts et al., 2002).
- Interruptions (temporary cessation of prescription filling) and distractions (external stimulus without cessation of prescription filling) are highly correlated with dispensing errors (Flynn et al., 1999). Error rates per half hour of 6.65 percent for interruptions and 6.55 percent for distractions were found, with incorrect instructions to the patient being the most common error. About 26 percent of pharmacists' time is spent dealing with issues (interruptions) related to third parties and miscellaneous administrative tasks (NACDS, 1999).
- Product labels are often read under less-than-ideal conditions, and the way a medication is packaged and labeled can have a significant impact on error rates. Problematic aspects of packaging and labeling include look-alike packaging, obscure placement of critical safety information, and print that is too small and lacks sufficient distinctions in contrast or boldness (Cohen, 2000; Phillips et al., 2001; IOM, 2000, 2004c; USP, 2004).
- Improper lighting, inadequate counter space, poor placement of telephones, and uncomfortable temperature and humidity create a work area that can negatively affect workflow from one task to another and contribute to errors caused by clutter or contamination (Cohen, 2000).
- Drug reference files, texts, and/or database systems may not be current, resulting in errors associated with outdated and incorrect information (Cohen, 2000). Constant updating of drug information is particularly critical to patient safety given the limited data available when medications enter the market and the amount of new data on medications already in use among the population.

Administering and Consumption

Nurses have primary responsibility for administering medications in acute care hospitals, in long-term care facilities, and during home care. In certain instances, a nursing assitant/technician may be permitted to administer selected medications (Munroe, 2003; Castle and Engberg, 2005). In many of these settings, the environment for nurses is demanding, characterized by long work hours, staffing shortages, high patient and staff turnover, and constant interruptions (O'Shea, 1999; IOM, 2004b; Jenkins and Elliott, 2004; Suzuki et al., 2005). Accurate administration of medications can be challenging in this environment.

Tasks associated with preparing medications for administration can range from simple retrieval of a unit dose from a ward-based automated dispensing system to reconstitution of a powder with a sterile diluent

(Cohen, 2000; Kastango, 2003; IOM, 2004b). Most medications are now administered in unit dose form to minimize the amount of compounding by nurses. Ideally, medications should be kept in the dispensing container and in their individual packages until they reach the bedside so as to decrease the risk of their being confused with another patient's drug. In addition, it is standard practice for the drug label to be read three times prior to administration—when obtaining the drug from the storage area; when preparing the dosage at the bedside; and after administration, when discarding the package (Cohen, 2000; Manias et al., 2005)—although there is some support for registered nurses' competence to perform single-checking (Jarman et al., 2002). Averting errors also requires careful attention to dosage and route when preparing medications. For example, pediatric and chemotherapy doses should indicate milligrams per kilogram (mg/kg) or milligrams per meter squared (mg/m^2) in order to leave little margin for error (Cohen, 2000). Nurses must also ensure that drug infusion or administration devices are functioning properly and programmed accurately to ensure that the dose and infusion rate are correct (Smetzer, 2001; Fields and Peterman, 2005; Nicholas and Agius, 2005). These nursing activities are indispensable to patient safety.

Perhaps most important, the nurse is often the last professional to evaluate the appropriateness of the medication that has been prescribed. In fact, a study of medication errors found that nurses were responsible for intercepting 86 percent of all errors made by physicians, pharmacists, and others involved in providing medications for patients (Leape et al., 1995). Nurses' involvement and vigilance during the preparation process is thus central to accurate medication administration.

Medication administration is founded on what are termed the "five rights"—the right drug, in the right dose, by the right route, at the right time, to the right patient (Manias et al., 2005; Nicholas and Agius, 2005; Schull, 2005; Manasse and Thompson, 2005). While achieving the five rights is essential to safe medication administration, more complex factors must also be considered to ensure positive outcomes. First, medications can be administered via a number of different routes and formulations—oral tablet, capsule, or liquid; intravenous solution; intramuscular injection; inhalant; eye/ear drops; topical cream or solution; transdermal patch; or other means—depending on the patient, drug, and condition. Without attention to this issue, for instance, a liquid intended for oral dosing might be administered intravenously. Excessive variations in dosing regimens (e.g., multiple sliding scales for insulin dosing, as needed), use of high-risk drugs (e.g., anticoagulants, narcotics), and the proliferation of new drugs and devices add significantly to the intricacies of the administration process (Greengold et al., 2003; USP, 2003). In addition, the severity of a patient's medical condition and the presence of comorbidities further increase the challenges to evaluating the safety and appropriateness of a medication that has been ordered (IOM, 2001). Relative to the other points along the medication-use continuum, the administration process has the fewest safeguards and fewest support mechanisms, and it often relies on a single health care professional for perfection (Cohen, 2000; IOM, 2003, 2004b).

Several inpatient facilities are beginning to implement bar code medication administration systems to increase assurance that the five rights are being achieved (IOM, 2002; Patterson, 2003; FR, 2004b; Burke et al., 2005). The bar codes placed on unit doses of medications are encoded with the patient's name, drug, dose, route, and time of administration. Bar code scanners (placed in each patient's room) are linked to computerized databases containing the patient's drug regimen. The database may be crosslinked to other health information systems, such as a patient identification master file, an order entry system, and/or the pharmacy database (FR, 2004b; Nicholas and Agius, 2005). The nurse scans the bar code on the medication package and the patient's identification wristband, allowing the system to determine whether there is a match. Following a confirmation signal, the nurse administers the medication. If there is an alert, the nurse stops the process from going forward, preventing a potential medication error. Because medication administration is a high-volume activity, bar code medication administration systems can provide needed support to nurses during clinical care. They also generate data for the medication administration record (MAR).

Maintenance of an accurate MAR is essential to safety and quality of care (IOM, 2004b). This record serves as a log of all medication-related activities for each patient. Entries are made immediately after a dose has been administered to minimize errors of omission (Cohen, 2000). MARs also document that medications were given in a timely manner for the correct indications. Expanded records are usually reserved for high-risk drugs (e.g., anticoagulants, cardiac drugs, insulin) so as to record important variables affecting administration (e.g., international normalized ratio [INR], used to measure prothrombin time). All medications are typically documented consistently in one place for ease of reference by the team of health care providers that may be caring for a patient. The MAR also serves as a reference in the event of a medication error (Gladstone, 1995; Wakefield et al., 1999). In some cases, third-party payers have reviewed the MAR to look for inconsistencies and gaps in treatment and to find evidence for denying payment.

The types of errors associated with administration-related mortality include (1) dosing errors (40.9 percent, 36.4 percent of which were overdoses); (2) incorrect drug (16 percent); and (3) incorrect route (9.5 percent) (Phillips et al., 2001). Causes of administration errors include miscommunications, miscalculations, workload/staffing problems, interruptions, rapid increases in knowledge and technology demands, and incomplete documentation (IOM, 2004b).

• Miscommunications during medication administration generally result from errors in transcribing oral or written orders (e.g., prescriber fails to insert a zero before a decimal point), reading product names (e.g., look-alike, sound-alike), or labeling (e.g., similar or misleading container labels) (Donohue and Needleman, 1998; Phillips et al., 2001). Commonly used abbreviations for drug names, dosage units, and references to timing of administration cause many medication errors (e.g., the abbreviation "U" for units of insulin can be read as a zero, leading to an overdose) (Cohen, 2000). Also, only the metric system should be used in the MAR, and apothecary symbols and terms that can easily be misinterpreted should be avoided.

• Miscalculations of medication dosages are often due to the complexity of drug protocols (e.g., for cancer chemotherapy), the need for speedy action in emergency situations, marketing of multiple concentrations of drug products, and the availability of highly concentrated drug products on nursing units (e.g., those that are intended only for compounding infusions but that might be given undiluted) (Phillips et al., 2001; Fields and Peterman, 2005).

• As noted above, the work environment for nurses can contribute to medication errors (O'Shea, 1999; IOM, 2004b; Jenkins and Elliott, 2004). As the numbers of available hospital beds and lengths of stay have decreased, patient turnover rates have risen (some by 40–50 percent in an 8- to 10-hour period), increasing the workload of hospital nurses even as funding reductions and resulting work environment dissatisfaction have led to inadequate staffing (Norrish and Rundall, 2001). High rates of nursing staff turnover (21.3 percent per year for hospitals and 56 percent for long-term care facilities) have adverse consequences for staffing levels, quality of care, and patient safety (AHCA, 2002; The HSM Group, 2002). Although most nursing shifts are 8–12 hours, mandatory overtime and double shifts contribute to nursing-related medication administration errors (IOM, 2004b).

• Distractions and interruptions as nurses carry out their primary patient care responsibilities increase the potential for adverse events, such as errors in patient identification as a nurse prepares doses for more than one patient. Many distractions and interruptions are associated with added tasks that nurses undertake during staffing shortages, such as delivering and receiving food trays, performing housekeeping tasks, transporting patients, and performing ancillary services (e.g., delivery of medical supplies, blood products) (IOM, 2004b). Distractions also result from the fact that patients hospitalized today have less stable health conditions than they did, on average, when longer hospital stays were the norm. Thus, nurses often must respond to the health crises of some patients, which distract them from timely and thoughtful medication administration to others.

• The growth of a rapidly expanding knowledge base in clinical care, drugs, devices, and health information technology is forcing changes in the work nurses are asked to perform (IOM, 2004b; Nicholas and Agius, 2005). Appropriate levels of training, continuing education, reconditioning of workflows, and support mechanisms are necessary to minimize medication-related errors (Gladstone, 1995). This includes improved familiarity with less common medications, attention to commonly used medications to which many patients are allergic (e.g., antibiotics, nonsteroidal anti-inflammatory drugs), and more vigilant follow-through on medications that require monitoring to ensure proper dosing (e.g., warfarin, lithium, digoxin) (Woods and Johnson, 2002). Technologies that provide ready access to this information are essential.

Self-Administration

From the perspective of consumers, the most common types of medication errors are associated with administration of wrong dosages; unnecessary medicating; adverse drug reactions, including drug–drug interactions; and nonadherence. Errors occur from overdosing or underdosing as a result of inadequate instructions and use of inconsistent or improper measuring devices. For example, the household teaspoon is the device used most frequently for measuring liquid medication for home administration, instead of a dosing syringe. Common errors also include misinterpreting instructions, confusing teaspoons with tablespoons on a medicine cup, and misreading a dosage chart when the weight is not typical for a particular age group (Madlon-Kay and Mosch, 2000). One study found that acetaminophen (Tylenol) dosing by parents was inaccurate 73 percent of the time, resulting in ineffective fever control and increased emergency room visits in two-thirds of cases (Gribetz and Crunley, 1987). A recent article reported that two infants died from suspected overdoses of an OTC cold medicine (Presecky, 2006). The cold medicine had been administered with a 1 mg eyedropper provided in the product package. The dosage for the infants was 0.2 mg (two-tenths of one dropper) but was misunderstood to mean 2 droppers full of medicine. The probability of medication dosing errors is greatly increased with high-risk medications that have complex dosing regimens, such as oral chemotherapy agents, oral anticoagulants, opioids, and insulin (Watzke et al., 2000; Grissinger et al., 2003; Hartigan, 2003). These drugs have narrower therapeutic indices, meaning there is less margin for error, and the consequences of error may be more devastating (Cohen, 2000). Many dosing errors could be avoided with the use of more accurate devices, such as oral dosing syringes; color coding of age–weight dosing zones, particularly for liquid medications administered to children; and better presentation of use information and safety warnings (Frush et al., 2004).

Other types of dosing errors are associated with the frequency or duration of treatment. One study found that only 38 percent of patients correctly administered medications when instructed to do so every 6 hours; most thought they were to consume the medication every 6 hours when awake and thus to take three rather than four doses (Madlon-Kay and Mosch, 2000). In other cases the prescriber may write "q6h," the abbreviation for every 6 hours, when intending that the patient take the medication three times per day. Additionally, unnecessary use of antibiotics for the wrong infections or when no infection is present and not taking all doses through the prescribed treatment duration are important factors contributing to antimicrobial resistance (Davey et al., 2002).

Monitoring for Effects

Monitoring (also referred to as assessment, evaluation, observation, and surveillance) involves obtaining and evaluating clinical indicators and other relevant information to determine a drug's effect in an individual patient (Knowlton and Penna, 2003). Monitoring for desired and undesired effects is a crucial step in the care process and in the prevention or detection of adverse drug events. In every setting in which care is delivered—ambulatory care sites, hospitals, schools, workplace health sites, home health care, and nursing homes—assessment and monitoring is a primary responsibility of licensed nurses (IOM, 2004b). Pharmacists also may play a role in assessing beneficial or adverse effects during inpatient care, as may patients (including family members) in ambulatory and self-care.

At its best, monitoring is individualized, taking into consideration that different patients may experience different therapeutic results and outcomes, and it is responsive, correcting the regimen if an adverse effect is found (Knowlton and Penna, 2003). Assessing the effect of medications can be accomplished through direct observation of the patient, use of monitoring devices, and/or information technology (e.g., predefined triggers in a laboratory database) (Forester et al., 2004; Manasse and Thompson, 2005). The type and frequency of patient monitoring activities vary by care setting, clinical condition, and other characteristics of the patient (IOM, 2004b).

In acute care hospitals, bedside monitoring of the patient's condition prior to, during, and following medical procedures such as initiation of new medications, surgery, or a course of medical therapy typically includes monitoring vital signs (i.e., temperature, heart rate and rhythm, breathing rate and character, blood pressure), airway, risk/presence of infection, fluid intake and output, electrolytes, and pain (Bulechek et al., 1994). In intensive care units, monitoring is more frequent, more often invasive, and technologically complex (IOM, 2004b). In long-term and home care, other patient characteristics are observed and evaluated to determine the response to medications, including cognition, communication, vision, mood and behavior patterns, psychosocial well-being, and ability to perform daily care activities (e.g., grooming, bathing). Results of patient monitoring and any adverse effects are documented in the patient's medical record. For nursing homes and home health services, these assessments must be completed by licensed nurses according to federally prescribed guidelines to comply with federal regulatory and reimbursement requirements (i.e., Medicare) (ANA, 1998; IOM, 2004b).

Medical devices designed for patient monitoring range from small, wearable devices that monitor a single physiological parameter, such as blood pressure, to complex devices (e.g., respiratory oximeters, electrocardiograms) that measure a variety of parameters and transmit them electronically to a central monitoring station. Changes in physiological responses detected with these devices can signal a nurse that the patient may be experiencing an adverse drug reaction. For example, a heart monitor may detect an inappropriate change in heart rate or rhythm after administration of a cardiac drug. Medication infusion devices, such as smart pumps and patient-controlled analgesia machines, go a step further and maintain a record not only of medications administered, but also of errors that may have occurred. In addition, telemedicine and remote patient monitoring devices that are connected to specialized computer modems and can reliably measure and transmit physiological data (e.g., blood pressure, heart rate, blood glucose level) are a growing method of care management supporting providers and patients in rural settings (inpatient, ambulatory, home/self-care) (Field and Grigsby, 2002).

The ability of pharmacists to monitor the effectiveness of drug therapy through computerized pharmacy and laboratory database systems has been an important advance in assessing patient responses to medications, especially in inpatient settings (Knowlton and Penna, 2003). Linkage of these systems enhances opportunities for improved monitoring through evaluation and review of drug appropriateness, drug dosages, drug–drug interactions, drug–allergy conflicts, drug blood serum concentrations, and metabolic responses, particularly for potent medications with narrow therapeutic indices (Armstrong, 2000; Knowlton and Penna, 2003; Schiff et al., 2003). Electronic medical records with event-driven surveillance systems are able to monitor patients around the clock and have been shown to detect some adverse drug events early enough to prevent their progression from mild or moderate to severe (Classen et al., 1991; Evans et al., 1991, 1994; Jha et al., 1998; Bates and Gawande, 2003). These systems monitor specific signals from laboratory results, medication orders, information on vital signs, drug levels, and text reports to identify patients experiencing possible adverse drug events. Pharmacists then follow up on high-risk patients. Patient monitoring could be further improved through the incorporation of linked pharmacy and laboratory data into electronic order entry and real-time decision-support technologies, although issues concerning alert mechanisms must be resolved if this potential is to be realized (Schiff et al., 2003). In addition, recognition of the benefits of the pharmacist's involvement in medication monitoring is extending beyond the inpatient setting to home health care, nursing homes, and community care (Knowlton and Penna, 2003).

It should be noted that susceptibility to adverse reactions is greatly increased in patients with multiple health conditions taking multiple medications. This is a growing problem for the elderly and others with chronic illnesses receiving care from several clinicians who may fail to coordinate medication treatment. On average, Medicare enrollees with chronic conditions are seen by eight different physicians or other providers during the course of a single year (Anderson and Knickman, 2001). Studies of medication errors among the elderly (Gurwitz et al., 2003, 2005) found that in both hospital and ambulatory care settings, monitoring errors were attributable to inadequate laboratory monitoring of drug therapies, or to a delayed response or failure to respond to signs and symptoms of drug toxicity (36 percent) or laboratory evidence of drug toxicity (37 percent) (Gurwitz et al., 2003, 2005). The most common preventable adverse effects from these monitoring errors were electrolyte/renal, gastrointestinal tract, hemorrhagic, and metabolic/endocrine events. Patient adherence was a contributing factor in 20 percent of the cases studied (Gurwitz et al., 2003). Another study of four primary care practices found that 25 percent of patients experienced an adverse drug event over a 3-month period (13 percent of these events were serious, 39 percent were preventable, and 6 percent were both serious and preventable) (Gandhi et al., 2003). The events were attributed to poor communication—the physician's failure to respond to symptoms reported by the patient or the patient's failure to report symptoms to the physician.

Using the methods noted above, the overarching goal of monitoring is the early detection of a downturn in a patient's health status or the occurrence of an adverse event and the initiation of activities to restore the patient's health (IOM, 2004b). Drugs may cause adverse effects in patients for a variety of reasons. For example, a drug may be highly potent and toxic at therapeutic doses, a drug may interact in an unforeseen way with another drug or a food product, a patient may have a particular sensitivity to a drug, a wrong drug or improper dosage may be administered, or a drug may be improperly manufactured (Noah and Brushwood, 2000). The signs and symptoms of an adverse reaction may be unpredictable (e.g., a skin rash or anaphylaxis); foreseeable (e.g., nausea with chemotherapy); or un-anticipated because they arise from errors in prescribing, dispensing, or administering (Noah and Brushwood, 2000). Regardless of the cause, as discussed above, nursing surveillance is critically important in preventing, identifying, and recovering from adverse events (IOM, 2004b). In summary, medication safety and monitoring depend on the following (Noah and Brushwood, 2000):

- Knowledge of results of laboratory tests that affect drug dosages.
- Knowledge of previously unrecognized adverse reactions.
- Knowledge of adverse reactions that were previously recognized and were thought to be preventable, but are in fact not being prevented.
- Knowledge of previously recognized, unpreventable adverse reactions that were thought to occur at acceptably low rates in light of the drug's anticipated benefit, but occur more frequently in practice than anticipated.

Health care providers can enhance patient safety by welcoming the involvement of patients and families, especially in monitoring care and responses to medications. There should be no place in the health care system where a surrogate is prevented from being present whenever a patient without full faculties is receiving medications.

Self-Monitoring

Self-monitoring of responses to OTCs, prescription medications, and dietary supplements is an important aspect of good self-care and self-management. Since most patients do not discuss their use of OTCs with their primary care provider, they rely on their own judgment and product labels for prescribing, administering, and monitoring their consumption of these products (Simaon and Winkle, 1997; Frank et al., 2001). The greatest concern with the use of OTCs is the possibility of interactions with other products, mainly prescription medications, that can produce an adverse reaction. Warnings about such interactions are often listed on product labels, but difficulty in understanding the labels can increase the probability of an error or adverse effect (Patel et al., 2002). Likewise, a growing literature documents interactions of complementary and alternative medicines (including dietary supplements) with OTCs and prescription drugs (D'Arcy, 1993; Calis and Young, 2004). Thus, active self-monitoring is necessary for those consuming these products to identify and prevent serious events.

Self-monitoring of physiological and psychological responses to prescription drugs is even more critical to the identification of adverse events. Insufficient self-monitoring and nonadherence to drug regimens are well-noted problems that can contribute to poor health outcomes, adverse events, and emergency room visits (Sawicki, 1999; Cummings et al., 2000). Some prescription medications have a particularly high propensity to drug and food interactions; examples are warfarin, an anticoagulant, and monamine oxidase (MAO) inhibitors, an (older) class of antidepressant. One study found an abundance of adverse interactions between warfarin and commonly used medications and foods such as anti-infective agents, lipid-lowering drugs, nonsteroidal anti-inflammatories, certain antidepressants, anabolic steroids, fish oil, mango, green tea, and grapefruit juice, to name a few (Holbrook et al., 2005). In total, 34 reports of major interactions were confirmed in the study, as were 41 highly probable and 38 probable causations. Likewise, a wide range of drug and food interactions have been reported with the use of MAO inhibitors (Livingston and Livingston, 1996; NLM, 2005). Dangerous reactions such as sudden high blood pressure may result when these agents are taken with certain drugs, foods, or drinks, such as antihypertensives, asthma medicines, other antidepressants, cheese, poultry, fish, sausage, overripe fruit, alcoholic beverages, and high amounts of caffeine (NLM, 2005). Individuals taking these medications have a difficult time adhering to their regimens without adequate education and support mechanisms.

A number of factors affect individuals' ability to engage in illness self-management such as their particular illness and life circumstances. Barriers to self-management generally fall into three categories: knowledge deficits (e.g., insufficient information, literacy issues); practical barriers (e.g., physiological, functional, or financial constraints); and attitudinal factors (e.g., personal beliefs, culture, values, and experiences). These barriers are discussed extensively in Chapter 4.

Conversely, several studies have noted certain individuals' ability, given adequate education, to participate successfully in self-care and disease management for various health conditions, including diabetes, which requires frequent self-monitoring of blood glucose levels to make adjustments in self-administered insulin therapy; depression, which requires self-assessment of changes in psychosocial affect resulting from prescribed medications; and cancer, which requires self-monitoring of adverse reactions to powerful chemotherapy agents (Grissinger et al., 2003; Ikesue et al., 2004; Schroeder et al., 2004). For example, self-monitoring of glucose levels and strict adherence to insulin therapy or oral hypoglycemic agents, along with extensive patient education, lead to major improvements in medical outcomes and substantial decreases in long-term complications of diabetes (Tamada et al., 1999). Similar positive results were found in initial studies of patients receiving oral anticoagulation therapy (Sawicki, 1999). Self-management support programs that emphasized use of portable capillary whole-blood analyzers for regular testing of prothrombin time, together with structured patient education, improved the accuracy of medication management and overall quality of life. However, additional studies are needed to assess the impact of such self-monitoring on bleeding and thromboembolic complications. Given the growing prevalence of chronic conditions in the U.S. population, investment in the development of well-designed programs to assist patients with self-monitoring is essential to achieving improvements in medication safety. (See Box 2-5 for a summary of key problems with provider processes.)

ADVERSE EVENT REPORTING AND SURVEILLANCE SYSTEMS

Health care providers and safety agencies use error and adverse event reporting programs to learn about potential safety risks and the circumstances of individual errors (Smetzer and Cohen, 2006). Currently, a wide range of external reporting programs are available (IOM, 2004c; Smetzer and Cohen, 2006). Some of the systems are voluntary, and others are mandatory; some receive data only on adverse events, while others receive reports on all medication errors. These reporting programs include the following:

- *Institutional error reporting programs* such as the Veterans Administration Patient Safety Reporting System and the U.S. Pharmacopeia's MedMARx Program.
- *Mandatory state reporting programs*, for which almost half of states require mandatory reporting of certain serious adverse events (Rosenthal and Booth, 2005).
- *Voluntary national reporting programs*, such as the U.S. Pharmacopeia–Institute for Safe Medication Practice Medication Errors Reporting Program and the FDA's MedWatch Program.

Reportable events include those due to practice-based errors (e.g., misadministered drug dosage), product safety issues (e.g., an adverse reaction to a drug), or hazardous situations (e.g., confusing labeling). All of these reporting systems currently utilize their own reporting formats. For a serious adverse event that occurs in a hospital, this means that several reports must be completed to meet the requirements for different reporting systems. The lack of a common reporting format and terminology is a significant factor that not only inhibits the reporting process, but also prevents comparison of data across health care organizations and pooling of data from different reporting programs. The IOM report, *Patient Safety: Achieving a New Standard for Care*, discussed extensively the need for common standards for patient safety reporting systems.

BOX 2-5
Summary of Key Problems with Provider Processes
Affecting Safety and Quality in the Medication-Use System

Prescribing
- Individual provider's insufficient knowledge of or experience with a medication
- Insufficient knowledge base for determination of benefits and risks of off-label prescribing
- Incomplete knowledge about the patient (e.g., incomplete history)
- Failure to assess potential drug–drug, drug–disease, or drug–lifestyle (e.g., alcohol or illegal drug consumption) interactions; failure to note allergies to medications
- Lack of linkages among providers (e.g., dose changed without notification of pharmacist)
- Insufficent responsiveness to pharmacist concerns or questions about a prescription

Transcribing
- Miscommunication among providers (e.g., illegible handwritten prescription, misunderstanding of verbal order)

Preparing and Dispensing
- Problems with sound-alike drug names and look-alike drug names and packaging
- Stressful and distracting work environments

Administration and Monitoring
- Lack of timely access to knowledge at the point of care (e.g., drug or patient history or laboratory information)
- Lapses in performance (e.g., memory, adherence to guidelines, slips) due to human factors
- Incorrect dosing due to confusion among medications
- Stressful and distracting work environments

Reporting
- Culture inimical to reporting; complex and time-consuming reporting procedures

Self-Care
- Inappropriate demand for medications that are not clinically necessary (e.g., antibiotics for the common cold)
- Insufficient understanding of medication instructions (e.g., language, literacy, or cognitive barriers; not reading instructions)
- Nonadherence to medication regimens
- Insufficient attention to interactions with other medications and products
- Insufficient self-monitoring for effectiveness and adverse effects
- Insufficient understanding about how to handle adverse effects

Institutional Reporting Systems

Many health care organizations have an internal incident reporting program, frequently managed by a patient safety officer or equivalent, who carries out analyses of the errors and determines the external programs to which the incident reports should be sent. Often, reports are made directly to one or more of the external programs by the patient or provider, bypassing the patient safety office.

Rates of reporting of events have been quite low (Leape, 2002). Providers' fear of discoverability during litigation and professional disciplinary action has been a major factor affecting their willingness to report (IOM, 2004c). This particular concern should be alleviated with the recent passage of the Patient Safety and Quality Improvement Act of 2005 (P.L. 109-41). The act promotes the establishment and use of voluntary patient safety reporting systems, peer review protection from report disclosure during legal proceedings, and protection of providers who report from professional retaliation. However, the legislation failed to set measurable goals and criteria for evaluating the reporting program's success or failure.

Evidence on the effectiveness of reporting programs is limited. There is anecdotal evidence that the Joint Commission on Accreditation of Health Care Organizations' Sentinel Event Reporting System and the U.S. Pharmacopeia–Institute for Safe Medication Practice Medication Errors Reporting Program have led to important safety improvements (Leape, 2002). The only reporting program whose effect on safety has been demonstrated by a controlled trial is the National Nosocomial Infection Survey (Haley et al., 1985). Many reporting programs distribute newsletters or advisories to alert providers of hazardous situations and possible preventive measures. The impact of these materials is not known (Leape, 2002). However, performance measurement is an important component of quality improvement programs, which include activities directly related to patient safety (IOM, 2001). The new legislation mentioned above is expected to increase physician participation in adverse event reporting systems, and subsequently the translation of findings into learning and improvement. This will facilitate assessment of the positive, neutral, or negative impact of reporting systems in the near term.

State Reporting Systems

About half of all states have passed legislation or regulations related to hospital reporting of adverse events; almost all of these reporting systems are mandatory. The development of state reporting systems is tracked by the National Academy for State Health Policy (NASHP, 2006). Each state reporting system takes a different approach as to what events must be reported and what type of information must be provided (Leape, 2002; IOM, 2004). The main reason for many of these reporting systems is to ensure accountability, although a number of state reporting systems also have a learning component (Rosenthal and Booth, 2005). Each system has the potential to improve patient safety through analysis of event reports and dissemination of best practices and lessons learned. For example, the Pennsylvania Patient Safety Authority regularly issues patient safety advisories (PPSA, 2006).

Evidence that mandatory reporting systems have led hospitals to introduce changes is largely anecdotal (Leape, 2002). Despite interest in analyzing the data from reporting systems and providing feedback that can be used to improve patient safety, states have found barriers to analysis and feedback (Rosenthal and Booth, 2005). Rates of reporting are low because hospitals fear the consequences of disclosure. Further, reporting is discouraged by the cumbersome and time-consuming nature of reporting systems (Leape, 2002). In addition, states often lack the clinical expertise to analyze the data. To address these barriers, in May 2005 the National Academy for State Health Policy convened a meeting of stakeholders in reporting systems to identify mechanisms and tools for improving reporting and feedback (Rosenthal and Booth, 2005).

Federal Reporting and Surveillance Systems

The FDA's spontaneous reporting system (the MedWatch program) collects information about adverse events associated with all marketed drugs. The system depends on voluntary reports submitted by clinicians and mandatory reports submitted by manufacturers (comprising patient/ clinician reports forwarded to the company) (Fontanarosa et al., 2004). While about 250,000 such reports are received annually, several shortcomings of the system have been described in government, academic, and press publications (FDA, 1999). The reliance on voluntary reports and the factors that discourage reporting (e.g., time pressures, fear of liability, and lack of perceived benefit) result in significant underreporting of adverse outcomes and thus the inability to calculate true rates of such events (Fontanarosa et al., 2004). The reports also suffer from poor data quality, often including inadequate documentation and detail, which limits the ability to establish causal relationships in the analysis of the events. The consumer version of the system, MedWatch Plus, is designed to collect direct reports from consumers who have experienced an adverse drug reaction (Behrman, 2005). A number of activities are under way to improve the reporting systems, the quality and interpretation of the data gathered, and the use of postmarket surveillance studies, thus helping to ensure the safety and efficacy of marketed medicines.

BOX 2-6
Centers for Disease Control and Prevention's
Active Surveillance Systems for Clinical Care

The CDC's adverse event surveillance systems include the National Health-care Safety Network (the successor to the National Nosocomial Infections Surveil-lance System, the Dialysis Surveillance Network, and the National Surveillance System for Health Care Workers) (Tokars et al., 2004) and the National Electronic Injury Surveillance System-Cooperative Adverse Drug Event Surveillance project (NEISS-CADES). Through NEISS-CADES, the CDC conducts nationally repre-sentative surveillance for adverse drug events (ADEs) treated in hospital emer-gency departments. The program is aimed at controlling or preventing injury by identifying and describing the public health burden of outpatient ADEs, generating hypotheses about risk factors for these events, and helping to design interventions for reducing medication errors in the outpatient setting.

Estimates for 2004 indicate that approximately 700,000 patients were treated in emergency rooms for an ADE, and approximately 100,000 were admitted or transferred to another facility (Budnitz, 2005). Early data indicate that unintentional overdoses were the most common cause of ADEs (39 percent), and that two drugs (i.e., warfarin and insulin) were associated with 16 percent of all ADEs and 33 percent of ADEs in patients over age 50 (Budnitz et al., 2005).

NEISS-CADES has several important limitations. First, the system is limited to ADEs occurring outside the hospital and to those that result in emergency room visits. Second, the system may fail to capture some serious outpatient ADEs (those treated in a care setting other than an emergency department) and may include nonserious events (as patients may use emergency departments for pri-mary health care) (Walls et al., 2002). Third, the system is designed for national surveillance and not for quality improvement by individual hospitals. Nonetheless, given the importance of monitoring the national health burden of ADEs as one aspect of medication safety and quality improvement, the continued operation and enhancement of NEISS-CADES could play an important role in monitoring the nation's progress toward reducing medication-related harm in the outpatient set-ting. The system's usefulness would be enhanced by identifying appropriate mea-sures of drug exposure, ensuring continued data quality, and developing mecha-nisms for timely data dissemination.

The Centers for Disease Control and Prevention (CDC) performs both active and passive surveillance of safety-related morbidity and mortality associated with vaccines, treatment of infectious diseases, and other aspects of health care. Adverse events involving vaccines are reported passively through the Vaccine Adverse Event Reporting System (VAERS), maintained by the CDC jointly with the FDA. Reporting is mandatory for manufactur-ers, and for health professionals for specified adverse events (see the Re-portable Events table posted at vaers.hhs.gov) associated with the following vaccines: tetanus; pertussis; measles, mumps, and rubella; rubella; inactivated polio; hepatitis B; hemophilus influenzae type B (polysaccharide); hemophilus influenzae type B (conjugate); varicella; and pneumococcal conjugate (IOM, 2004c). From its establishment in 1990 through the end of 2001, VAERS had received over 128,000 reports (CDC, 1999).

Gaps in scientific knowledge about the possible adverse effects of vaccines and in the capacity to evaluate such effects scientifically prompted the CDC to initiate the Vaccine Safety Datalink (VSD) project in 1990 (Medstat, 2002). This project involves partnerships with several large HMOs to conduct high-quality scientific evaluations of important safety questions related to immunization. The CDC also has a number of reporting and surveillance systems for evaluating the prevalence of adverse events in clinical settings (see Box 2-6).

REFERENCES

AAMC (Association of American Medical Colleges). 2005. *Drug Development Science: Obstacles and Opportunities for Collaboration Among Academia, Industry, and Government.* Washington, DC: FDA.

Abrams T. 2005. *FDA, Division of Drug Marketing, Advertising, and Communications. Submission to the IOM Committee on Identifying and Preventing Medication Errors.* Washington, DC: FDA.

Allan EL, Barker KN, Malloy MJ, Heller WM. 1995. Dispensing errors and counseling in community practice. *American Pharmacy* NS35(12):25–33.

Allinson TT, Szeinbach SL, Schneider PJ. 2005. Perceived accuracy of drug orders transmitted orally by telephone. *American Journal of Health System Pharmacists* 62(1):78–83.

AHCA (American Health Care Association). 2002. *Results of the 2001 AHCA Nursing Position Vacancy and Turnover Survey.* Washington, DC: AHCA.

ANA (American Nurses Association). 1998. *Standards of Clinical Nursing Practice.* Washington, DC: ANA.

Anderson G, Knickman JR. 2001. Changing the chronic care system to meet people's needs. *Health Affairs* 20(6):146–160.

Angell M. 2004. *The Truth About Drug Companies.* New York: Random House.

Armstrong EP. 2000. Electronic prescribing and monitoring are needed to improve drug use. *Archives of Internal Medicine* 160(18):2713–2714.

Avorn J. 2004. *Powerful Medicines: The Benefits, Risks, and Costs of Prescription Drugs.* New York: Vintage Books, Random House.

Bates DW, Gawande AA. 2003. Improving safety with information technology. *New England Journal of Medicine* 348(25):2526–2534.

Bates DW, Cullen DJ, Laird N, Petersen LA, Small SD, Servi D, Laffel G, Sweitzer BJ, Shea BF, Hallisey R, Vander Vliet M, Nemeskal R, Leape LL. 1995. Incidence of adverse drug events and potential adverse drug events. Implications for prevention. ADE Prevention Study Group. *Journal of the American Medical Association* 274(1):29–34.

Behrman RE. 2005. *Adverse Reactions: Information in, Information out.* [Online]. Available: http://www.iom.edu/CMS/3740/24155/29378.aspx [accessed February 6, 2006].

Bekelman JE, Li Y, Gross GP. 2003. Scope and impact of financial conflicts of interest in biomedical research. *Journal of the American Medical Association* 289(4):454–465.

Berndt ER, Gottschalk AHB, Strobeck MW. 2005. *Opportunities for Improving the Drug Development Process: Results from a Survey of Industry and the FDA.* Cambridge, MA: National Bureau of Economic Research.

Bero LA, Rennie D. 1996. Influences on the quality of published drug studies. *International Journal of Technology Assessment in Health Care* 12(20):209–237.

Blumenthal D. 2004. Doctors and drug companies. *New England Journal of Medicine* 351(18):1885–1890.

Bobb A, Gleason K, Husch M, Feinglass J, Yarnold PR, Noskin GA. 2004. The epidemiology of prescribing errors. *Archives of Internal Medicine* 164(7):785–792.

Bodenheimer T. 2000. Clinical investigators and the pharmaceutical industry. *New England Journal of Medicine* 42(20):1540–1543.

Boyd CM, Darer J, Boult C, Fried LP, Boult L, Wu AW. 2005. Clinical practice guidelines and quality of care for older patients with multiple comorbid diseases: Implications for pay for performance. *Journal of the American Medical Association* 294(6): 716–724.

Brennan TA, Gawande A, Thomas E, Studdert D. 2005. Accidental deaths, saved lives, and improved quality. *New England Journal of Medicine* 353(13):1405–1409.

Brennan TA, Rothman DJ, Blank L, Blumenthal D, Chimonas SC, Cohen JJ, Goldman J, Kassirer JP, Kimball H, Naughton J, Smelser N. 2006. Health industry practices that create conflicts of interest: A policy proposal for academic medical centers. *Journal of the American Medical Association* 295(4):429–433.

Buchanan TL, Barker KN, Gibson JT, Jiang BC, Pearson RE. 1991. Illumination and errors in dispensing. *American Journal of Hospital Pharmacy* 48(10):2137–2145.

Budnitz D. 2005. *The CDC's National Electronic Injury Surveillance System: Cooperative Adverse Drug Event Surveillance Project.* Washington, DC: IOM Committee on Identifying and Preventing Medication Errors.

Budnitz DS, Pollock DA, Mendelsohn AB, Weidenbach KN, McDonald AK, Annest JL. 2005. Emergency department visits for outpatient adverse drug events: Demonstration for a national surveillance system. *Annals of Emergency Medicine* 45(2):197–206.

Bulechek G, McCloskey J, Titler M, Denehey J. 1994. Nursing interventions used in practice. *American Journal of Nursing* 94(10):59–66.

Burke KG, Mason DJ, Alexander M, Barnsteiner JH, Rich VL. 2005. Making medication administration safe: Report challenges nurses to lead the way. *American Journal of Nursing* 28(Suppl. 2):2–3.

Califf RM. 2004. Defining the balance of risk and benefit in the era of genomics and proteomics. *Health Affairs* 23(1):77–87.

Califf RM, DeMets DL. 2002a. Principles from clinical trials relevant to clinical practice: Part I. *Circulation* 106:1015–1021.

Califf RM, DeMets DL. 2002b. Principles from clinical trials relevant to clinical practice: Part II. *Circulation* 106:1172–1175.

Califf RM, Gibbons RJ, Brindis RG, Smith SC. 2002. Integrating quality into the cycle of therapeutic development. *Journal of the American College of Cardiology* 40(11):1895–1901.

Calis KA, Young LR. 2004. Clinical analysis of adverse drug reactions: A primer for clinicians. *Hospital Pharmacy* 39(7):697–712.

Carney SL, Nair KR, Sales MA, Walsh J. 2001. Pharmaceutical industry-sponsored meetings: Good value or just a free meal? *Internal Medicine Journal* 31(8):488–491.

Castle NG, Engberg J. 2005. Staff turnover and quality of care in nursing homes. *Medical Care* 43(6):616–626.

CDC (Centers for Disease Control and Prevention). 1999. *FDA on VAERS.* [Online]. Available: http://www.cdc.gov/nip/vacsafe/concerns/hepB/fdatest.htm#Limitations [accessed January 11, 2006].

Chew LD, O'Young TS, Hazlet TK, Bradley KA, Maynard C, Lessler D. 2000. A physician survey of the effect of drug sample availability on physicians' behavior. *Journal of General Internal Medicine* 15(7):478–483.

Chimonas S, Rothman DJ. 2005. New federal guidelines for physician-pharmaceutical industry relations: The politics of policy formation. *Health Affairs* 24(4):949–960.

Chopra SS. 2003. Industry funding of clinical trials: Benefit or bias? *Journal of the American Medical Association* 290(1):113–114.

Christensen ML, Helms RA, Chesney RW. 1999. Is pediatric labeling really necessary? *Pediatrics* 104(3 Pt. 2):593–597.

Chung RS, Taira DA, Noh C. 2003. Alternate financial incentives in multitiered formulary systems to improve accountability for outcomes. *Journal of Managed Care Pharmacy* 9(4):360–365.

Classen DC, Pestotnik SL, Evans RS, Burke JP. 1991. Computerized surveillance of adverse drug events in hospital patients. *Journal of the American Medical Association* 266(20):2847–2851.

Cohen MR. 2000. *Medication Errors: Causes, Prevention, and Risk Management*. Sudbury, MA: Jones and Bartlett Publishers.

Cohen MR. 2005. *Overview of the Institute for Safe Medication Practice and Reported Adverse Drug Events*. Huntingdon Valley, PA: Institute of Safe Medication Practice.

Coyle SL. 2002. Physician–industry relations: Part 1: Individual physicians. *Annals of Internal Medicine* 136(5):396–402.

Cropper CM. 2005. Counter intelligence. *BusinessWeek*. [Online]. Available: http://www.businessweek.com/@@1N2NgIUQOPQ*bx0A/magazine/content/05_21/b3934126_mz070.htm [accessed June 7, 2006].

Cummings SR, Palermo L, Browner W, Marcus R, Wallace R, Pearson J, Blackwell T, Eckert S, Black D. 2000. Monitoring osteoporosis therapy with bone densitometry: Misleading changes and regression to the mean. *Journal of the American Medical Association* 283(10):1318–1321.

D'Arcy PF. 1993. Adverse reactions and interactions with herbal medicines. Part 2. Drug interactions. *Adverse Drug Reactions and Toxicological Reviews* 12:147–162.

Davey P, Pagliart C, Hayes A. 2002. The patient's role in the spread and control of bacterial resistance to antibiotics. *Clinical Microbiology and Infectious Disease* 8(Suppl. 2):43–68.

Davis NM. 1996. Performance lapses as a cause of medication errors. *Hospital Pharmacy* 31:1524–1527.

Davis NM, Cohen MR. 1994. Ten steps for ensuring dispensing accuracy. *American Pharmacy* NS34(7):22–23.

Dean B, Schachter M, Vincent C, Barber N. 2002. Prescribing errors in hospital inpatients: Their incidence and clinical significance. *Quality Safety Health Care* 11(4):340–344.

Deyo RA. 2004. Gaps, tensions, and conflicts in the FDA approval process: Implications for clinical practice. *Journal of the Board of Family Practice* 17(2):142–149.

Dick A, Keady S, Mohamed F, Brayley S, Thomson M, Lloyd BW, Heuschkel R, Afzal NA. 2003. Use of unlicensed and off-label medications in pediatric gastroenterology with a review of the commonly used formularies in the U.K. *Aliment Pharmacology and Therapeutics* 17:571–575.

Donohue SM, Needleman SM. 1998. Potential cause of medication administration error. *Anesthiology* 89(3):800–803.

Evans RS, Pestotnik SL, Classen DC, Bass SB, Menlove RL, Gardner RM, Burke JP. 1991. Development of a computerized adverse drug event monitor. *Proceedings of the Annual Symposium on Computer Applications in Medical Care* 23–27.

Evans RS, Pestotnik SL, Classen DC, Horn SD, Bass SB, Burke JP. 1994. Preventing adverse drug events in hospitalized patients. *The Annals of Pharmacotherapy* 28(4):523–527.

FDA (U.S. Food and Drug Administration). 1994. *Specific Requirements on Content and Format of Labeling for Human Prescription Drugs. Revision of Pediatric Use Subsection in the Labeling. Final Rule Edition*. CFR Part 201 [Docket No. 92N-0165]. Rockville, MD: FDA.

FDA. 1998. *The CDER Handbook*. Rockville, MD: U.S. Department of Health and Human Services.

FDA. 1999. *From Test Tube to Patient: Improving Health Through Human Drugs*. Rockville, MD: FDA.

FDA. 2003. *FDA's Review Process for New Drug Applications: A Management Review*. Rockville, MD: U.S. Department of Health and Human Services.

FDA. 2004a. *2004 Report to the Nation: Improving Public Health Through Human Drugs*. Rockville, MD: FDA.

FDA. 2004b. *Guidance for Industry Information Program on Clinical Trials for Serious or Life-Threatening Diseases and Conditions*. Rockville, MD: FDA.

Fialova D, Topinkova E, Gambassi G, Finne-Soveri H, Jomsson PV, Carpenter I, Schroll M, Onder G, Sorbye LW, Wagner C, Reissigova J, Bernabei R. 2005. Potentially inappropriate medication use among elderly home care patients in Europe. *Journal of the American Medical Association* 293(11):1348–1358.

Fick DM, Maclean JR, Rodriguez NA, Short L, Vanden Heuvel R, Waller JL, Rogers RL. 2004. A randomized study to decrease the use of potentially inappropriate medications among community-dwelling older adults in a Southeastern managed care organization. *American Journal of Managed Care* 10(11):761–768.

Field MJ, Grigsby J. 2002. Telemedicine and remote patient monitoring. *Journal of the American Medical Association* 288(4):423–425.

Fields M, Peterman J. 2005. Intravenous medication safety system averts high-risk medication errors and provides actionable data. *Nursing Administration Quarterly* 29(1):78–87.

Flynn EA, Barker KN, Gibson JT, Pearson RE, Berger BA, Smith LA. 1999. Impact of interruptions and distractions on dispensing errors in an ambulatory care pharmacy. *American Journal of Health System Pharmacists* 56(13):1319–1325.

Flynn EA, Barker KN, Carnahan BJ. 2003. National observational study of prescription dispensing accuracy and safety in 50 pharmacies. *Journal of the American Pharmaceutical Association* 43(2):191–200.

Fontanarosa PB, Rennie D, DeAngelis CD. 2004. Postmarketing surveillance-lack of vigilance, lack of trust. *Journal of the American Medical Association* 292(21):2647–2650.

Forester AJ, Halil RB, Tierney MG. 2004. Pharmacist surveillance of adverse drug events. *American Journal of Health System Pharmacists* 61(14):1466–1472.

FR (Federal Register). 2004a. *Report on the Performance of Drug and Biologics Firms in Conducting Postmarketing Commitment Studies*. Washington, DC: U.S. Department of Health and Human Services.

FR. 2004b. *Bar Code Label Requirements for Human Drug Products and Biological Products: Final Rule*. Washington, DC: National Archives and Records Administration.

FR. 2006. *Requirements on Content and Format of Labeling for Human Drug and Biological Products and Draft Guidances and Two Guidances for Industry on the Content and Format of Labeling for Human Prescription Drug and Biological Products: Final Rule and Notices*. Washington, DC: National Archives and Records Administration.

Frank C, Godwin M, Verma S, Kelly A, Birenbaum A, Seguin R, Anderson J. 2001. What drugs are our frail elderly patients taking? Do drugs they take or fail to take put them at increased risk of interactions and inappropriate medication use? *Canadian Family Physician* 47:1198–1204.

Frush KS, Luo X, Hutchinson P, Higgins JN. 2004. Evaluation of a method to reduce over-the-counter medication dosing error. *Archives of Pediatric Medicine* 158:620–624.

Gandhi TK, Weingart SN, Borus J, Seger AC, Peterson J, Burdick E, Seger DL, Shu K, Federico F, Leape LL, Bates DW. 2003. Adverse drug events in ambulatory care. *New England Journal of Medicine* 348(16):1556–1564.

GAO (Government Accountability Office). 2004. *Internet Pharmacies: Some Pose Safety Risks for Consumers*. Washington, DC: GAO.

Gladstone J. 1995. Drug administration errors: A study into the factors underlying the occurrence and reporting of drug errors in a district general hospital. *Journal of Advanced Nursing* 22:628–637.

Golden AG, Preston RA, Barnett SD, Llorente M, Hamdan K, Silverman MA. 1999. Inappropriate medication prescribing in homebound older adults. *Journal of the American Geriatrics Society* 47(8):948–953.

Goodman B. 2001. Do drug company promotions influence physician behavior? *Western Journal of Medicine* 174:232–233.

Greengold NL, Shane R, Schneider P, Flynn E, Elashoff J, Hoying CL, Barker K, Bolton LB. 2003. The impact of dedicated medication nurses on the medication administration error rate. *Archives of Internal Medicine* 163(19):2359–2367.

Gribetz B, Crunley SA. 1987. Underdosing of acetaminophen by parents. *Pediatrics* 80: 630–633.

Grissinger M, Kroon L, Prenna P. 2003. Misadventures in insulin therapy: Are your members at risk? *Journal of Managed Care Pharmacy* 9(Suppl. 3).

Groves KEM, Sketris I, Tett SE. 2003. Prescription drug samples: Does this marketing strategy counteract policies for quality use of medicines? *Journal of Clinical Pharmacy and Therapeutics* 28:259–271.

Gurwitz JH, Field TS, Avorn J, McCormick D, Jain S, Eckler M, Benser M, Edmondson AC, Bates DW. 2000. Incidence and preventability of adverse drug events in nursing homes. *American Journal of Medicine* 109(2):87–94.

Gurwitz JH, Field TS, Harrold LR, Rothschild J, Debellis K, Seger AC, Cadoret C, Fish LS, Garber L, Kelleher M, Bates DW. 2003. Incidence and preventability of adverse drug events among older persons in the ambulatory setting. *Journal of the American Medical Association* 289(9):1107–1116.

Gurwitz JH, Field TS, Judge J, Rochon P, Harrold LR, Cadoret C, Lee M, White K, LaPrino J, Mainard JF, DeFlorio M, Gavendo L, Auger J, Bates DW. 2005. The incidence of adverse drug events in two large academic long-term care facilities. *American Journal of Medicine* 118(3):251–258.

Haley RW, Culver DH, White JW, Morgan WM, Emori TG, Munn VP, Hooton TM. 1985. The efficacy of infection surveillance and control programs in preventing nosocomial infections in U.S. hospitals. *American Journal of Epidemiology* 121(2):182–205.

Hanlon JT, Fillenbaum GG, Schmader KE, Kuchibhatla M, Horner RD. 2000a. Inappropriate drug use among community-dwelling elderly. *Pharmacotherapy* 20(5): 575–582.

Hanlon JT, Shrimp LA, Semla TP. 2000b. Recent advances in geriatrics: Drug-related problems in the elderly. *Annals of Pharmacotherapy* 34:360–365.

Hartigan K. 2003. Patient education: The cornerstone of successful oral chemotherapy treatment. *Clinical Journal of Oncology Nursing* 7(6):21–24.

Holbrook AM, Pereira JA, Labris R, McDonald H, Douketis JD, Crowther M, Wells PS. 2005. Systematic overview of warfarin and its drug and food interactions. *Archives of Internal Medicine* 165(10):1095–1106.

Horsky J, Kuperman GJ, Patel VL. 2005. Comprehensive analysis of a medication dosing error related to CPOE. *Journal of the American Medical Informatics Association* 12(4): 377–382.

HPA (Health Policy Alternatives, Inc.). 2003. *Pharmacy Benefit Managers: Tools for Managing Drug Benefit Costs, Quality, and Safety*. Washington, DC: Pharmaceutical Care Management Association.

The HSM Group. 2002. *Acute Care Hospital Survey of RN Vacancy and Turnover Rates*. Chicago, IL: American Organization of Nurse Executives.

Hubal R, Day RS. 2006. Understanding the frequency and severity of side effects: Linguistic, numeric, and visual representations. In: Bickmore T, Green N, Editors. *Argumentation for Consumers of Healthcare: Papers From the 2006 Spring Symposium*. Technical Report SS-06-01. Menlo Park, CA: American Association of Artificial Intelligence.

Husakamp HA, Deverka PA, Epstein AM, Epstein RS, McGuigan KA, Frank RG. 2003. The effect of incentive-based formularies on prescription-drug utilization and spending. *New England Journal of Medicine* 349(23):2224–2232.

Ikesue H, Ishida M, Uchida M, Harada M, Haro T, Mishima K, Itoh Y, Kotsubo K, Yoshikawa M, Oishi R. 2004. Monitoring for potential adverse drug reactions in patients receiving chemotherapy. *American Journal of Health System Pharmacy* 61(22):2366–2369.

IMS Health. 2004. *Total U.S. Promotional Spending by Type, 2003*. [Online]. Available: http://www.imshealth.com/ims/portal/front/articleC/0,2777,6599_44304752_44889690,00.html [accessed June 7, 2006].

IOM (Institute of Medicine). 2000. *To Err Is Human: Building a Safer Health System*. Washington, DC: National Academy Press.

IOM. 2001. *Crossing the Quality Chasm: A New Health System for the 21st Century*. Washington, DC: National Academy Press.

IOM. 2002. *Leadership by Example: Coordinating Government Roles in Improving Health Care Quality*. Washington, DC: The National Academies Press.

IOM. 2003. *Priority Areas for National Action: Transforming Health Care Quality*. Washington, DC: The National Academies Press.

IOM. 2004a. *Health Literacy: A Prescription to End Confusion*. Washington, DC: The National Academies Press.

IOM. 2004b. *Keeping Patients Safe: Transforming the Work Environment of Nurses*. The National Academies Press.

IOM. 2004c. *Patient Safety: Achieving a New Standard for Care*. Washington, DC: The National Academies Press.

IOM. 2006. *Developing a Registry of Pharmacologic and Biologic Clinical Trials*. Washington, DC: The National Academies Press.

Jarman H, Jacobs E, Zielinski V. 2002. Medication study supports registered nurses' competence for single checking. *Internal Journal of Nursing Practice* 8(6):330–335.

Jenkins R, Elliott P. 2004. Stressors, burnout and social support: Nurses in acute mental health settings. *Journal of Advanced Nursing* 48(6):622–631.

Jha AK, Kuperman GJ, Teich JM, Leape L, Shea B, Rittenberg E, Burdick E, Seger DL, Vander Vliet M, Bates DW. 1998. Identifying adverse drug events: Development of a computer-based monitor and comparison with chart review and stimulated voluntary report. *Journal of the American Medical Informatics Association* 5(3):305–314.

Jong GW, Vulto AG, de Hoog M, Schimmel KJM, Tibboel D, van den Anker JN. 2001. A survey of the use of off-label and unlicensed drugs in a Dutch children's hospital. *Pediatrics* 108(5):1089–1093.

Kastango ES. 2003. *Compounding Sterile Preparations*. Bethesda, MD: American Society of Health System Pharmacists.

Katz D, Caplan AL, Merz JF. 2003. All gifts large and small: Toward an understanding of the ethics of pharmaceutical industry gift-giving. *American Journal of Bioethics* 3(3):39–46.

Kenny R. 2001. *Introduction to Compliance with FDA Labeling and Advertising Requirements.* [Online]. Available: http://www.ehcca.com/presentations/PharmaReg1/203_1.pdf [accessed June 30, 2005].

Klein DF, Thase ME, Endicott J, Adler L, Glick I, Kalai A, Leventer S, Mattes J, Ross P, Bystritsky A. 2002. Improving clinical trials. *Archives of General Psychiatry* 59(3):272–278.

Knowlton CH, Penna RP. 2003. *Pharmaceutical Care.* 2nd ed. Bethesda, MD: American Society of Health System Pharmacists.

Koppel R, Metlay JP, Cohen A, Abaluck B, Localio AR, Kimmel SE, Strom BL. 2005. Role of computerized physician order entry systems in facilitating medication errors. *Journal of the American Medical Association* 293(10):1197–1203.

Kos M. 2005. Satisfaction with pharmacotherapy for approved and off-label indications: A Delphi study. *Annals of Pharmacotherapy* 39(4):649–654.

Landon BE, Reschovsky JD, Blumenthal D. 2004. Physicians' views of formularies: Implications for Medicare drug benefit design. *Health Affairs* 23(1):218–226.

Leape LL. 2002. Reporting of adverse events. *New England Journal of Medicine* 347(20):1633–1638.

Leape LL, Bates DW, Cullen DJ, Cooper J, Demonaco HJ, Gallivan T, Hallisey R, Ives J, Laird N, Laffel G, Nemeskal R, Petersen L, Porter K, Servi D, Shea B, Small S, Sweitzer B, Thompson B, Vander Vliet M. 1995. Systems analysis of adverse drug events. *Journal of the American Medical Association* 274(1):35–43.

Lee PY, Alexander KP, Hammill BG, Pasquali SK, Peterson ED. 2001. Representation of elderly persons and women in published randomized trials of acute coronary syndromes. *Journal of the American Medical Association* 286(6):708–713.

Leonard EM. 1994. Quality assurance and the drug development process: An FDA perspective. *Quality Assurance* 3:178–186.

Lesar TS, Briceland LL, Delcoure K, Parmalee JC, Masta-Gornic V, Pohl, H. 1990. Medication prescribing errors in a teaching hospital. *Journal of the American Medical Association* 263(17):2329–2334.

Lesar TS, Briceland L, Stein D. 1997. Factors related to errors in medication prescribing. *Journal of the American Medical Association* 277(4):312–317.

Levy R. 1994. The role and value of pharmaceutical marketing. *Archives of Family Medicine* 3:327–332.

Lifshitz M, Gavrilov V, Gorodischer R. 2001. Off-label and unlicensed use of antidotes in pediatric patients. *European Journal of Clinical Pharmacology* 56:839–841.

Livingston MG, Livingston HM. 1996. Monamine oxidase inhibitors. An update on drug interactions. *Drug Safety* 14(4):219–227.

Loder EW, Biondi DM. 2004. Off-label prescribing of drugs in specialty headache practice. *Headache* 44(7):636–641.

Loucks M. 2003. *Department of Justice Investigations and the Pharmaceutical Industry.* Washington, DC: Fourth Annual Pharmaceutical Regulatory and Compliance Congress and Best Practices Forum.

Madlon-Kay DJ, Mosch FS. 2000. Liquid medication dosing errors. *Journal of Family Practice* 49(8):741–744.

Maguire P. 2001. *Samples: Cost-Driver or Safety Net?* [Online]. Available: http://www.acponline.org/journals/news/jan01/drugsamples.htm [accessed August 21, 2005].

Manasse HR, Thompson KK. 2005. *Medication Safety: A Guide for Health Care Facilities.* Bethesda, MD: American Society of Health System Pharmacists.

Manias E, Aitken R, Dunning T. 2005. How graduate nurses use protocols to manage patients' medications. *Journal of Clinical Nursing* 14:935–944.

March JS, Silva SG, Compton S, Shapiro M, Califf R, Krishnan R. 2005. The case for practical clinical trials in psychiatry. *American Journal of Psychiatry* 162(5):836–846.

Martin EW. 1978. *Hazards of Medications*. Philadelphia, PA: J.B. Lippincott Company.
Medstat. 2002. *Implementation Planning Study for the Integration of Medical Event Reporting Input and Data Structure for Reporting to AHRQ, CDC, CMS, and FDA*. Final Report: Volume 2–Appendixes. Rockville, MD: AHRQ.
Moore TJ, Psaty BM, Furberg CD. 1998. Time to act on drug safety. *Journal of the American Medical Association* 279:1571–1573.
Moynihan R. 2003. Who pays for the pizza? Redefining the relationships between doctors and drug companies. 2: Disentanglement. *British Medical Journal* 326:1193–1196.
Munroe DJ. 2003. Assisted living issues for nursing practice. *Geriatric Nursing* 24(2): 99–105.
Murphy D. 2005. *Pediatric Drug Development and Medication Errors*. Washington, DC: IOM Committee on Identifying and Preventing Medication Errors.
NABP (National Association of Boards of Pharmacy). 2004. *Survey of Pharmacy Law*. Mount Pleasant, IL: NAPB.
NACDS (National Association of Chain Drug Stores). 1999. *Pharmacy Activity Cost and Productivity Study*. Alexandria, VA: NACDS.
NASHP (National Academy for State Health Policy). 2006. *Patient Safety Toolbox for States*. [Online]. Available: http://www.pstoolbox.org/_docdisp_page.cfm?LID=6BC2AB7D-6F1E-4DF2-AD20DAE18001147B [accessed, June 7, 2006].
NCI (National Cancer Institute). 2004. *Q&A: Off-Label Drugs*. [Online]. Available: http://www.nci.nih.gov/clinicaltrials/learning/approval-process-for-cancer-drugs/page5 [accessed June 29, 2005].
Nicholas PK, Agius CR. 2005. Toward safer IV medication administration. *American Journal of Nursing* 105(3):25–30.
Nies AS. 2001. Principles of therapeutics. In: Hardman JG, Limbird LE, Gilman AG, *Goodman and Gilman's The Pharmacological Basis of Therapeutics*. 10th ed. New York: McGraw Hill.
NIHCMREF (National Institute for Health Care Management and Research and Educational Foundation). 2002. *Prescription Drug Expenditures in 2001: Another Year of Escalating Costs*. Washington, DC: NIHCMREF.
NLM (National Library of Medicine). 2005. *MedlinePlus: Antidepressants, Monamine Oxidase Inhibitors (MAO) (Systemic)*. [Online]. Available: http://www.nlm.nih.gov/medlineplus/druginfo/uspdi/202054.html [accessed August 30, 2005].
Noah BA, Brushwood DB. 2000. Adverse drug reactions in elderly patients: Alternative approaches to postmarket surveillance. *Journal of Health Law* 33(3):383–454.
Norrish B, Rundall T. 2001. Hospital restructuring and the work of registered nurses. *Milbank Quarterly* 79(1):55.
NPSF (National Patient Safety Foundation). 1997. *National Patient Safety Foundation at the AMA: Public Opinion of Patient Safety Issues Research Findings*. Louis Harris and Associates.
NRC (National Research Council). 1995. *Standards, Conformity Assessment, and Trade*. Washington, DC: National Academy Press.
NRC. 2004. *Health and Medicine: Challenges for the Chemical Sciences in the 21st Century*. Washington, DC: The National Academies Press.
Nunn AJ. 2003. Making medicines that children can take. *Archives of Disease in Childhood* 88(5):369–371.
O'Shea E. 1999. Factors contributing to medication errors: A literature review. *Journal of Clinical Nursing* 8:496–504.
Patel VL, Branch T, Arocha JF. 2002. Errors in interpreting quantities as procedures: The case of pharmaceutical labels. *International Journal of Medical Informatics* 65(3): 193–211.

Patterson ES. 2003. Addressing human factors in bar code medication administration systems. *Hospital Pharmacy* 38(11):S16–S17.

Pedersen CA, Schneider PJ, Scheckelhoff DJ. 2003. ASHP national survey of pharmacy practice in hospital settings: Dispensing and administration—2002. *American Journal of Health System Pharmacists* 60(1):52–68.

Petersen M. 2000, November 15. Growing opposition to free drug samples. *New York Times.* Business.

Phillips J, Beam S, Brinker A, Holquist C, Honig P, Lee LY, Pamer C. 2001. Retrospective analysis of mortalities associated with medication errors. *American Journal of Health System Pharmacists* 58:1835–1841.

Poole SG, Dooley MJ. 2004. Off-label prescribing in oncology. *Supportive Care in Cancer* 12(5):302–305.

PPSA (Pennsylvania Patient Safety Authority). 2006. *Patient Safety Authority.* [Online]. Available: http://www.psa.state.pa.us/psa/site [accessed June 7, 2006].

Presecky W. 2006, February 25. FDA joins probe after 2 infants die in Kane. *Chicago Tribune.*

Psaty BM, Furberg CD, Ray WA, Weiss NS. 2004. Potential for conflict of interest in the evaluation of suspected adverse drug reactions: Use of cerivastatin and risk of rhabdomyolysis. *Journal of the American Medical Association* 292(21):2622–2631.

Ringold DJ, Santell JP, Schneider PJ. 1999. ASHP national survey of pharmacy practice in acute care settings: Dispensing and administration. *American Journal of Health System Pharmacists* 57(19):1759–1775.

Roberts DE, Spencer MG, Burfield R, Bowden S. 2002. An analysis of dispensing errors in U.K. hospitals. *Internal Journal of Pharmacy Practice* 10(Supplement):R6.

Rochon PA, Gurwitz JH, Simms RW, Fortin PR, Felson DT, Minaker KL, Chalmers TC. 1994. A study of manufacturer-supported trials of nonsteroidal anti-inflammatory drugs in the treatment of arthritis. *Archives of Internal Medicine* 154:157–163.

Rosenthal J, Booth M. 2005. *Maximizing the Use of State Adverse Event Data to Improve Patient Safety.* Portland, ME: National Academy for State Health Policy.

Rothman K, Michels K. 1994. The continuing unethical use of placebo controls. *New England Journal of Medicine* 331(6):394–398.

RSW (Roper Starch Worldwide). 2001. *Self-Care in the New Millennium.* Washington, DC: Consumer Healthcare Products Association.

Sawicki PT. 1999. A structured teaching and self-management program for patients receiving oral anticoagulation: A randomized controlled trial. *Journal of the American Medical Association* 281(2):145–150.

Schiff GD, Klass D, Peterson J, Shah G, Bates DW. 2003. Linking laboratory and pharmacy: Opportunities for reducing errors and improving care. *Archives of Internal Medicine* 163(8):893–900.

Schondelmeyer S. 2005. Community Pharmacy Perspectives on Preventing Medication Errors at the July 6, 2005, Meeting of the IOM Committee on Identifying and Preventing Medication Errors, Washington, DC.

Schroeder K, Fahey T, Ebrahim S. 2004. How to improve adherence to blood pressure-lowering medication in ambulatory care? *Archives of Internal Medicine* 164(7): 722–732.

Schull PD. 2005. *Five Rights Still Resound. Nursing Spectrum.* [Online]. Avaliable: http://community.nursingspectrum.com/MagazineArticles/article.cfm?AID=17801 [accessed June 7, 2006].

Shrank WH, Young HN, Ettner SL, Glassman P, Asch SM, Kravitz RL. 2005. Do the incentives in 3-tiered pharmaceutical benefit plans operate as intended? Results from a physician leadership survey. *American Journal of Managed Care* 11(1):16–22.

Simaon HK, Winkle DA. 1997. Over-the-counter medications: Do parents give what they intend to give? *Archives of Pediatrics and Adolescent Medicine* 151(7):654–656.

Smalley W, Shatin D, Wysowski DK, Gurwitz J, Andrade SE, Goodman M, Chan KA, Platt R, Schech SD, Ray W. 2000. Contraindicated use of cisapride: Impact of Food and Drug Administration regulatory action. *Journal of the American Medical Association* 284(23):3036–3039.

Smetzer J. 2001. Safer medication management. *Nursing Management* 32(12):44–48.

Smetzer J, Cohen MR. 2006. *Medication Error Reporting Systems in Medication Errors*. 2nd ed. Washington, DC: American Pharmacists Association.

Smith PC, Araya-Guerra R, Bublitz C, Parnes B, Dickinson LM, Van Vorst R, Westfall JM, Pace WD. 2005. Missing clinical information during primary care visits. *Journal of the American Medical Association* 293(5):565–571.

Steinbrook R. 2004. Public registration of clinical trials. *New England Journal of Medicine* 351(4):315–317.

Strom BL. 2004. Potential conflict of interest in the evaluation of suspected adverse drug reactions. *Journal of the American Medical Association* 292(21):2643–2646.

Studdert DM, Mello MM, Brennan TA. 2004. Financial conflicts of interest in physicians' relationships with the pharmaceutical industry: Self-regulation in the shadow of federal prosecution. *New England Journal of Medicine* 351(18):1891–1900.

Suzuki K, Ohida T, Kaneita Y, Yokoyama E, Uchiyama M. 2005. Daytime sleepiness, sleep habits and occupational accidents among hospital nurses. *Journal of Advanced Nursing* 52(4):445–453.

Svarstad BL, Bultman DC, Mount JK. 2004. Patient counseling provided in community pharmacies: Effects of state regulation, pharmacist age, and business. *Journal of the American Pharmaceutical Association* 44(1):22–29.

Szefler SJ, Whelan GJ, Leung DY. 2006. Black box warning: Wake-up call or overreaction? *Journal of Allergy and Clinical Immunology* 117(1):26–29.

Taira DA, Iwane KA, Chung RS. 2003. Prescription drugs: Elderly enrollee reports of financial access, receipt of free samples, and discussion of generic equivalents related to type of coverage. *American Journal of Managed Care* 9(4):305–312.

Tamada JA, Garg S, Jovanovic L, Pitzer KR, Fermi S, Potts RO. 1999. Noninvasive glucose monitoring: Comprehensive clinical results. *Journal of the American Medical Association* 282(19):1839–1844.

Teutsch SM, Berger ML, Weinstein MC. 2005. Comparative effectiveness: Asking the right questions, choosing the right method. *Health Affairs* 24(1):128–132.

Thomas CP. 2003. Incentive-based formularies. *New England Journal of Medicine* 349(23): 2186–2188.

Tokars JI, Richards C, Andrus M, Klevens M, Curtis A, Horan T, Jernigan J, Cardo D. 2004. The changing fact of surveillance for health care-associated infections. *Clinical Infectious Diseases* 39:1347–1352.

University of Utah. 2006. *Chapter 1: Testing and Marketing: Drug Development*. [Online]. Available at: http://www.pharmacy.utah.edu/pharmtox/common_meds/ICM1.html [accessed June 5, 2006].

USP (U.S. Pharmacopeia). 2003. *Summary of Information Submitted to MedMarx in the Year 2002*. Rockville, MD: USP.

USP. 2004. *MedMarx 5th Anniversary Data Report: A Chartbook of 2003 Findings and Trends 1999–2003*. Rockville, MD: USP.

Vincent C. 2001. *Clinical Risk Management: Enhancing Patient Safety*. 2nd ed. London, UK: BMJ Books.

Wagner AK, Chan KA, Dashevsky I, Raebel MA, Andrade SE, Lafata JE, Davis RL, Gurwitz JH, Soumerai SB, Platt R. 2006. FDA drug prescribing warnings: Is the black box half empty or half full? *Pharmacoepidemiology and Drug Safety* 15(6):369–386.

Wakefield DS, Wakefield BJ, Borders T, Uden-Holman T, Blegen M, Vaughn T. 1999. Understanding and comparing differences in reported medication administration error rates. *American Journal of Medical Quality* 14(2):73–80.

Walls CA, Rhodes KV, Kennedy JJ. 2002. The emergency department as usual source of medical care: Estimates from the 1998 National Health Interview Survey. *Academic Emergency Medicine* 9(11):1140–1145.

Walters PG. 1992. FDA's new drug evaluation process: A general overview. *Journal of Public Health and Dentistry* 52:333–337.

Watzke HH, Forberg E, Svolba G, Jimenez-Boj E, Krinninger B. 2000. A prospective controlled trial comparing weekly self-testing and self-dosing with the standard management of patients on stable oral anticoagulation. *Thrombosis and Haemostasis* 83(5):661–665.

Wazana A. 2000. Physicians and the pharmaceutical industry: Is a gift ever just a gift? *Journal of the American Medical Association* 283(3):373–380.

Weatherby LB, Walker AM, Fife D, Vervaet P, Klausner MA. 2001. Contraindicated medications dispensed with cisapride: Temporal trends in relation to the sending of "Dear doctor" letters. *Pharmacoepidemiology and Drug Safety* 10:210–218.

Weatherby LB, Nordstrom BL, Fife D, Walker AM. 2002. The impact of wording in "Dear doctor" letters and in black box labels. *Clinical Pharmacology and Therapeutics* 72(6):735–742.

Wilkes MS, Bell RA, Kravitz RL. 2000. Direct-to-consumer prescription drug advertising: Trends, impact, and implications. *Health Affairs* 19:110–128.

Woods A, Johnson SD. 2002. Executive summary: Toward a taxonomy of nursing practice errors. *Nursing Management* 33(10):45–48.

3

Medication Errors: Incidence and Cost

CHAPTER SUMMARY

Medication error rates are important for gauging the scope of the problem, setting priorities for prevention strategies, and measuring the impact of those strategies. This chapter summarizes the evidence base on rates of medication errors; preventable adverse drug events; and failure to prescribe medications for which the evidence supports the ability to reduce morbidity and mortality in hospital, nursing home, and ambulatory settings. An understanding of the costs of medication errors is important as well to inform decisions about the implementation of strategies designed to reduce the risk of medication errors. This chapter also summarizes the evidence base on these costs.

As noted in Chapter 1, the committee's charge encompassed developing estimates of the incidence, severity, and costs of medication errors and evaluating alternative approaches to reducing such errors in different settings. To this end, the committee commissioned papers summarizing the salient peer-reviewed literature in the areas of hospital care, nursing home care, ambulatory care, pediatric care, psychiatric care, and use of over-the-counter (OTC) and complementary and alternative medications.[1] The au-

---

[1]The authors of the papers are as follows: for hospital care, Harvey J. Murff, MD, MPH, Vanderbilt University; for nursing home care, Ginette A. Pepper, PhD, RN, FAAN, University of Utah College of Nursing; for ambulatory care, Grace M. Kuo, PharmD, MPH, Baylor

thors were asked to review this literature from the last 10 years[2] (and earlier major studies if still relevant). Where possible, the five steps in the medication-use process were to be analyzed separately. Special attention was to be given to errors that arise during transfers between care settings, for example, from hospital to ambulatory care. In addition, the authors were asked to identify the approaches to reducing medication errors recommended by major health care organizations and to evaluate each approach in terms of the evidence/process used by these organizations to justify it. In addition, a paper was commissioned to review the non-peer-reviewed literature for approaches to reducing medication errors.[3] The authors of the commissioned papers were encouraged to use a modified search strategy as described by Smeaton and colleagues (2002). They were also encouraged to search the following databases: MEDLINE, CINAHL (Cumulative Index to Nursing and Allied Health Literature), PsycINFO, IPA (International Pharmaceutical Abstracts), Science Citation Index, and Dissertation Abstracts. The authors tailored these suggestions to their own requirements. In summary, the study focused on English-language articles published in the period 1995–2005, augmented by earlier important studies and studies published after the literature reviews had been completed. The majority of studies reviewed were conducted in the United States. Where relevant, when there were no or few U.S. studies for a particular setting or study category, foreign studies are cited in the report, with the country of origin noted.

Drawing on these commissioned papers, this chapter summarizes the committee's findings on the incidence and costs of medication errors (more detail on incidence is given Appendix C). Chapter 5 summarizes the committee's findings on prevention strategies as part of the recommended action agendas for each care setting (more detail on these strategies is given in Appendix D).

INCIDENCE

The extent of the research on the incidence of medication errors and adverse drug events (ADEs) varies greatly across care settings (see Appendix C); Box 3-1 summarizes the difficulties encountered by the committee

---

College of Medicine; for pediatric care, Marlene R. Miller, MD, MSc, Karen A. Robinson, MSc, Lisa H. Lubornski, PhD, Michael L. Rinke, BA, and Peter J. Pronovost, MD, PhD, The Johns Hopkins University; for psychiatric care, Benjamin C. Grasso, MD, The Institute for Self-Directed Care; and for OTC and complementary and alternative medications, Albert I. Wertheimer, MBA, PhD and Thomas M. Santella, BS, Temple University.

[2] The pediatric care paper examined peer-reviewed journals over the last 5 years.

[3] Authored by Eta Berner, EdD, University of Alabama at Birmingham, and Richard Maisiak, PhD, MSPH, consultant.

BOX 3-1
Difficulties in Synthesizing the Evidence on Incident Rates

Since the publication of *To Err Is Human: Building a Safer Health System* (IOM, 2000), there has been a rapid growth in contributions to the field of patient safety. As with any emerging discipline, synthesizing the results of this research is challenging because of the heterogeneity of study definitions and error identification methodologies.

Significant confusion exists about the most fundamental issue in quantifying medication errors. One broad definition of medication errors is any inappropriate use of a drug, regardless of whether that use resulted in harm (Nebeker et al., 2004). Other definitions include only medication errors that have the potential to produce harm, or "clinically significant medication errors" (Lesar et al., 1997). Thus a medication error that could never be executed, such as a prescription to give orally a medication that comes only in parenteral form, would be excluded. As discussed previously, medication use also involves various stages, including selecting and procuring the drug by the pharmacy, prescribing and selecting the drug for the patient, preparing and dispensing the drug, administering the drug, and monitoring the patient for effect, and many studies have focused on errors occurring during only one of these stages.

Contributing to the heterogeneity of the patient safety literature are the varying methodologies used to identify errors. The incidence rates found in the literature depend dramatically on the particular detection method used. Although many such methods exist, those most commonly employed include direct observation, chart review, computerized monitoring, and voluntary reporting (Murff et al., 2003) (see Chapter 5 for more detail). Many studies have established that voluntary reporting results in marked underestimation of rates of medication errors and ADEs (Allan and Barker, 1990; Cullen et al., 1995; Jha et al., 1998; Flynn et al., 2002). Voluntary reporting rates are generally low because of such factors as time pressures, fear of punishment, and lack of a perceived benefit (Cullen et al., 1995). Improvements in internal reporting have been achieved in nonpunitive reporting environments (Rozich and Resar, 2001), but these rates still vastly underestimate the true incidence.

A large study comparing direct observation, chart review, and incident reporting found that direct observation identified the greatest number of errors (Flynn et al., 2002). Earlier it had been established that automated surveillance could detect ADEs at a much higher rate than voluntary reporting. A comparison of automated surveillance, chart review, and voluntary reporting found that of the 617 ADEs detected, chart review identified 65 percent, automated surveillance 45 percent, and voluntary reporting 4 percent (Jha et al., 1998). In this study, only 12 percent of all ADEs detected were identified by both chart review and computerized surveillance (Jha et al., 1998).

Several studies have noted that different methods of detection appear more suited to identifying different types of medication-related problems (O'Neil et al., 1993; Jha et al., 1998), suggesting that the method selected should depend on the area of interest (again, see Chapter 5 for more detail). In conclusion, the incidence rates found in the patient safety literature depend dramatically on the particular detection method used.

A further confounding factor is that medication error rates are quoted in varying ways—errors per order/dose/opportunity, errors per 1,000 patient-days, and errors per 1,000 patient admissions. Rates of preventable ADEs are cited in a similar manner—preventable ADEs per 1,000 patient-days and per 1,000 patient admissions.

in synthesizing this heterogeneous evidence base. Hospital care is the setting with the most extensive research. Studies have estimated the rate of ADEs incurred in hospitals and error rates at each stage of the medication-use process. There is also an extensive literature on errors of omission in prescribing—failure to prescribe medications in appropriate situations.

Other care settings are much less well researched. For nursing home care, there are estimates of the rates of ADEs incurred while in a nursing home, plus a few studies on error rates at various stages of the medication-use process.[4] Little attention has been paid to errors of omission in the nursing home population. For ambulatory care, a modest amount of research has been carried out, spread thinly over a large number of topics—ADE and error rates at various stages of the medication-use process, and omissions of effective therapies in specific populations. Similarly for pediatric care, a modest amount of research has been carried out, again thinly spread over a wide range of topics.

For the remaining care settings considered in this report, little or no research has been conducted on ADE and error rates. Of the limited number of studies relating to self-care, most addressed adherence issues. No study was found on medication error rates in the school setting. Just two studies were found on medication error rates in psychiatric care. Finally, there has been hardly any research on medication errors relating to OTC medications, and no study was found on error rates associated with complementary and alternative medications.

The discussion in this section is based on a large number of studies reviewed by the committee. It first addresses the incidence of medication errors in general, and then the incidence of three specific categories of medication errors—preventable ADEs, underutilization of medications, and overutilization of medications.

Incidence of Medication Errors

Hospitals

As noted, hospital care is the most researched setting for medication error incidence rates, although no study was identified that addressed medi-

---

[4]There have been many studies of inappropriate prescribing for the elderly in nursing homes, ambulatory care, and home health care, based on such criteria as the Beers criteria (Beers et al., 1991) and subsequent updates/extensions (Beers, 1997). The committee did not include these studies in its synthesis since the causal link between inappropriate prescribing and poor health outcomes has not been documented.

cation errors in the selection and procurement of drugs by the hospital pharmacy.

Medication errors occur in all stages of the medication-use process, most frequently at the prescribing and administration stages. Several U.S. studies using differing definitions of error and methods of error identification found that rates of prescribing errors for adults in hospitals varied considerably (see Table 3-1). Prescribing errors occurred at rates of 12.3–1,400.00 per 1,000 patient admissions (Bates et al., 1995a; Lesar et al., 1997; Lesar, 2002; LaPointe and Jollis, 2003; Winterstein et al., 2004). Such errors occurred at rates of 0.6–53.0 per 1,000 orders (Lesar et al., 1990; Bates et al., 1995a; Lesar et al., 1997; Lesar, 2002). And in studies that evaluated prescribing errors per opportunity for error, rates of 1.5–9.9 per 100 opportunities were found (Dean et al., 2002; van den Bemt et al., 2002; Bobb et al., 2004; Lisby et al., 2005).

Errors rates depend on the thoroughness of the error detection methods that are used (Gandhi et al., 2000). Most of the above studies used less comprehensive error detection methods, such as spontaneous reports by pharmacists after review of written orders (Lesar et al., 1997; Lesar, 2002), prompted reporting (Winterstein et al., 2004), and reporting by a clinical pharmacist participating in patient care (LaPointe and Jollis, 2003). The study that found by far the highest rate (Bates et al., 1995a) used much more comprehensive detection methods—chart review, including review of written medication orders by a dedicated trained reviewer, in addition to prompted reporting from nurses and pharmacists. This study found a rate of 1,400 prescribing errors per 1,000 patient admissions or 0.3 prescribing errors per patient per day. Of the errors identified, 7.5 percent were adjudged serious—preventable or potential ADEs. By comparison, a study (Kaushal et al., 2001) using similar error detection methods in pediatric units identified 405 prescribing errors per 1,000 patient admissions or 0.1

TABLE 3-1 Error Rates in Hospitals

Prescribing errors	Per 1,000 admissions 12.3–1,400 (5 studies)
	Per 1,000 orders 0.61–53 (4 studies)
	Per 100 opportunities for error 1.5–9.9 (4 studies)
Administration errors	Per 100 opportunities/doses 2.4–11.1 (5 studies)

prescribing error per patient per day. In this study, 19.5 percent of the errors were adjudged serious—preventable or potential ADEs.

Turning to medication administration errors, according to several international studies, administration errors (excluding wrong-time errors) are frequent, with error rates per dose ranging from 2.4 to 11.1 percent (Dean et al., 1995; Taxis et al., 1999; Barker et al., 2002; Tissot et al., 2003; Lisby et al., 2005). The U.S. study in this group found an administration error rate of 11 percent, excluding wrong-time errors (Barker et al., 2002). This study employed an observation-based method for detecting medication administration errors that has been used by the Centers for Medicare and Medicaid Services (CMS) for almost 20 years as a quality indicator for nursing homes. It was carried out in Colorado and Georgia in 36 different facilities (12 accredited hospitals, 12 nonaccredited hospitals, and 12 skilled nursing facilities). There was no significant difference in error rates (regardless of whether wrong-time errors were included) by type of facility. For the 36 facilities, the administration error rate (excluding wrong-time errors) ranged from 0 to 26 percent, with 8.3 percent as the median value. The 36 institutions studied were selected at random primarily from the Atlanta, Georgia, metropolitan statistical area and the Denver-Boulder-Greeley, Colorado, consolidated statistical area. Each facility had to agree to participate in the study. Twenty-six selected facilities declined to take part in the study. Most did not give reasons for not wishing to participate; of those that did, many expressed concerns about poor scores and wanting to improve their performance first (Barker et al., 2002). Thus the authors concluded that the error rates reported likely represent a lower bound.

A study in five intensive care units (ICUs) in U.S. tertiary teaching facilities (Calabrese et al., 2001) found an administration error rate of 3.3 percent—lower than that reported in the above study. The ICU study identified administration errors for a group of high-alert medications using a similar observational technique. The authors of this study commented that the rates they obtained were lower than those found in a comparable French ICU study (Tissot et al., 1999), and suggested that this difference might be due to varying methods of observation and pharmacist participation in patient care in the U.S. study. The committee believes these results—while the best available for large ICUs in the United States—are not generalizable to non-ICU hospital care and that the study by Barker and colleagues (2002) represents the best estimate of administration error rates in U.S. hospitals for non-ICU care.

Much higher rates of administration errors were observed in two studies that focused on intravenous medications—34 per 100 in a joint U.K./German study (Wirtz et al., 2003) and 49 per 100 in a U.K. study (Taxis and Barber, 2003).

On the basis of the Barker et al. (2002) study and assuming a patient in

TABLE 3-2 Error Rates in Nursing Homes

Administration errors	Per 100 opportunities/doses
	6 (Cooper et al., 1994)
	12.2 (Barker et al., 1982)
	14.7 (Barker et al., 2002)
	20 (Baldwin, 1992)

the hospital receives 10 doses of medication per day,[5] a typical patient would be subject to one administration medication error per day. These data, taken together with the results of the above studies, which identified 0.1 prescribing error per patient per day (Kaushal et al., 2001) and 0.3 prescribing error per patient per day (Bates et al., 1995a), as well as plus the fact that medication errors occur in other stages of the medication-use process (e.g., errors in the prescribing and administration stages accounted for 77 percent of medication errors [Leape et al., 1995]), suggest to the committee that about one medication error occurs per patient per day in hospital care.

Nursing Homes

There is little information on rates of dispensing errors in nursing homes, since this function generally is outsourced. According to the available data (see Table 3-2), medication administration errors appear to occur in nursing homes at a rate of 6–20 per 100 doses (Barker et al., 1982, 2002; Baldwin, 1992; Cooper et al., 1994). The two main studies in this area, published 20 years apart, both used the same error detection method (direct observation) and reported similar error rates—12 errors per 100 doses (Barker et al., 1982), and 15 errors per 100 doses (Barker et al., 2002) (in both cases excluding doses administered at the wrong time). Excluding wrong-time errors, omission of an ordered medication is generally the most common type of drug administration error in nursing homes. Given that administration error rates are higher in nursing homes than in hospitals, it

---

[5]Rates of doses dispensed in hospital are rarely quoted in the literature. At MountainView Hospital, Las Vegas, Nevada, dose rates increased steadily at about 10 percent per year over the period 2002–2006 (Wood and Nam, 2005). During this period, the average numbers of doses dispensed per patient per day were 13.6 (January 2002), 13.3 (July 2002), 15.8 (January 2003), 15.1 (July 2003), 16.8 (January 2004), 16.3 (July 2004), 19.5 (January 2005), 18.0 (July 2005), and 22.1 (January 2006). The committee also carried out a small survey of eight community and teaching hospitals in Pennsylvania, Michigan, Ohio, and Minnesota. Based on 2005 or 2006 data, for the three community hospitals, the results were 24.4, 20.6, and 12.2 doses per patient per day; and for the teaching hospitals, the results were 25.8, 29.7, 32.8, 22.3, and 20.9 doses per patient per day. These data suggest that the assumption of 10 doses per patient per day is a conservative one.

is likely that per day, nursing home patients are more likely to experience a medication error than are hospital patients. Monitoring errors are probably the most common type of error in the nursing home setting, but are much more difficult to identify, and no study in this area was found. Because a typical medication pass in long-term care exceeds 2 hours, it is impossible for the nurse to deliver all medications within 1 hour of the scheduled time; thus wrong-time errors are predictably high in this setting. Finally, transitions from the nursing home to other settings are a time of high risk for adverse effects due to prescribing or transcription errors.

Ambulatory Care

For the purposes of this study, the committee examined medication error rates in six different settings within the ambulatory care domain: (1) the interface between care settings, for example, from hospital care to outpatient clinic; (2) the ambulatory clinic; (3) the community pharmacy; (4) the home care setting; (5) self-care; and (6) the school setting. In general, there is little or no understanding of incidence rates in all these areas.

Error rates in ambulatory clinics have been thinly researched (see Table 3-3). One study found that 21 percent of prescriptions in these settings

TABLE 3-3 Error Rates in Ambulatory Clinics

Prescription writing errors	Percentage of prescriptions containing at least one prescription writing error 21 (Shaughnessy and Nickel, 1989)
Errors in an ambulatory hemodialysis unit	Percentage of patients subject to prescribing errors 97.7 (Manley et al., 2003b)
	Medication-related problems per patient per month 0.45 (Manley et al., 2003a)
Errors in an ambulatory chemotherapy unit	Percentage of doses containing an error 3 (Gandhi et al., 2005)
Errors in dispensing samples	Percentage of labels with usual dosage not present 12 (Dill and Generali, 2000)
	Percentage of labels that referred user to enclosed prescribing information that was absent 17 (Dill and Generali, 2000)
Documentation errors	Current medications per patient missing from patient record 0.37 (Wagner and Hogan, 1996) 0.89 (Bedell et al., 2000)
	Percentage of prescription renewals missing from patient record 15 (Ernst et al., 2001)

TABLE 3-4 Errors by Community and Mail Order Pharmacies

Community pharmacy: telephoned prescription errors	Percentage of telephoned prescriptions containing an error 12.4 (Camp et al., 2003)
Community pharmacy: dispensing errors	Percentage of prescriptions erroneously dispensed 1.7 (Flynn et al., 2003) 3.4 (Buchanan et al., 1991) 12.5 (Kistner et al., 1994) 24 (Allan et al., 1995)
Mail order pharmacy: dispensing errors	Percentage of prescriptions erroneously dispensed 0.075 (Teagarden et al., 2005)

contained at least one prescription writing error (Shaughnessy and Nickel, 1989). Two studies found high rates of medication errors in ambulatory hemodialysis units (Manley et al., 2003a,b). Extrapolating the findings of the study with the lower rate (Manley et al., 2003a) to the 246,000 U.S. hemodialysis patients, nearly 111,000 medication-related problems occur to these patients each month. In an ambulatory chemotherapy clinic, a medication error rate of 3.0 percent was found (Gandhi et al., 2005). Another study (Dill and Generali, 2000) found a lack of adequate documentation provided with drug samples available for administration to patients in an ambulatory clinic. Finally, three studies (Wagner and Hogan, 1996; Bedell et al., 2000; Ernst et al., 2001) found high rates of medication documentation errors.

Regarding community pharmacies (see Table 3-4), one study (Camp et al., 2003) found that 12.4 percent of telephoned prescriptions contained an error in the information provided by the person calling in the prescription. Four studies examining dispensing errors and using the same error detection method found a wide range of prescription dispensing error rates—1.7 to 24 percent. One study conducted in a hospital-based outpatient pharmacy found the rate of dispensing errors to be 12.5 percent (Kistner et al., 1994). Another small-scale study found a 24 percent dispensing error rate (Allan et al., 1995). In a study at a high-volume outpatient pharmacy, the error rate was found to be 3.4 percent (Buchanan et al., 1991). These three studies published in the period 1991–1995, reported much higher error rates than a more recent study reflecting the likely improvements in dispensing systems and technology over time. This more recent, large-scale study of both new prescriptions and prescription refills found an error rate of 1.7 percent (Flynn et al., 2003). This dispensing error rate translates to approximately 4 errors per 250 prescriptions per pharmacy per day, or an estimated 51.5 million errors during the filling of 3 billion prescriptions each year. One study of medication errors at Medco Health Solutions, Inc., a large mail order pharmacy, carried out by Medco employees, found a dispensing error rate of 0.075 percent—16 dispensing errors among 21,252 prescriptions (Teagarden et al., 2005).

Self-care studies have focused mainly on adherence rates, which are generally low. An early study found adherence rates for prescribed medications of 50 percent (Sackett and Snow, 1979). A more recent meta-analysis of 328 studies reporting on adherence to medication regimens found an adherence rate of 79.4 percent (DiMatteo, 2004). Adherence rates appear to vary according to the number of doses taken per day (Cramer et al., 1989).

Pediatric Care

It has become clear that the prescription, dispensing, and administration of medications account for a substantial portion of the preventable medical errors that occur with children (Kaushal et al., 2001, 2004). Children are uniquely vulnerable to medication errors: all pediatric medication doses need to be based on body-size parameters (e.g., weight, body mass index) and the state of organ development; children are much less able than adults to double-check their own medications; and the wide range of appropriate doses for any given medication based on the child's size gives the "average" dose little predictability for those doing the administering. Accurate pediatric medication administration requires knowledge of the child's precise weight; proper conversion of pounds to kilograms; the correct choice of appropriate preparations and concentrations; and the ability to measure and administer doses properly, particularly for liquid medications.

An inpatient study covering all types of medications carried out at two urban teaching hospitals reported a rate of medication order errors of 4.2 percent, or 405 prescribing errors per 1,000 pediatric patients (Kaushal et al., 2001). Using a broader definition of medication error, a French study reported a higher rate—24.0 percent (Fontan et al., 2003). Also using a broader definition, a still higher rate was observed in a pediatric ICU—30.0 percent (Potts et al., 2004).

Rates of administration errors were estimated to be 0.72 per 100 orders (or 7.0 per 100 admissions, or 19.8 per 1,000 patient days) for all types of medication in a pediatric inpatient setting (Kaushal et al., 2001) and 23.0 per 100 opportunities for error in a pediatric nephrology ward (Fontan et al., 2003).

There have been two pediatric emergency department studies. One of these, conducted in a Canadian hospital, estimated that 100.0 prescribing

TABLE 3-5 Errors in Hospital Pediatric Care

Medication ordering errors	**Percentage of prescriptions containing an error** 4.2 (Kaushal et al., 2001) 24 (Fontan et al., 2003)
Medication ordering errors in pediatric intensive care	**Percentage of prescriptions containing an error** 30 (Potts et al., 2004)
Administration errors	**Per 100 orders** 0.72 (Kaushal et al., 2001)
Administration errors in pediatric nephrology units	**Per 100 opportunities for error** 23 (Fontan et al., 2003)
Emergency department prescribing errors	**Per 1,000 patients** 100 (Kozer et al., 2002)
Emergency department administration errors	**Per 1,000 patients** 39 (Kozer et al., 2002)
Emergency department acetaminophen doses ordered outside recommended range	**Per 100 doses ordered** 22 (Losek, 2004)

errors and 39.0 administration errors occurred in the emergency department per 1,000 pediatric patients (Kozer et al., 2002). The other study found that 22.0 percent of acetaminophen doses ordered were outside the recommended 10–15 milligrams/kilogram recommendation for these patients (Losek, 2004). (See Table 3-5 for a summary of errors in hospital pediatric care).

Finally, a recent study found that potential medication errors occur frequently in outpatient pediatric clinics (McPhillips et al., 2005). In a sample of new prescriptions for 22 common medications, approximately 15 percent of children were dispensed a medication with a potential dosing error.

Psychiatric Care

Many studies of medication errors associated with psychotropic medications either were conducted as part of larger general medical–surgical studies or other ADE-reporting databases, or were restricted to geriatric populations in nonpsychiatric restricted settings, such as nursing homes and ambulatory clinics. The one major study devoted exclusively to medication errors in psychiatric care found a very high rate of errors in a state psychiatric hospital—2,194 errors over 1,448 patient days, or an error rate of 1.5 errors per patient day (Grasso et al., 2003).

Use of Over-the-Counter and Complementary and Alternative Medications

The committee could only find three studies in the peer-reviewed literature addressing incidence rates for medication errors arising from the use of OTC drugs. These studies (Li et al., 2000; McErlean et al., 2001; Goldman and Scolnik, 2004) showed that parents using OTC medications to treat children with fever often administer an incorrect dosage. One study of 118 caregivers treating their children with a fever reducer revealed that incorrect doses were given 47 percent of the time; another study of 248 caregivers found that 12 percent gave an overdose and 41 percent an underdose; and a third study found that of 200 patients treated for fever by a parent, 51 percent received the wrong dose. Moreover, these studies indicated that a misdose often resulted in a continued fever and an eventual trip to the emergency department.

Despite the paucity of data on OTC-related error rates, there is a growing body of literature documenting adverse OTC drug–disease and OTC drug–drug interactions. Some examples are presented in Box 3-2.

The committee could find no studies of medication error rates associated with complementary and alternative medications. There is, however, an emerging literature indicating that these medications have the potential for adverse interactions with prescription drugs (D'Arcy, 1993; Calis and Young, 2004). In particular, these types of products can interfere with the metabolism and elimination of other drugs in the body. St. John's Wort, an herbal product commonly used to treat depression, is an example. Studies have found that St. John's Wort impacts an enzyme that ultimately increases the oxidation of drugs (Bailey and Dresser, 2004). This action limits the bioavailability of some drugs, resulting in serious adverse effects. Specifically, studies have shown that St. John's Wort can increase organ rejection and increase the viral load in HIV patients by limiting the effects of prescription medications (Piscitelli et al., 2000; Ruschitzka et al., 2000).

Error Rates: Much More Needs to Be Done

Where incidence rates have been measured systematically, medication errors have been found to be common and to occur at unacceptably high levels. Reasonably well-researched stages of the medication-use process include prescribing, dispensing, and administering in hospitals; prescribing in ambulatory clinics; dispensing in community pharmacies; and medication adherence in self-care.

BOX 3-2
Examples of Adverse OTC Drug–Disease
and OTC Drug–Drug Interactions

Drug–Disease Interactions
- Cough syrup and diabetes. Because most OTC cough syrups contain large quantities of sugar, an unknowing diabetic patient could go into diabetic shock.
- Ibuprofen and other nonsteroidal anti-inflammatory drugs (NSAIDs). NSAIDs increase blood pressure in hypertensive individuals. Moreover, chronic NSAID use can counteract the effects of beta-blockers, thiazide diuretics, and other medications (Houston, 1991; Espino and Lancaster, 1992).
- Acetaminophen and ibuprofen can result in kidney damage for those with congestive heart failure and renal impairment. Prostaglandins are critical to proper renal functioning in these individuals, and NSAIDs suppress prostaglandin synthesis (Bakris and Kern, 1989).

Drug–Drug Interactions
- NSAIDs. These drugs can cause gastric bleeding. Many adults self-medicate with OTC NSAIDs to treat osteoarthritis, a practice known to cause gastric ulceration. When NSAIDs are combined with antacids or H_2 antagonists, the risk of hospitalization for serious gastrointestinal bleeding is increased (Bradley et al., 1991; Singh et al., 1996).
- Calcium supplements. When calcium supplements are combined with products such as aspirin, erythromycin, or bisacodyl (i.e., Dulcolax), gastric irritation results. Additionally, calcium supplements reduce the bioavailability of other medications, such as levothyroxine, ciproflaxin, phenytoin, and digoxin, and limit the absorption of such nutrients as iron, thiamin, zinc, and B_{12} (D'Arcy and McElnay, 1987).
- Aspirin and coumadin. Because both aspirin and coumadin are blood thinners, there is an acute possibility of too much anticoagulation when they are taken together.
- Too much acetaminophen. Many OTC and prescription medicines contain acetaminophen. An unassuming patient may self-treat a cold with both Advil Cold® or some other cough/cold medication and regular Tylenol without realizing that this constitutes a double dose of acetaminophen. It has been well documented that overuse of acetaminophen leads to hepatotoxicity (liver damage), which can lead to liver failure.
- Antacids. These medications interfere with the effects of some HIV drugs (Piscitelli and Gallicano, 2001).

When it is possible to compare the results of more than one study, estimates of error rates vary greatly. Much but not all of this variation can be explained by differing definitions and identification methods. Even when the definition of error is standardized and the same identification method is used, substantial variation in administration error rates by institution are found (Barker et al., 2002). Taking this variability into account, however, the underlying error rates are unacceptably high.

Over the past decade, much scholarly activity and sizable government resources have been directed at determining the extent and scope of medication errors. Nonetheless, there remain broad aspects of the medication-use process for which we have little or no understanding of error rates. These include the selection and procurement of medications, monitoring of the effectiveness of medications in all care settings, medication use in schools, self-care, medication use in psychiatric care, and the use of OTC and complementary and alternative medications. The committee concludes that greater effort is needed to identify medication errors in most care settings, both to measure the extent and scope of such errors and to assess the impact of error prevention strategies.

Preventable Adverse Drug Events

ADEs, defined as any injury due to medication (Bates et al., 1995b), are common in hospitals, nursing homes, and ambulatory care. ADEs that are associated with a medication error are considered preventable (see the detailed discussion in Chapter 1). This section presents findings from the literature on the incidence of preventable ADEs.

Hospitals

Three major studies[6] examined the incidence of preventable ADEs occurring during hospitalization (see Table 3-6). In chronological order, their findings are as follows:

• 1.2 preventable ADEs per 100 admissions at LDS Hospital, Salt Lake City, Utah (Classen et al., 1997). Extrapolating these results nationally and assuming 32 million admissions annually, 380,000 hospital patients in America would experience a preventable ADE annually.
• 1.8 preventable ADEs per 100 nonobstetric admissions at Brigham and Women's Hospital, Boston, Massachusetts (Bates et al., 1995b). Extrapolating these results nationally and assuming 25 million nonobstetrical admissions annually, 450,000 hospital patients in America would experience a preventable ADE annually.
• 5.7 preventable ADEs per 1,000 patient days at Brigham and Women's Hospital, Boston, Massachusetts (Jha et al., 1998).

---

[6]The committee also reviewed three other studies on the incidence of preventable ADEs occurring during hospitalization. In two studies the sample sizes were too small (Senst et al., 2001; Forster et al., 2004), and the third study used a much broader definition of preventable ADEs than that in other studies (Nebeker et al., 2005).

TABLE 3-6 Rates of Preventable ADEs in Hospitals

Study	Preventable ADE Rate	Proportion of ADEs Preventable (No. of ADEs in study)	ADE Rate
Classen et al., 1997	1.2 per 100 admissions	About 50% (2,227)	2.4 per 100 admissions
Bates et al., 1995b	1.8 per 100 admissions	28% (247)	6.5 per 100 admissions
	3.2 per 1,000 patient-days		11.5 per 1,000 patient-days
Jha et al., 1998	5.7 per 1,000 patient-days	27% (617)	21 per 1,000 patient-days

NOTE: ADE rates usually are not reported in the medical literature by categories such as renal failure, hypotension, or bleeding. On the other hand, severity levels are often quoted—for example, mild (self-limited); moderate (requiring treatment); severe (life-threatening, disabling, or markedly prolonging hospitalization) (Classen et al., 1991); or fatal, life-threatening, serious, or significant (Bates et al., 1995b).

In the study at LDS Hospital (Classen et al., 1997), ADEs were identified using computerized surveillance of medical records through the use of various automated signals (for example, drug stop orders, antidote orders) plus voluntary reporting. Among the 2,227 ADE patients, 42 percent of the ADEs arose from excessive dosage of a drug for a patient's weight and calculated renal function, 4.6 percent from drug interactions, and 1.5 percent from known drug allergies. All these ADEs were thought to be potentially preventable, particularly through the application of computer-based programs that monitor drug use for appropriate selection and dosage.

In the first Brigham and Women's Hospital study (Bates et al., 1995b), ADEs were identified by stimulated self-reports by nurses and pharmacists and daily review of charts by nurse investigators. Relative to the LDS Hospital study, this study reported a higher ADE incidence rate (6.5 ADEs per 100 nonobstetric admissions versus 2.4 ADEs per 100 admissions) and a lower proportion of ADEs identified as preventable (28 percent versus almost 50 percent). Among the preventable events (preventable ADEs and potential ADEs) in the first study at Brigham and Women's Hospital (Bates et al., 1995b), 49 percent of primary errors occurred in the ordering stage, 11 percent in the transcription stage, 14 percent in the dispensing stage, and 26 percent in the administration stage. The leading types of ordering errors—wrong dose, known allergy, wrong frequency, and drug–drug interactions—were all thought to be potentially preventable by computerized order checking. The data in this study were analyzed further. For the 70 preventable ADEs and 194 potential ADEs, a systems analysis group found 334 errors associated with these 264 events. The group identified the proximal causes of these errors (Leape et al., 1995) (see Table 3-7). These proximal causes cut across multiple stages; most errors occurred in the ordering (39 percent) and drug administration (38 percent) stages. Lack of knowledge of the drug was the most common proximal cause (22 percent), followed by lack of knowledge of the patient (14 percent) and rule violations (10 percent).

The systems group then identified the system failures that led to the proximal causes (see Table 3-8). The seven most common system failures (defects in drug knowledge dissemination, dose and identity checking, the availability of patient information, order transcription, the allergy defense system, medication order tracking, and interservice communications) all have in common impaired access to information. This group of system failures accounted for 78 percent of the errors identified.

In the second Brigham and Women's Hospital study (Jha et al., 1998), ADEs were identified using a combination of the methods of the LDS Hospital study and the first Brigham and Women's Hospital study—computerized surveillance of medical records, chart review, and voluntary reporting. Relative to the first Brigham and Women's Hospital study, this second study reported a higher preventable ADE incidence rate (5.7 per 1,000 patient days versus 3.2 per 1,000 patient days) and a similar proportion of ADEs identified as preventable (27 percent versus 28 percent). This study demonstrated that the types of ADEs found by chart review and computer surveillance are different despite some overlap, with the chart-based approach also finding 45 percent more ADEs. In this study, 25 percent of the ADEs identified by the computer monitor were preventable; for chart review, this proportion was 27 percent. Moreover, the computer monitor used in the second Brigham and Women's Hospital study found ADEs at a higher rate than the computer monitor used in the LDS Hospital study because it was more sensitive (i.e., able to detect milder ADEs) and contained rules for identifying a wider range of ADEs. A key insight from the second Brigham and Women's Hospital study was that the three detection methods used in the study—computerized surveillance of medical records, chart review, and voluntary reporting—complemented each other in identifying preventable and potential ADEs.

The committee believes the key messages from this series of studies are as follows:

• The estimates of about 400,000 preventable ADEs occurring annually in U.S hospitals, derived from the LDS Hospital study (Classen et al., 1997) and the first Brigham and Women's study (Bates et al., 1995b), are likely

TABLE 3-7 Distribution of Errors by Proximal Cause and Stage

Proximal Cause	Ordering % (No.)	Transcription and Verification % (No.)	Dispensing % (No.)	Administration % (No.)	All % (No.)
Lack of knowledge of the drug	36 (47)	15 (6)	0 (0)	15 (19)	22 (72)
Lack of information about the patient	24 (31)	10 (4)	0 (0)	10 (13)	14 (48)
Rule violations	19 (25)	0 (0)	16 (6)	2 (2)	10 (33)
Slips and memory lapses	11 (14)	0 (0)	0 (0)	12 (15)	9 (29)
Transcription errors	0 (0)	73 (29)	0 (0)	0 (0)	9 (29)
Faulty drug identity checking	0 (0)	0 (0)	29 (11)	10 (13)	7 (24)
Faulty interaction with other services	1 (1)	0 (0)	8 (3)	10 (13)	5 (17)
Faulty dose checking	0 (0)	0 (0)	8 (3)	10 (13)	5 (16)
Infusion pump and parenteral delivery problems	0 (0)	0 (0)	0 (0)	13 (16)	5 (16)
Inadequate monitoring	8 (11)	0 (0)	0 (0)	3 (4)	4 (15)
Drug stocking and delivery problems	0 (0)	0 (0)	29 (11)	0 (0)	3 (11)
Preparation errors	0 (0)	0 (0)	11 (4)	5 (6)	3 (10)
Lack of standardization	0 (0)	0 (0)	0 (0)	6 (8)	2 (8)
Unclassified	1 (1)	3 (1)	0 (0)	3 (4)	2 (6)
TOTALS*	100 (130)	100 (40)	100 (38)	100 (126)	100 (334)

*Percentages do not add to 100% due to rounding.

SOURCE: Leape et al, 1995.

TABLE 3-8 Distribution of Errors by System Failure

System Failure	Errors Attributed	
	%	No.
Drug knowledge dissemination	29	98
Dose and identity checking	12	40
Patient information availability	11	37
Order transcription	9	29
Allergy defense	7	24
Medication order tracking	5	18
Interservice communication	5	17
Device use	4	12
Standardization of doses and frequencies	4	12
Standardization of drug distribution within unit	3	11
Standardization of procedures	3	10
Preparation of intravenous medications	2	6
Transfer/transition procedures	1	4
Conflict resolution	1	4
Others	4	12
TOTALS	100	334

SOURCE: Leape et al., 1995.

lower bounds since the second Brigham and Women's study (Jha et al., 1998), using more comprehensive detection methods, reported higher rates.

• A high proportion of preventable ADEs are caused by system errors that could be eliminated by computerized provider order entry (CPOE).

• Sophisticated decision-support tools that address dosing, prophylaxis, and patient monitoring, among other issues, must be built into CPOE systems.

Nursing Homes

Two studies estimated the incidence of preventable ADEs in long-term care (see Table 3-9). Their findings were as follows:

TABLE 3-9 Rates of Preventable ADEs in Nursing Homes

Study	Preventable ADE Rate per Patient Month	Proportion of ADEs Preventable (No. of ADEs in study)	ADEs per 100 Admissions
Gurwitz et al., 2000	0.01	51% (546)	0.02
Gurwitz et al., 2005	0.04	42% (815)	0.1

- 0.01 preventable ADE per resident-month (Gurwitz et al., 2000).
- 0.04 preventable ADE per resident-month (Gurwitz et al., 2005).

In the first study, carried out in 18 community-based nursing homes in Massachusetts, ADEs were identified by voluntary reporting and review of the record of each nursing home resident by two nurses and one pharmacist, performed every 6 weeks. In the second study, carried out in two large academic long-term care facilities, one in Connecticut and one in Ontario, Canada, ADEs were identified by a pharmacist's monthly review of patient records. Medical records were also targeted for review using computer-generated signals (for example, abnormal serum levels), and administrative incident reports were reviewed as well for any indication of an ADE. This second study identified a much higher rate of ADEs than the first study. The authors suggested this difference could be attributed to the enhanced approach to identification of ADEs in the second study, although they thought the estimates from this study were still conservative since the study relied solely on information in medical records; there was no direct assessment of residents, which likely would have led to the identification of additional events.

The committee believes the second Gurwitz et al. study provides a better estimate of preventable ADE rates in the long-term care population. Applying the findings of this study to an average nursing home in the United States (bed size 105), 50 preventable ADEs (Gurwitz et al., 2005) would occur annually in the nursing home setting; applying the findings to the entire 1.6 million nursing home population in the United States, 800,000 (Gurwitz et al., 2005) preventable ADEs would occur each year in these settings. These figures are likely conservative, however, given the much higher ADE incident rates published in two other studies—0.44 ADEs per patient-month or 115 ADEs per 100 admissions (Gerety et al., 1993) and 134 ADEs per 100 admissions (Cooper, 1999). (Neither of these studies quoted the proportion of ADEs considered preventable.)

In one of the two nursing home studies by Gurwitz and colleagues (2000), of the 464 preventable ADEs and potential ADEs identified, 315 occurred in the ordering stage. Among those 315 errors, wrong dose (for example, excessive dose for an elderly patient) occurred in 63 percent of cases, followed by prescription of a drug for which there was a well-established interaction with another drug, which occurred in 22 percent of cases. The other Gurwitz et al. (2005) nursing home study found similar results. Among the 338 preventable ADEs identified, 198 occurred in the ordering stage. Of these prescribing errors, the most common were wrong dose (48 percent), wrong drug choice (38 percent), and known interaction (12 percent).

Ambulatory Care

In a large study of Medicare enrollees, Gurwitz and colleagues (2003) found 5 ADEs per 100 patient-years and 1.4 preventable ADEs per 100 patient-years. The study took place in a large New England multispecialty ambulatory practice providing health care for more than 30,000 persons aged 65 and over. In total, 1,523 ADEs were identified, 421 of which were adjudged preventable (28 percent). ADEs were identified using multiple methods: reporting from health care providers, review of hospital discharge summaries, review of emergency department notes, computer-generated signals, free-text review of electronic clinical notes, and review of administrative incident reports of medication errors. Generalizing these results to the population of all Medicare enrollees, the authors estimated that 530,000 preventable ADEs occur among the 38 million enrollees (Gurwitz et al., 2003).

Another study, which contacted patients directly, found a much higher rate of ADEs but a lower proportion adjudged preventable. In a study (Gandhi et al., 2003) carried out in four primary care practices in Boston, of the 661 patients who had received at least one prescription during a 4-week period and who responded to a survey, 181 ADEs were identified (27 per 100 patients). Many more ADEs were identified by surveying the patients than by reviewing charts: of the 181 ADEs, 166 (92 percent) were identified by surveying patients, 50 (28 percent) by reviewing charts, and 35 (19 percent) by both means. Of the 181 ADEs identified, 20 were considered preventable (11 percent).

In a study on ADEs in ambulatory care (Gandhi et al., 2003), of the 20 preventable ADEs identified, 9 were due to the selection of an inappropriate dose, 2 to wrong dose, and 2 to wrong frequency of dose. It was considered that CPOE, including checking of dosages, interactions with other drugs, and allergies to the drug, could have prevented 7 of the 20 preventable ADEs. In a study of ADEs among elderly patients in the ambulatory setting (Gurwitz et al., 2003), of the 421 preventable ADEs identified, 246 were found in the prescribing stage. Among these prescribing errors, 46 percent involved wrong drug/wrong therapeutic choice and 41 percent wrong dose. (See Table 3-10 for rates of preventable ADEs in ambulatory care.)

Summary

In total, the committee estimates that at least 1.5 million preventable ADEs occur each year in the United States:

TABLE 3-10 Rates of Preventable ADEs in Ambulatory Care

Study	Preventable ADE Rate	Proportion of ADEs Preventable (No. of ADEs in study)	ADE Rate
Gurwitz et al., 2003	1.4 per 100 patient-years	28% (1,523)	5 per 100 patient-years
Gandhi et al., 2003	5.4 per 100 patients	20% (181)	27 per 100 patients

• Preventable ADEs occurring in hospitals—Classen and colleagues (1997) projected 380,000 occurring annually and Bates and colleagues (1995b) 450,000. These are likely underestimates given the higher preventable ADE rate found in another study using more comprehensive ADE identification methods (Jha et al., 1998).

• Preventable ADEs occurring in long-term care—Gurwitz and colleagues (2005) projected 800,000—again likely an underestimate given the higher ADEs rates of other studies (Gerety et al., 1993; Cooper, 1999).

• Preventable ADEs among outpatient Medicare patients—Gurwitz and colleagues (2003) projected 530,000.

Underutilization and Overutilization of Medications

Both underutilization of medications (the failure to prescribe medications for which there is an evidence base for reduction in morbidity and mortality) and overutilization of medications (prescribing of medications for which there is no evidence base for reduction in morbidity and mortality) are common in hospitals, nursing homes, and the ambulatory setting. The committee found well-documented evidence of inadequate treatment for acute coronary syndromes, heart failure, chronic coronary disease, atrial fibrillation, bacterial infection prophylaxis, and thrombosis prophylaxis in hospitals. Underutilization of medications in nursing homes and assisted-living facilities relative to national standards is best documented for pain management, congestive heart failure, and use of anticoagulants in stroke prevention and atrial fibrillation, but there is also limited evidence for deficits in use of medications for depression, myocardial infarction prophylaxis, and treatment of osteoporosis. Overutilization of medication is best documented in the treatment of colds, upper respiratory infections, and bronchitis by antibiotics.

Underutilization of Medications in Hospitals

For hospital care, three broad classifications of studies were identified: on treatment of acute coronary syndromes, on antibiotic prophylaxis for surgical patients, and on thromboembolic prophylaxis for surgical patients (see Table 3-11). Seven studies addressed acute myocardial infarction. Within the first 24 hours of hospitalization for a myocardial infarction, 85–93 percent had received aspirin (Sanborn et al., 2004; Granger et al., 2005; Roe et al., 2005), and 66–78 percent beta-blockers (Sanborn et al., 2004; Granger et al., 2005; Roe et al., 2005). Among patients discharged with a diagnosis of acute myocardial infarction, aspirin was prescribed for 53–93 percent of ideal candidates (those with no known contraindication), beta-blockers for 53–83 percent of ideal candidates, and angiotensin converting enzyme (ACE) inhibitors for 59–83 percent of ideal candidates (Alexander et al., 1998; Petersen et al., 2001, 2003; Krumholz et al., 2003; Sanborn et al., 2004; Granger et al., 2005; Roe et al., 2005). Rates of prophylaxis for bacterial infections among surgical patients ranged from 70 to 98 percent (Heineck et al., 1999; Vaisbrud et al., 1999; Gupta et al., 2003; van Kasteren et al., 2003; Bedouch et al., 2004; Quenon et al., 2004). Rates of thromboembolic prophylaxis varied greatly—from 5 to 81 percent (Ageno et al., 2002; Ahmad et al., 2002; Aujesky et al., 2002; Campbell et

TABLE 3-11 Underutilization of Medications in Hospitals

Patients discharged with diagnosis of acute myocardial infarction	Percentage of patients given aspirin within 24 hours of hospitalization 85–93 (3 studies)
	Percentage of patients prescribed aspirin at discharge 53–93 (6 studies)
	Percentage of patients given beta-blockers within 24 hours of hospitalization 66–78 (3 studies)
	Percentage of patients prescribed beta-blockers at discharge 53–83 (6 studies)
	Percentage of patients prescribed angiotensin converting enzyme (ACE) inhibitors at discharge 51–73 (6 studies)
Rates of antibiotic prophylaxis in surgical studies	Percentage of procedures for which patients prescribed antibiotics 70–98 (6 studies)
Rates of thromboembolic prophylaxis in surgical studies	Percentage of procedures for which thromboembolic prophylaxis carried out 5–90 (9 studies)

al., 2001; Freeman et al., 2002; Learhinan and Alderman, 2003; Scott et al., 2003; Tan and Tan, 2004; Chopard et al., 2005).

Underutilization of Medications in Nursing Homes

In a study of residents over age 65 in assisted-living facilities, 62 percent of those with congestive heart failure were not receiving an ACE inhibitor; of those with a history of myocardial infarction, 60.5 percent were not receiving aspirin, and 76 percent were not receiving beta-blockers; of those with a history of stroke, 37.5 percent were not receiving an anticoagulant or antiplatelet product; and of those with osteoporosis, 61 percent were not receiving calcium supplements (Sloane et al., 2004). In a second study of nursing home residents, only 53 percent of ideal candidates with atrial fibrillation were receiving warfarin (McCormick et al., 2001). A third study showed that only 25 percent of nursing home residents with congestive heart failure had been prescribed an ACE inhibitor (Gambassi et al., 2000). A fourth study showed that only 55 percent of residents identified as depressed had received antidepressants (Brown et al., 2002).

Inadequate pain management is well documented in nursing homes, with 45–80 percent of residents experiencing unrelieved pain (AGS, 2002). Results of cross-sectional studies indicate that 26 percent of nursing home residents overall and 30 percent of those with a cancer diagnosis have daily pain, and approximately 25 percent of these patients receive no analgesics (Bernabei et al., 1998; Won et al., 1999, 2004).

Underutilization of Medications in Ambulatory Care

A number of studies have examined underutilization of medications in ambulatory care. A major U.S. study of both inpatient and outpatient care carried out during 1998–2000 found high levels of errors of omission generally: across a wide range of acute and chronic conditions, patients received 55 percent of recommended care (McGlynn et al., 2003). Regarding the use of medications in particular, 69 percent of patients received recommended care; of those presenting with myocardial infarction, however, only 45 percent of ideal candidates received beta-blockers and 61 percent aspirin.

Analysis of the results of three phases of the National Health and Nutrition Examination Survey shows that rates of hypertension control, although improving, continue to be low (Hajjar and Kotchen, 2003). Of those with hypertension in the 1988–1991 phase of the survey, 52 percent received treatment, and 25 percent achieved control of their hypertension; in the 1991–1994 phase, 52 percent received treatment, and 23 percent achieved control; and in the 1999–2000 phase, 58 percent received treatment, and 31 percent achieved control.

One study found that the outpatient use of evidence-based therapies for coronary artery disease is increasing, but remains suboptimal (Newby et al., 2006). The proportion of patients reporting use (consistently or inconsistently) of aspirin, beta-blockers, and lipid-lowering agents increased over time, and in the last year (2002) of the study, the use of aspirin was 83 percent, of beta-blockers 61 percent, and of lipid-lowering agents 63 percent. Rates of consistent use were, however, much lower: for aspirin 71 percent of patients, for beta-blockers 46 percent, and for lipid-lowering agents 43 percent.

Overutilization of Medications

Overutilization of medications represents an important problem and is best documented in the treatment of colds, upper respiratory infections, and bronchitis by antibiotics. These infections are common diagnoses in the ambulatory care setting. Such infections are overwhelmingly viral in origin and do not respond to antibiotics (Arroll and Kenealy, 2002; Thomas and Arroll, 2000). Nevertheless, patients are often prescribed antibiotics for these diseases, thereby being exposed to ADEs; increased antibiotic resistance results as well. Although prescribing of unnecessary drugs has not always been considered a medication error (but rather overuse), clearly the problem exists and represents a major opportunity for improvement.

For example, using National Ambulatory Medical Care Survey data for 1992, a study found that 51 percent of adult patients diagnosed as having colds, 52 percent of adult patients diagnosed as having upper respiratory tract infections, and 66 percent of adult patients diagnosed as having bronchitis were treated with antibiotics (Gonzales et al., 1997). A parallel study on antibiotic prescribing for children using the same dataset found similar results: antibiotics were prescribed for 44 percent of patients with colds, 46 percent of patients with upper respiratory tract infections, and 75 percent of patients with bronchitis (Nyquist et al., 1998). A third study, using National Ambulatory Medical Care Survey data for 1996, found that in the emergency department, antibiotics were prescribed for 24 percent of patients with common colds and upper respiratory tract infections and 42 percent of patients with bronchitis (Stone et al., 2000).

Results of later studies indicate that the prescribing of antimicrobials for respiratory tract infections has declined somewhat. Again using National Ambulatory Medical Care Survey data for the period 1989–1990 to 1999–2000 for respiratory tract infections, the prescribing of antimicrobials for children and adolescents decreased from 67 to 38 prescriptions per 100 office visits, and the visit-based prescription rate decreased from 72 to 61 per 100 visits (McCaig et al., 2002). Similarly for adults, the prescribing of antibiotics for acute respiratory infections fell from 60 percent of outpatient office visits during 1995–1996 to 49 percent of office visits during the 2001–2002 (Roumie et al., 2005). The general issue of overuse of medications in patients with other conditions is also undoubtedly important, but this is perhaps the best-documented case.

Impact of Formularies on Medication Safety

In an effort to control the costs of pharmaceuticals, managed care organizations have established formularies—schedules of prescription drugs that will be paid for by a health insurance plan and dispensed through participating pharmacies. Often patients taking prescription drugs switch from one managed care organization to another, resulting in the need to switch to another formulary. This sometimes involves patients changing their medications. Moreover, there can be difficulties in the handoffs between managed care organizations, which can result in patients having periods of time off their medications. Formulary changes may also be required when a patient moves from an outpatient to an inpatient and then back to an outpatient setting. In this situation, a recent study found a minimal effect of the hospital formulary on postadmission use of proton pump inhibitors and statins as compared with preadmission use in a privately insured managed care population (Sun et al., 2005).

Limited research has been carried out on the impact of the use of formularies and formulary switching on medication safety. A major review of studies of interventions to improve drug use in managed care organizations found evidence for the effectiveness of several interventions but little understanding of longer-term efficacy and safety issues (Pearson et al., 2003). An editorial in a psychiatric journal commented that Medicaid preferred drug lists had been rapidly implemented across the nation, but studies analyzing the impact of these lists on patients had not kept pace (Elam et al., 2005). In the case of psychotropic drugs, however, concerns have been raised about the use of overly restrictive formularies. Studies have shown that the failure to respond to one selective serotonin reuptake inhibitor or the occurrence of severe side effects does not mean the patient will have the same experience with another such drug (Huskamp, 2003). The committee believes the impact of the use of formularies and formulary switching on medication safety is an area that requires further research.

COSTS

The costs of medication errors have been much less well researched than incidence rates. The committee could find no studies on the costs of ADEs relating to pediatric and psychiatric care or to the use of OTC and complementary and alternative medications. Most of the cost studies that have been carried out relate to ADEs associated with hospital care. This group of studies has examined both the costs of ADEs experienced in hospitals and the costs of emergency room visits or hospital admissions that are attributable to an earlier ADE. A few studies have examined the costs of ADEs in nursing home and ambulatory care. Some studies have used cost models of the health care delivery system to estimate annual national costs attributable to drug-related morbidity and mortality in ambulatory care.

Hospitals

As noted, hospital-related studies fall into two categories—those addressing the costs of ADEs experienced while in the hospital, and those addressing the costs of emergency room visits and hospital admissions that can be attributable to earlier ADEs.

Costs of ADEs Experienced in Hospitals

Only one study was found that estimated the extra hospital costs of a preventable ADE occurring in a hospital. This study, carried out in 1993 within the Adverse Drug Events Prevention Study, found that after adjusting[7] for patient comorbidities and case mix, the additional length of stay associated with a preventable ADE was 4.6 days, with an increase in total cost of $5,857 (Bates et al., 1997). From these data, the authors estimated that in a 700-bed teaching hospital, preventable ADEs resulted in an additional cost of $2.8 million per year (Bates et al., 1997).

Costs of Emergency Room Visits and Hospital Admissions Attributable to Prior ADEs

A few studies have estimated the hospital/emergency room costs and the proportion of hospital admissions and emergency room visits attributable to an earlier preventable ADE.

In a study at a tertiary hospital, a computer-based monitoring program was used to identify admissions that may have been associated with an ADE. Among 3,238 admissions, 1.4 percent were found to be due to an ADE (Jha et al., 2001). Of these ADEs, 28 percent were preventable. Estimated costs were $10,375 per preventable ADE; annual costs to the hospital were $1.2 million per year for all preventable ADEs.

---

[7]Adjusting for patient comorbidities and case mix is rarely completely successful, but it is the best possible approach since patients cannot be randomized to have or not have an ADE.

Based on data on patients who presented in 1994 at the emergency department of a 560-bed teaching hospital, the costs of treating those with a preventable ADE experienced previously were $308 for those who were not hospitalized and $2,752 for those who were (Dennehy et al., 1996). The study found that 4 percent of all emergency department visits (50 of 1,260) were due to prior ADEs; of these ADEs, 66 percent were judged preventable.

In one study of 253 patients presenting to an emergency department, 71 (28 percent) made their visit because of an ADE (Tafreshi et al., 1999). Of these 71 visits, 50 (70.4 percent) were judged to be due to a preventable ADE. The average cost to the institution was approximately $1,444 for each preventable medication-related visit.

Costs of Medication Errors in Nursing Homes

A study of medication problems in one nursing home provided information on the costs of ADEs in the nursing home setting (Cooper, 1987). That study reported two cases of antibiotic-related errors (omission and known drug allergy) that resulted in hospitalizations costing $3,923 and more than $5,000, respectively. It was further reported (GAO, 2000) that preventable errors in that nursing home cost up to $340,942 over a 2-year period.

Costs of Medication Errors in Ambulatory Care

Only one study was found that addressed the cost of ADEs in ambulatory care. In a study carried out from July 1999 to June 2000, the estimated increased costs (relative to costs incurred in a matched comparison group) associated with ADEs and preventable ADEs among older adults in the ambulatory care setting were $1,310 and $1,983, respectively. Inpatient stays accounted for 71 percent of the additional costs for ADEs and 62 percent of the additional cost for preventable ADEs. Based on the study's cost estimates and rates of ADEs, the annual costs related to ADEs and preventable ADEs in 1,000 older adults would be $65,631 and $27,365, respectively (Field et al., 2005).

Overall Costs of Preventable Medication Errors

In summary, our understanding of the cost of medication errors is very incomplete. Most of what we know relates to additional health care costs associated with preventable ADEs, which represent the injuries caused by errors:

• Hospitals—Classen and colleagues (1997) projected 380,000 preventable ADEs occurring annually and Bates and colleagues (1995b)

450,000; these are likely underestimates given the higher rates of another study (Jha et al., 1998). There is one estimate of the extra costs of inpatient care for a preventable ADE—$5,857 (Bates et al., 1997); this figure excludes health care costs outside the hospital and is derived from 1993 cost data. Assuming conservatively an annual incidence of 400,000 preventable ADEs, each incurring extra hospital costs of $5,857, gives a total cost of $2.3 billion (1993 dollars) or $3.5 billion[8] (2006 dollars).

• Long-term care—Gurwitz and colleagues (2005) projected an annual incidence of 800,000 preventable ADEs—again likely an underestimate given the higher ADE rates of earlier studies (Gerety et al., 1993; Cooper, 1999). However, there is no estimate of the health care costs for this group of preventable ADEs.

• Ambulatory care—The best estimate derives from a study (Field et al., 2005) of the costs of ADEs in older adults, which estimated the annual cost of preventable ADEs for all Medicare enrollees aged 65 and older. The cost per preventable ADE was $1,983, and the national annual costs were estimated to be $887 million in 2000. These figures include the costs of inpatient stays (62 percent of the total cost), emergency department visits (6 percent), outpatient care and physician fees (28 percent), and prescribed medicines (4 percent). The national estimate is almost certainly conservative because the detection approach used did not include direct patient contact, which identifies many more ADEs than other approaches.

In addition to the likelihood of being underestimates, the above estimates have some important omissions. First, the costs of some highly common medication errors, such as drug use without a medically valid indication and failure to receive drugs that should have been prescribed, were excluded from the Medicare study of ambulatory ADEs (Field et al., 2005). Moreover, the costs of morbidity and mortality arising from the lack of adherence to the drug regimen were not assessed. Second, all the cost studies omitted other important costs—lost earnings, the costs of not being able to carry out household duties (lost household production), and compensation for pain and suffering. Third, few data are available for any setting regarding the costs of medication errors that do not result in harm. While no injury is involved, these errors often create extra work, and the costs involved may be substantial. For example, one estimate suggested that a 700-bed hospital has 300,000 medication errors per year, each of which creates approximately 20 minutes of extra work for providers—mainly nurses and pharmacists (Bates et al., 1995a). Near-misses may also cost

---

[8]The producer price index for general medical and surgical hospitals increased by 49.4 percent between 1993 and 2006 (BLS, 2006).

more than medication errors with little potential for harm, although this possibility has not been assessed formally.

Limited Understanding of the Costs of Medication Errors

Very few studies have examined the costs of medication errors in individual care settings; rather, studies have focused mainly on the additional hospital costs of ADEs. One study (Bates et al., 1997) used cost data that are now more than 10 years old. There has been one study of the health care costs of treating preventable ADEs occurring in ambulatory care.

There are large gaps in our understanding of the costs of medication errors. No studies have been conducted on (1) the costs of medication errors in pediatric and psychiatric care, (2) the costs associated with errors involving OTC and complementary and alternative medications, (3) the costs of medication errors not considered ADEs, (4) the costs of the failure to receive drugs that should have been prescribed, (5) the costs of over-utilization of drugs (for example, antibiotics), and (6) the costs associated with nonadherence to prescribed drugs in the ambulatory setting. Finally, we have limited understanding of the economic and social costs of medication errors borne by patients and their families.

CONCLUSION

On the basis of the information currently available about the various types of medication errors, the committee acknowledges that it is impossible to formulate a fully comprehensive set of corrective medication error strategies. For example, there is a need to better define the impact on the incidence of errors in the medication-use stage of system problems in the research and development, regulatory review, and distribution/marketing stages (for example, inadequate information about dosages for special populations, look-alike/sound-alike drug names). In addition, the impact of underutilization of medications for the treatment of acute coronary syndromes, for antibiotic prophylaxis, and for thrombosis prophylaxis is not well understood. The area best understood is the incidence of preventable ADEs in various care settings—especially in the hospital, but also in nursing homes and in ambulatory care for adults—where significant problems and their causes have been identified. More research is needed to evaluate the impact of upstream problems on the incidence of errors in the use of medications, as well as the impact of the underutilization of medications.

REFERENCES

Ageno W, Squizzato A, Ambrosini F, Dentali F, Marchesi C, Mera V, Steidl L, Venco A. 2002. Thrombosis prophylaxis in medical patients: A retrospective review of clinical practice patterns. *Haematologica* 87(7):746–750.

AGS (American Geriatrics Society). 2002. The management of persistent pain in older persons. *Journal of the American Geriatrics Society* 50(Suppl. 6):S205–S224.

Ahmad HA, Geissler A, MacLellan D. 2002. Deep venous thrombosis prophylaxis: Are guidelines being followed? *ANZ Journal of Surgery* 72(5):331–334.

Alexander KP, Peterson ED, Granger CB, Casas AC, Van de Werf F, Armstrong PW, Guerci A, Topol EJ, Califf RM. 1998. Potential impact of evidence-based medicine in acute coronary syndromes: Insights from GUSTO-IIb. Global use of strategies to open occluded arteries in acute coronary syndromes trial. *Journal of the American College of Cardiology* 32(7):2023–2030.

Allan EL, Barker KN. 1990. Fundamentals of medication error research. *American Journal of Hospital Pharmacy* 47(3):551–571.

Allan EL, Barker KN, Malloy MJ, Heller WM. 1995. Dispensing errors and counseling in community practice. *American Pharmacy* NS35(12):25–33.

Arroll B, Kenealy T. 2002. Antibiotics for the common cold. *The Cochrane Database of Systematic Reviews* Issue 3. Art. No. CD000247.

Aujesky D, Guignard E, Pannatier, Cornuz J. 2002. Pharmacological thromboembolic prophylaxis in a medical ward: Room for improvement. *Journal of General Internal Medicine* 17(10):788–791.

Bailey DG, Dresser K. 2004. Natural products and adverse drug interactions. *Canadian Medical Association Journal* 170(10):1531–1532.

Bakris G, Kern S. 1989. Renal dysfunction resulting from NSAIDs. *American Family Physician* 40:199–204.

Baldwin VR. 1992. An analysis of subjective and objective indicators of quality of care in North Carolina homes for the aged. *Dissertation Abstracts Online.*

Barker KN, Mikeal RL, Pearson RE, Illig NA, Morse ML. 1982. Medication errors in nursing homes and small hospitals. *American Journal of Hospital Pharmacy* 39:987–991.

Barker KN, Flynn EA, Pepper GA, Bates DW, Mikeal RL. 2002. Medication errors observed in 36 health care facilities. *Archives of Internal Medicine* 162(16):1897–1903.

Bates DW, Boyle DL, Vander Vliet MB, Schneider J, Leape L. 1995a. Relationship between medication errors and adverse drug events. *Journal of General Internal Medicine* 10(4): 100–205.

Bates DW, Cullen DJ, Laird N, Petersen LA, Small SD, Servi D, Laffel G, Sweitzer BJ, Shea BF, Hallisey R, Vander Vliet M, Nemeskal R, Leape LL. 1995b. Incidence of adverse drug events and potential adverse drug events. Implications for prevention. ADE Prevention Study Group. *Journal of the American Medical Association* 274:29–34.

Bates DW, Spell N, Cullen DJ, Burdick E, Laird N, Petersen LA, Small SD, Sweitzer BJ, Leape L. 1997. The costs of adverse drug events in hospitalized patients. Adverse Drug Events Prevention Study Group. *Journal of the American Medical Association* 277(4):307–311.

Bedell SE, Jabbour S, Goldberg R, Glaser H, Gobble S, Young-Xu Y, Graboys TB, Ravid S. 2000. Discrepancies in the use of medications: Their extent and predictors in an outpatient practice. *Archives of Internal Medicine* 160(14):2129–2134.

Bedouch P, Labarere J, Chirpaz E, Allenet B, Lepape A, Fourny M, Pavese P, Girardet P, Merloz P, Saragaglia D, Calop J, Francois P. 2004. Compliance with guidelines on antibiotic prophylaxis in total hip replacement surgery: Results of a retrospective study of 416 patients in a teaching hospital. *Infection Control and Hospital Epidemiology* 25(4):302–307.

Beers MH. 1997. Explicit criteria for determining potentially inappropriate medication use by the elderly. An update. *Archives of Internal Medicine* 157(14):1531–1536.

Beers MH, Ouslander JG, Rollingher I, Reuben DB, Brooks J, Beck JC. 1991. Explicit criteria for determining inappropriate medication use in nursing home residents. *Archives of Internal Medicine* 151(9):1825–1832.

Bernabei R, Gambassi G, Lapane K. 1998. Management of pain in elderly patients with cancer. SAGE Study Group. Systematic Assessment of Geriatric Drug Use via Epidemiology. *Journal of the American Medical Association* 279:1877–1882.

BLS (Bureau of Labor Statistics). 2006. *Producer Price Indexes*. [Online]. Available: http://www.bls.gov/ppi [accessed June 5, 2006].

Bobb A, Gleason K, Husch M, Feinglass J, Yarnold PR, Noskin GA. 2004. The epidemiology of prescribing errors. *Archives of Internal Medicine* 164(7):785–792.

Bradley JD, Brandt KD, Katz BP, Kalasinski LA, Ryan SI. 1991. Comparison of an anti-inflammatory dose of ibuprofen, an analgesic dose of ibuprofen, and acetaminophen in the treatment of patients with osteoarthritis of the knee. *New England Journal of Medicine* 325(2):87–91.

Brown MN, Lapane KL, Luisi AF. 2002. The management of depression in older nursing home residents. *Journal of the American Geriatrics Society* 50:69–76.

Buchanan TL, Barker KN, Gibson JT, Jiang BC, Pearson RE. 1991. Illumination and errors in dispensing. *American Journal of Hospital Pharmacy* 48(10):2137–2145.

Calabrese AD, Erstad BL, Brandl K, Barletta JF, Kane SL, Sherman DS. 2001. Medication administration errors in adult patients in the ICU. *Intensive Care Medicine* 27(10):1592–1598.

Calis KA, Young LR. 2004. Clinical analysis of adverse drug reactions: A primer for clinicians. *Hospital Pharmacy* 39(7):697–712.

Camp SC, Hailemeskel B, Rogers TL. 2003. Telephone prescription errors in two community pharmacies. *American Journal of Health-System Pharmacy* 60(6):613–614.

Campbell SE, Walke AE, Grimshaw JM, Campbell MK, Lowe GD, Harper D, Fowkes FG, Petrie JC. 2001. The prevalence of prophylaxis for deep vein thrombosis in acute hospital trusts. *International Journal for Quality in Health Care* 13(4):309–316.

Chopard P, Dorffler-Melly J, Hess U, Wuillemin WA, Hayoz D, Gallino A, Bachli EB, Canova CR, Isenegger J, Rubino R, Bounameaux H. 2005. Venous thromboembolism prophylaxis in acutely ill medical patients: Definite need for improvement. *Journal of Internal Medicine* 257(4):352–357.

Classen DC, Pestotnik SL, Evans RS, Burke JP. 1991. Computerized surveillance of adverse drug events in hospital patients. *Journal of the American Medical Association* 266:2847–2851.

Classen DC, Pestotnik SL, Evans RS, Lloyd JF, Burke JP. 1997. Adverse drug events in hospitalized patients. Excess length of stay, extra costs, and attributable mortality. *Journal of the American Medical Association* 277(4):301–306.

Cooper JW. 1987. Adverse drug reactions and interactions in a nursing home. *Nursing Homes and Senior Citizen Care* 36(4):7–11.

Cooper JW. 1999. Adverse drug reaction-related hospitalizations of nursing facility patients: A 4-year study. *Southern Medical Journal* 92(5):485–490.

Cooper S, Zaske D, Hadsall R, Freemont D, Fehr S, Suh D. 1994. Automated medication packaging for long-term care facilities: An evaluation. *The Consultant Pharmacist* 9(1): 58–70.

Cramer JA, Mattson RH, Prevey ML, Scheyer RD, Ouellette VL. 1989. How often is medication taken as prescribed? A novel assessment technique. *Journal of the American Medical Association* 261(22):3273–3277.

Cullen DJ, Bates DW, Small SD, Cooper JB, Nemeskal AR, Leape LL. 1995. The incident reporting system does not detect adverse drug events: A problem for quality improvement. *The Joint Commission Journal on Quality Improvement* 21(10):541–548.

D'Arcy PF. 1993. Adverse reactions and interactions with herbal medicines. Part 2. Drug interactions. *Adverse Drug Reactions and Toxicological Reviews* 12:147–162.

D'Arcy PF, McElnay JC. 1987. Drug-antacid interactions: Assessment of clinical importance. *Drug Intelligence in Clinical Pharmacy* 21(7/8):607–617.

Dean B, Schachter M, Vincent C, Barber N. 2002. Prescribing errors in hospital inpatients: Their incidence and clinical significance. *Quality and Safety in Health Care* 11(4): 340–344.

Dean BS, Allan EL, Barber ND, Barker KN. 1995. Comparison of medication errors in an American and a British hospital. *American Journal of Health-System Pharmacy* 52(22): 2543–2549.

Dennehy CE, Kishi DT, Louie C. 1996. Drug-related illness in emergency department patients. *American Journal of Health-System Pharmacy* 53(12):1422–1426.

Dill JL, Generali JA. 2000. Medication sample labeling practices. *American Journal of Health-System Pharmacy* 57(22):2087–2090.

DiMatteo MR. 2004. Variations in patients' adherence to medication recommendations: A qualitative review of 50 years of research. *Medical Care* 42(3):200–209.

Elam L, Murawski MM, Childs S, Vanable JW. 2005. Patient Safety Forum: Do state Medicaid preferred drug lists affect patient safety? *Psychiatric Services* 56(8):1012–1016.

Ernst ME, Brown GL, Klepser T, Kelly MW. 2001. Medication discrepancies in an outpatient electronic medical record. *American Journal of Health-System Pharmacy* 58(21):2072–2075.

Espino DV, Lancaster MC. 1992. Neutralization of the effects of captopril by the use of ibuprofen in elderly women. *Journal of the American Board of Family Practice* 5(3): 319–321.

Field TS, Gilman BH, Subramanian S, Fuller JC, Bates DW, Gurwitz JH. 2005. The costs associated with adverse drug events among older adults in the ambulatory setting. *Medical Care* 43(12):1171–1176.

Flynn EA, Barker KN, Pepper GA, Bates DW, Mikeal RL. 2002. Comparison of methods for detecting medication errors in 36 hospitals and skilled-nursing facilities. *American Journal of Health-System Pharmacy* 59(5):436–446.

Flynn EA, Barker KN, Carnahan BJ. 2003. National observational study of prescription dispensing accuracy and safety in 50 pharmacies. *Journal of the American Pharmaceutical Association* 43(2):191–200.

Fontan JE, Maneglier V, Nguyen VX, Loirat C, Brion F. 2003. Medication errors in hospitals: Computerized unit dose drug dispensing system versus ward stock distribution system. *Pharmacy World and Science* 25(3):112–117.

Forster AJ, Asmis TR, Clark HD, Al Saied G, Code CC, Caughey SC, Baker K, Watters J, Worthington J, van Walraven C. 2004. Ottawa Hospital Patient Safety Study: Incidence and timing of adverse events in patients admitted to a Canadian teaching hospital. *Canadian Medical Association Journal* 170(8):1235–1240.

Freeman C, Todd C, Camilleri-Ferrante C, Laxton C, Murrell P, Palmer CR, Parker M, Payne B, Rushton N. 2002. Quality improvement for patients with hip fracture: Experience from a multi-site audit. *Quality and Safety in Health Care* 11(3):239–245.

Gambassi G, Forman DE, Lapane KL, Mor V, Sgadari A, Lipsitz LA, Bernabei R, on behalf of The SAGE Study Group. 2000. Management of heart failure among very old persons living in long term care: Has the voice of trials spread? *American Heart Journal* 139(1): 85–89.

Gandhi TK, Seger DL, Bates DW. 2000. Identifying drug safety issues: From research to practice. *International Journal for Quality in Health Care* 12(1):69–76.

Gandhi TK, Weingart SN, Borus J, Seger AC, Peterson J, Burdick E, Seger DL, Shu K, Federico F, Leape LL, Bates DW. 2003. Adverse drug events in ambulatory care. *New England Journal of Medicine* 348(16):1556–1564.

Gandhi TK, Bartel SB, Shulman LN, Verrier D, Burdick E, Cleary A, Rothschild JM, Leape LL, Bates DW. 2005. Medication safety in the ambulatory chemotherapy setting. *Cancer* 104(11):2477–2483.

GAO (Government Accounting Office). 2000. *Adverse Drug Events: The Magnitude of Health Risk Is Uncertain Because of Limited Incidence Data.* Washington, DC: GAO.

Gerety MB, Cornell JE, Plichta DT, Eimer M. 1993. Adverse events related to drugs and drug withdrawal in nursing home residents. *Journal of the American Geriatrics Society* 41(12): 1326–1332.

Goldman RD, Scolnik D. 2004. Underdosing of acetaminophen by parents and emergency department utilization. *Pediatric Emergency Care* 20(2):89–93.

Gonzales R, Steiner JF, Sande MA. 1997. Antibiotic prescribing for adults with colds, upper respiratory tract infections, and bronchitis by ambulatory care physicians. *Journal of the American Medical Association* 278(11):901–904.

Granger CB, Steg PG, Peterson E, Lopez-Sendon J, Van de Werf F, Kline-Rogers E, Allegrone J, Dabbous OH, Klein W, Fox KA, Eagle KA, GRACE Investigators. 2005. Medication performance measures and mortality following acute coronary syndromes. *The American Journal of Medicine* 118(8):858–865.

Grasso BC, Genest R, Jordan CW, Bates DW. 2003. Use of chart and record reviews to detect medication errors in a state psychiatric hospital. *Psychiatric Services* 54(5):677–681.

Gupta N, Kaul-Gupta R, Carstens MM, Franga D, Martindale RG. 2003. Analyzing prophylactic antibiotic administration in procedures lasting more than four hours: Are published guidelines being followed? *The American Surgeon* 69(8):669–673.

Gurwitz JH, Field TS, Avorn J, McCormick D, Jain S , Eckler M, Benser M, Edmondson AC, Bates DW. 2000. Incidence and preventability of adverse drug events in nursing homes. *The American Journal of Medicine* 109(2):87–94.

Gurwitz JH, Field TS, Harrold LR, Rothschild J, Debellis K, Seger AC, Cadoret C, Fish LS, Garber L, Kelleher M, Bates DW. 2003. Incidence and preventability of adverse drug events among older persons in the ambulatory setting. *Journal of the American Medical Association* 289(9):1107–1116.

Gurwitz JH, Field TS, Judge J, Rochon P, Harrold LR, Cadoret C, Lee M, White K, LaPrino J, Mainard JF, DeFlorio M, Gavendo L, Auger J, Bates DW. 2005. The incidence of adverse drug events in two large academic long-term care facilities. *The American Journal of Medicine* 118(3):251–258.

Hajjar I, Kotchen TA. 2003. Trends in prevalence, awareness, treatment, and control of hypertension in the United States, 1988–2000. *Journal of the American Medical Association* 290(2):199–206.

Heineck I, Ferreira MB, Schenkel EB. 1999. Prescribing practice for antibiotic prophylaxis for 3 commonly performed surgeries in a teaching hospital in Brazil. *American Journal of Infection Control* 27(3):296–300.

Houston MC. 1991. Nonsteroidal anti-inflammatory drugs and antihypertensives. *American Journal of Medicine* 190(Suppl. 5A):42S–47S.

Huskamp HA. 2003. Managing psychotropic drug costs: Will formularies work? *Health Affairs* 22(5):84–96.

IOM (Institute of Medicine). 2000. *To Err Is Human: Building a Safer Health System.* Washington, DC: National Academy Press.

Jha AK, Kuperman GJ, Teich JM, Leape L, Shea B, Rittenberg E, Burdick E, Seger DL, Vander Vliet M, Bates DW. 1998. Identifying adverse drug events: Development of a computer-based monitor and comparison with chart review and stimulated voluntary report. *Journal of the American Medical Informatics Association* 5(3):305–314.

Jha AK, Kuperman GJ, Rittenberg E, Teich JM, Bates DW. 2001. Identifying hospital admissions due to adverse drug events using a computer-based monitor. *Pharmacoepidemiology and Drug Safety* 10(2):113–119.

Kaushal R, Bates DW, Landrigan C, McKenna KJ, Clapp MD, Federico F, Goldmann DA. 2001. Medication errors and adverse drug events in pediatric inpatients. *Journal of the American Medical Association* 285(16):2114–2120.

Kaushal R, Jaggi T, Walsh K, Fortescue EB, Bates DW. 2004. Pediatric medication errors: What do we know? What gaps remain? *Ambulatory Pediatrics* 4(1):73–81.

Kistner UA, Keith MR, Sergeant KA, Hokanson JA. 1994. Accuracy of dispensing in a high-volume, hospital-based outpatient pharmacy. *American Journal of Hospital Pharmacy* 51(22):2793–2797.

Kozer E, Scolnik D, Macpherson A, Keays T, Shi K, Luk T, Koren G. 2002. Variables associated with medication errors in pediatric emergency medicine. *Pediatrics* 110(4): 737–742.

Krumholz HM, Chen J, Rathore SS, Wang Y, Radford MJ. 2003. Regional variation in the treatment and outcomes of myocardial infarction: Investigating New England's advantage. *American Heart Journal* 146(2):242–249.

LaPointe NM, Jollis JG. 2003. Medication errors in hospitalized cardiovascular patients. *Archives of Internal Medicine* 163(12):1461–1466.

Leape LL, Bates DW, Cullen DJ, Cooper J, Demonaco HJ, Gallivan T, Hallisey R, Ives J, Laird N, Laffel G, Nemeskal R, Petersen L, Porter K, Servi D, Shea B, Small S, Weitzer B, Thompson B, Vander Vliet M. 1995. Systems analysis of adverse drug events. *Journal of the American Medical Association* 274(1):35–43.

Learhinan ER, Alderman CP. 2003. Venous thromboembolism prophylaxis in a South Australian teaching hospital. *The Annals of Pharmacotherapy* 37(10):1398–1402.

Lesar TS. 2002. Prescribing errors involving medication dosage forms. *Journal of General Internal Medicine* 17(8):579–587.

Lesar TS, Briceland LL, Delcoure K, Parmalee JC, Masta-Gornic V, Pohl H. 1990. Medication prescribing errors in a teaching hospital. *Journal of the American Medical Association* 263(17):2329–2334.

Lesar TS, Lomaestro BM, Pohl H. 1997. Medication-prescribing errors in a teaching hospital. A 9-year experience. *Archives of Internal Medicine* 157(14):1569–1576.

Li SF, Lacher B, Crain EF. 2000. Acetaminophen and ibuprofen dosing by parents. *Pediatric Emergency Care* 16(6):394–397.

Lisby M, Nielsen LP, Mainz J. 2005. Errors in the medication process: Frequency, type, and potential clinical consequences. *International Journal for Quality in Health Care* 17(1): 15–22.

Losek JD. 2004. Acetaminophen dose accuracy and pediatric emergency care. *Pediatric Emergency Care* 20(5):285–288.

Manley HJ, Drayer DK, Muther RS. 2003a. Medication-related problem type and appearance rate in ambulatory hemodialysis patients. *BMC Nephrology* 22:4–10.

Manley HJ, McClaran ML, Overbay DK, Wright MA, Reid GM, Bender WL, Neufeld TK, Hebbar S, Muther RS. 2003b. Factors associated with medication-related problems in ambulatory hemodialysis patients. *American Journal of Kidney Diseases* 41(2):386–393.

McCaig LF, Besser RE, Hughes, JM. 2002. Trends in antimicrobial prescribing rates for children and adolescents. *Journal of the American Medical Association* 287(23):3096–3102.

McCormick D, Gurwitz JH, Goldberg RJ, Becker R, Tate JP, Elwell A, Radford AJ. 2001. Prevalence and quality of warfarin use for patients with atrial fibrillation in the long term care setting. *Archives of Internal Medicine* 161:2458–2463.

McErlean MA, Bartfield JM, Kennedy DA, Gilman EA, Stram RL, Raccio-Robak N. 2001. Home Antipyretic use in children brought to the emergency department. *Pediatric Emergency Care* 17(4):249–251.

McGlynn EA, Asch SM, Adams J, Keesey J, Hicks J, DeCristofaro A, Kerr EA. 2003. The quality of health care delivered to adults in the United States. *New England Journal of Medicine* 348(26):2635–2645.

McPhillips HA, Stille CJ, Smith D, Hecht J, Pearson J, Stull J, Debellis K, Andrade S, Miller MR, Kaushal R, Gurwitz J, Davis RL. 2005. Potential medication dosing errors in outpatient pediatrics. *The Journal of Pediatrics* 147(6):761–767.

Murff HJ, Patel VL, Hripcsak G, Bates DW. 2003. Detecting adverse events for patient safety research: A review of current methodologies. *Journal of Biomedical Informatics* 36(1–2):131–143.

Nebeker JR, Barach P, Samore MH. 2004. Clarifying adverse drug events: A clinician's guide to terminology, documentation, and reporting. *Annals of Internal Medicine* 140(10):795–801.

Nebeker JR, Hoffman JM, Weir CR, Bennett CL, Hurdle JF. 2005. High rates of adverse drug events in a highly computerized hospital. *Archives of Internal Medicine* 165(10):1111–1116.

Newby LK, LaPointe NMA, Chen AY, Kramer JM, Hammill BG, DeLong ER, Muhlbaier LH, Califf RM. 2006. Long-term adherence to evidence-based secondary prevention therapies in coronary artery disease. *Circulation* 113(2):203–212.

Nyquist AC, Gonzales R, Steiner JF, Sande MA. 1998. Antibiotic prescribing for children with colds, upper respiratory tract infections, and bronchitis. *Journal of the American Medical Association* 279(11):875–877.

O'Neil AC, Petersen LA, Cook EF, Bates DW, Lee TH, Brennan TA. 1993. Physician reporting compared with medical-record review to identify adverse medical events. *Annals of Internal Medicine* 119(5):370–376.

Pearson SA, Ross-Degnan D, Payson A, Soumerai SB. 2003. Changing medication use in managed care: A critical review of the available evidence. *American Journal of Managed Care* 9(11):715–731.

Petersen LA, Normand SL, Leape L, McNeil BJ. 2001. Comparison of use of medications after acute myocardial infarction in the Veterans Health Administration and Medicare. *Circulation* 104(24):2898–2904.

Petersen LA, Normand SL, Druss BG, Rosenheck RA. 2003. Process of care and outcome after acute myocardial infarction for patients with mental illness in the VA health care system: Are there disparities? *Health Services Research* 38(1 Pt. 1):41–63.

Piscitelli SC, Gallicano KD. 2001. Interactions among drugs for HIV and opportunistic infections. *New England Journal of Medicine* 344(13):984–986.

Piscitelli SC, Burstein AH, Chaitt D, Alfaro RM, Falloon J. 2000. Indinavir concentrations and St. John's Wort. *Lancet* 355:547–548.

Potts AL, Barr FE, Gregory DF, Wright L, Patel NR. 2004. Computerized physician order entry and medication errors in a pediatric critical care unit. *Pediatrics* 113(1 Pt. 1):59–63.

Quenon JL, Eveillard M, Vivien A, Bourderont D, Lepape A, Lathelize M, Jestin C. 2004. Evaluation of current practices in surgical antimicrobial prophylaxis in primary total hip prosthesis: A multicentre survey in private and public French hospitals. *The Journal of Hospital Infection* 56(3):202–207.

Roe MT, Parsons LS, Pollack CV, Canto JG, Barron HV, Every NR, Rogers WJ, Peterson ED. 2005. Quality of care by classification of myocardial infarction: Treatment patterns for ST-segment elevation vs. non-ST-segment elevation myocardial infarction. *Archives of Internal Medicine* 165(14):1630–1636.

Roumie CL, Halasa NB, Grijalva CG, Edwards KM, Zhu Y, Dittus RS, Griffin MR. 2005. Trends in antibiotic prescribing for adults in the United States—1995 to 2002. *Journal of General Internal Medicine* 20(8):697–702.

Rozich JD, Resar RK. 2001. Medication safety: One organizations approach to the challenge. *Journal of Clinical Outcomes Management* 8(10):27–34.

Ruschitzka F, Meier PJ, Turina M, Luscher T, Noll G. 2000. Acute heart transplant rejection due to Saint John's Wort. *Lancet* 355:548–549.

Sackett DL, Snow, JC. 1979. *Compliance in Health Care.* Baltimore, MD: Johns Hopkins University Press.

Sanborn TA, Jacobs AK, Frederick PD, Every NR, French WJ. 2004. Comparability of quality-of-care indicators for emergency coronary angioplasty in patients with acute myocardial infarction regardless of on-site cardiac surgery (report from the National Registry of Myocardial Infarction). *The American Journal of Cardiology* 93(11):1335–1339.

Scott IA, Denaro CP, Flores JL, Bennett CJ, Hickey AC, Mudge AM, Atherton J. 2003. Quality of care of patients hospitalized with congestive heart failure. *Internal Medicine Journal* 33(4):140–151.

Senst BL, Achusim LE, Genest RP, Consentino LA, Ford CC, Little JA, Raybon SJ, Bates DW. 2001. Practical approach to determining costs and frequency of adverse drug events in a health care network. *American Journal of Health-System Pharmacy* 58(12):1126–1132.

Shaughnessy AF, Nickel RO. 1989. Prescription-writing patterns and errors in a family medicine residency program. *The Journal of Family Practice* 29(3):290–295.

Singh G, Ramey DR, Morfeld D, Shi H, Haroum HT, Fries JF. 1996. Gastrointestinal tract complications of nonsteroidal anti-inflammatory drug treatment in rheumatoid arthritis: A prospective observational cohort study. *Archives of Internal Medicine* 156:1530–1536.

Sloane PD, Gruber-Baldini AL, Zimmerman S, Roth M, Watson L, Boustani M, Magaziner J, Hebel JR. 2004. Medication undertreatment in assisted living settings. *Archives of Internal Medicine* 164(18):2031–2037.

Smeaton L, Sheikh A, Avery A, Royal S, Hurwitz B, Dewey M. 2002. Interventions for reducing preventable drug-related hospital admissions or preventable drug-related morbidity in primary care (Protocol). *The Cochrane Database of Systematic Reviews* Issue 4. Art. No.: CD003942. DOI: 10.1002/14651858.CD003942.

Stone S, Gonzales R, Maselli J, Lowenstein SR. 2000. Antibiotic prescribing for patients with colds, upper respiratory tract infections, and bronchitis: A national study of hospital-based emergency departments. *Annals of Emergency Medicine* 36(4):320–327.

Sun BC, Bates DW, Sussman A. 2005. Effects of a hospital formulary on outpatient drug switching. *Journal of Clinical Outcomes Management* 12(9):459–463.

Tafreshi MJ, Melby MJ, Kaback KR, Nord TC. 1999. Medication-related visits to the emergency department: A prospective study. *The Annals of Pharmacotherapy* 33(12):1252–1257.

Tan LH, Tan SC. 2004. Venous thromboembolism prophylaxis for surgical patients in an Asian hospital. *ANZ Journal of Surgery* 74(6):455–459.

Taxis K, Barber N. 2003. Ethnographic study of incidence and severity of intravenous drug errors. *British Medical Journal* 326(7391):684.

Taxis K, Dean B, Barber N. 1999. Hospital drug distribution systems in the UK and Germany: A study of medication errors. *Pharmacy World and Science* 21(1):25–31.

Teagarden JR, Nagle B, Aubert RE, Wasdyke C, Courtney P, Epstein RS. 2005. Dispensing error rate in a highly automated mail-service pharmacy practice. *Pharmacotherapy* 25(11):1629–1635.

Thomas MG, Arroll B. 2000. "Just say no"—reducing the use of antibiotics for colds, bronchitis and sinusitis. *New Zealand Medical Journal* 113(1113):287–289.

Tissot E, Cornette C, Demoly P, Jacquet M, Barale F, Capellier G. 1999. Medication errors at the administration stage in an intensive care unit. *Intensive Care Medicine* 25(4): 353–359.

Tissot E, Cornette C, Limat S, Mourand JL, Becker M, Etievent JP, Dupond JL, Jacquet M, Woronoff-Lemsi MC. 2003. Observational study of potential risk factors of medication administration errors. *Pharmacy World and Science* 25(6):264–268.

Vaisbrud V, Raveh D, Schlesinger Y, Yinnon AM. 1999. Surveillance of antimicrobial prophylaxis for surgical procedures. *Infection Control and Hospital Epidemiology* 20(9): 610–613.

van den Bemt PM, Postma MJ, van Roon EN, Chow MC, Fijn R, Brouwers JR. 2002. Cost-benefit analysis of the detection of prescribing errors by hospital pharmacy staff. *Drug Safety* 25(2):135–143.

van Kasteren ME, Kullberg BJ, de Boer AS, Mintjes-de Groot J, Gyssens IC. 2003. Adherence to local hospital guidelines for surgical antimicrobial prophylaxis: A multicentre audit in Dutch hospitals. *The Journal of Antimicrobial Chemotherapy* 51(6):1389–1396.

Wagner MM, Hogan WR. 1996. The accuracy of medication data in an outpatient electronic medical record. *Journal of the American Medical Informatics Association* 3(3):234–244.

Winterstein AG, Johns TE, Rosenberg EI, Hatton RC, Gonzalez-Rothi R, Kanjanarat P. 2004. Nature and causes of clinically significant medication errors in a tertiary care hospital. *American Journal of Health-System Pharmacy* 61(18):1908–1916.

Wirtz V, Taxis K, Barber ND. 2003. An observational study of intravenous medication errors in the United Kingdom and in Germany. *Pharmacy World and Science* 25(3):104–111.

Won A, Lapane K, Gambassi G, Bernabei R, Mor V, Lipsitz LA. 1999. Correlates and management of nonmalignant pain in the nursing home. SAGE Study Group. Systematic assessment of geriatric drug use via epidemiology. *Journal of the American Geriatrics Society* 47:936–942.

Won AB, Lapane KL, Vallow S, Schein J, Morris JN, Lipsitz LA. 2004. Persistent nonmalignant pain and analgesic prescribing patterns in elderly nursing home residents. *Journal of the American Geriatrics Society* 52(6):867–874.

Wood W, Nam B. 2005. Using workload measures as a management tool to increase pharmacy full-time equivalents. *ASHP Midyear Clinical Meeting* P-259D.

Part II

Moving Toward a Patient-Centered, Integrated Medication-Use System

TRANSFORMING THE MEDICATION-USE SYSTEM

Medication safety as a strategic goal and core value of health care is essential at all levels of the health care system—that of patient/consumer in terms of both self-management and relationship–partnership with the provider; that of provider microsystems (e.g., small units of care); that of systems, products, and stakeholders that support the consumer, the consumer–provider relationship, and provider microsystems; and that of the environment, which includes research, regulatory, and legal factors important to the function of each of the other levels and the system as a whole (Leape et al., 1998). From this perspective, medication safety becomes everyone's responsibility. All individuals, departments, committees, teams, and services apply safety principles in their work (CIHSP, 2001). Management provides necessary resources, incentives, and rewards for optimal safety performance. There is openness, including with patients and families, regarding errors and problems. Safety decisions are made by those in the best position to protect the patient, regardless of rank or hierarchy (CIHSP, 2001). At the heart of all care is patient- and family-centeredness encompassing the qualities of compassion; empathy; and responsiveness to the needs, values, and expressed preferences of the individual (IOM, 2001). This new system, then, is different in attitude, culture, design, and operation (Christopherson, 2004) from the health care system whose deficiencies were highlighted in the *Quality Chasm* report (IOM, 2001).

Given these deficiencies, the *Quality Chasm* report called for profound changes and a paradigm shift away from a paternalistic, provider-centric system. The report outlined 10 new rules to guide the transition to a health care system that would better meet patients' needs (IOM, 2001, p. 8–9):

1. *Care based on continuous healing relationships.* Patients should receive care whenever they need it and in many forms, not just face-to-face visits. This rule implies that the health care system should be responsive at all times (24 hours a day, every day) and that access to care should be provided over the Internet, by telephone, and by other means in addition to face-to-face visits.

2. *Customization based on patient needs and values.* The system of care should be designed to meet the most common types of needs, but have the capability to respond to individual patient choices and preferences.

3. *The patient as the source of control.* Patients should be given the necessary information and the opportunity to exercise the degree of control they choose over health care decisions that affect them. The health system should be able to accommodate differences in patient preferences and encourage shared decision making.

4. *Shared knowledge and the free flow of information.* Patients should have unfettered access to their own medical information and to clinical knowledge. Clinicians and patients should communicate effectively and share information.

5. *Evidence-based decision making.* Patients should receive care based on the best available scientific knowledge. Care should not vary illogically from clinician to clinician or from place to place.

6. *Safety as a system property.* Patients should be safe from injury caused by the care system. Reducing risk and ensuring safety require greater attention to systems that help prevent and mitigate errors.

7. *The need for transparency.* The health care system should make information available to patients and their families that allows them to make informed decisions when selecting a health plan, hospital, or clinical practice, or choosing among alternative treatments. This should include information describing the system's performance on safety, evidence-based practice, and patient satisfaction.

8. *Anticipation of needs.* The health system should anticipate patient needs, rather than simply reacting to events.

9. *Continuous decrease in waste.* The health system should not waste resources or patient time.

10. *Cooperation among clinicians.* Clinicians and institutions should actively collaborate and communicate to ensure an appropriate exchange of information and coordination of care.

These rules serve as the basis for the discussion of medication safety and quality improvement in this report. Applying these rules, the committee developed a new vision of a patient-centered, integrated medication-use system. This model, outlined in Table II-1, is intended to engender new expectations and actions on the part of those involved at all levels of the system by conceptualizing important factors that influence the current and the envisioned, safe state. More in-depth discussion of specific actions that can be taken to achieve the safe state is presented in Chapters 4 through 8.

TABLE II-1 Transforming the Medication-Use System: Where We Are and Where We Want to Be

Reality: Where We Generally Are	Vision: Where We Want to Be
Patient and Community Experiences	
The health system is provider-centric and provider-directed.	The health system is patient-centered; patients are listened to and respected as informed, engaged full partners and the source of control.
The patient experience is highly variable; minimum expectations are not consistently met.	Specific patient rights and expectations are honored across the health system and applied specifically and consistently to the medication-use process.
Providers focus on patient medications in the context of an encounter.	Patient health and satisfaction are the focus, optimized through self-care, self-management, and the continuum of care.
Self-management issues include nonadherence, knowledge deficits, practical barriers, and attitudinal barriers.	Through supportive interventions, education, patient contracts, and behavioral change, patients are skilled in managing wellness, along with their acute, chronic, and disability needs.
Families and caregivers are not generally recognized or supported.	Families and caregivers are encouraged to be full participants in care.
Patients, families, providers, and pharmacies lack a single accurate patient medication record.	Each patient has a single electronic medication record. The patient, all providers, and pharmacies work from this record. All medications are reconciled against this record.
Over-the-counter (OTC) drugs and dietary supplements are not considered medications for purposes of the medication record.	Medications, OTCs, and dietary supplements are part of the medication record and patient care.

continued

TABLE II-1 continued

Reality: Where We Generally Are	Vision: Where We Want to Be
Medication education is not a high priority, nor is it provided according to literacy levels.	Education is a priority, with verbal counseling and materials the patient can understand, and with sensitivity to culture and lifestyle.
Medication instructions are variable, presented with too much information, difficult to read, and inadequate.	Medication instructions are standardized, focused, comprehensive, and useful, and designed to maximize safety.
Staffing levels prevent providers from giving careful care, making respectful inquiries, and educating the patient.	Staffing calculations and expectations allow for careful care, respectful inquiries, and patient education.
The patient's medication experience is one of fragile processes, inconsistency, defects, and waste.	The medication-use process produces for the patient consistently high reliability and performance.
Patients are unclear about where to go for additional medication information and answers to questions.	Providers and pharmacies provide around-the-clock telephone and Internet resources to answer medication questions.
Patients are unclear on expectations for reporting complications and on how to report and resolve complications when they occur.	Clinicians provide appropriate instructions and encouragement to patients for reporting of adverse side effects. Resources to address complications from prescriptions are available around the clock.
Patients do not receive clear explanations on what to do if an adverse event or unanticipated medication outcome occurs.	After experiencing an adverse event or unanticipated medication outcome, patients, as well as families as appropriate, receive support, with their concerns addressed.
Patients feel distanced from health care staff and organizations and get few answers when a medication error occurs.	Patients, and families as appropriate, receive truth and support, being told what happened, why, what to expect, and what is being done to prevent a recurrence, as well as a statement of regret or apology.
Patients lack mechanisms to report medication errors for accountability or learning purposes.	Reporting systems with multiple options capture reports of medication errors from patients and families.
Patients do not experience a system that is organized for care across multiple settings or during care transitions.	The system is patient-centered, with active support across transitions of care. In partnership with the patient, a clinician is responsible for coordination of care, and in this case, medication management.

TABLE II-1 continued

Reality: Where We Generally Are	Vision: Where We Want to Be
Patients on chronic therapy may not be subject to appropriate monitoring for toxicities and side effects.	Patients receive appropriate monitoring (laboratory tests) to detect any harm resulting from chronic administration of medications.
Requests for renewals of medications are cumbersome and unreconciled.	Patients have easy access to telephone and Internet-based prescription renewals with concurrent reconciliation.
Patients are dependent on clinicians for medication safety alerts.	Safety alerts are communicated directly to patients, and follow-up measures are taken.

Organizational and Microsystem-Based Medication-Use Processes

Professional autonomy drives variability.	Medications are customized to patient needs and values.
Medication safety is an individual responsibility.	Medication safety is a system property.
Safety can be overridden by volume and time pressures.	Providing safe care is always the highest priority.
Secrecy is necessary.	Transparency is necessary.
Staffing is based on historical trends and budgetary considerations.	Staffing is based on workload and the complexity of patients needs.
Medication orders are largely paper-based.	Medication orders are computer-based, with decision support.
The safety of medication orders depends on the vigilance of the ordering physician, nurses, pharmacists, and others. Systems to validate the total medication management plan are not in place or not consistently used. Patients may be taking medications no longer needed or therapeutic duplications, or may not be taking medications on an optimum administration schedule.	All clinicians have immediate access to complete patient information and point-of-care reference information. The ordering process is guided by medication knowledge bases and other decision-support tools. Reconciliation is ongoing. In addition to being reviewed at the time of each prescribing event, a patient's medication regimen is reviewed at least every X months to minimize therapeutic duplications, drug interactions, unnecessary treatments, and the like.
Medication communications are unstructured and often oral.	Medication communications are inter-disciplinary and structured and include the patient.

continued

TABLE II-1 continued

Reality: Where We Generally Are	Vision: Where We Want to Be
Orders called into pharmacies are oral and error-prone.	All prescriptions are written and received in pharmacies electronically (e-prescribing), with appropriate decision support available in pharmacy computer systems.
The medication administration record is typically paper-based, incomplete, and broadly inaccessible.	A single electronic medication administration record is broadly accessible.
The incidence of near-misses, adverse drug events, and medication errors is generally unknown by setting.	All settings know their specific incidence of near-misses, adverse drug events, and medication errors through improved monitoring.
Learning with regard to medication errors, when it does occur, is limited to a single setting.	There is dissemination and diffusion of organizational learning from errors, with reporting to national agencies.
Reports of medication errors lead to punitive responses.	Reporting stimulates learning in a fair and just culture.
The impact of medication management on health outcomes is unknown.	Studies are conducted of medication management's impact on outcomes, by setting, both individually and collectively.
Processes supporting medication management have evolved over time, with multiple steps and high complexity.	The medication management process is carefully designed, using principles and tools such as lean reliability and six-sigma, to produce reliable results 100 percent of the time.
Medication management improvement activities are focused on pharmacy quality assurance.	Medication management quality improvement activities are interdisciplinary and systemwide, and include the patient's experience.
The focus of care coordination and medication management is on transitions into and out of one setting.	Care coordination embraces the whole experience of medication care.
Medication selection may be driven by cost rather than by optimization of therapy.	The approach to health care expenses and decisions to treat is holistic, based on what is best for the patient.
The focus of medication management is cost reduction.	The focus of medication management is waste reduction.

TABLE II-1 continued

Reality: Where We Generally Are	Vision: Where We Want to Be
Environmental Context for Medication-Use Processes	
Patients experience disjointed care, with confusing/contradictory medication management.	Medication treatment management programs are supported with incremental funding.
Adoption of electronic medical records and e-prescribing continues to be slow.	Financial incentives and baseline e-prescribing standards rapidly accelerate adoption.
Commercial pharmacy quality assurance and improvement activities are voluntary and inconsistent.	Medication management/pharmacy quality assurance and quality improvement are mandatory in all settings.
Medication safety education is fragmented and inconsistently delivered to the interdisciplinary team.	Stakeholders develop and disseminate standardized interdisciplinary medication education safety programs.
Direct-to-consumer marketing can result in misleading claims about the effectiveness of medications.	Clinicians and patients have the information they need to make informed decisions about medications. Manufacturers agree to curb claims in their advertising.
Medication information resources are scattered and disjointed.	Consumer-based resource centers for medication and safety information are widely distributed.
Drug naming, labeling, and information sheet development are complex and confusing and lead to errors.	A focused research agenda is aimed at determining what strategies and tactics can improve understanding and reduce errors.
The legal environment discourages transparency, reporting, and learning, as well as appropriate responses to claims.	All components of the medication-use system, including the patient, consider the current legal and claims system fair and just.
Some adverse medication events with harm are unavoidable—"the cost of doing business."	A concerted effort is made to reduce, minimize, or mitigate harm by reconsidering current treatment plans, dosing levels, and/or use of adjunctive therapy.

NOTE: This table is organized around the chain of effect in improving health care quality as identified by Berwick (2002).

MAKING THE VISION A REALITY:
AN OVERVIEW OF THE REMAINDER OF THE REPORT

The committee believes a key step in improving the safety of the medication-use process is establishing a strong patient–provider partnership. Chapter 4 provides guidance on ways for both patient and the provider to strengthen this partnership. In addition, the chapter recommends ways of improving the information infrastructure available to the patient.

Chapter 5 contains the committee's recommendations on short- and long-term system changes that health care organizations can make in the medication-use process in three settings—the inpatient, nursing home, and outpatient—and in care transitions.

Pharmaceutical, medical device, and health information technology companies represent the chief product-related industry sectors of the medication-use system. Chapter 6 provides an action agenda for design improvements to the information products and medical devices produced by these industries, focused on improving medication safety.

The committee uncovered enormous gaps in the knowledge base regarding medication errors. In Chapter 7, the committee proposes an applied research agenda for the safe use of medications across all care settings, covering research methodologies, incidence rates, costs of medication errors, reporting systems, and testing of error prevention strategies.

Finally, health care delivery is shaped by legislators, regulators, accreditors, and payers. Chapter 8 proposes ways for these stakeholders to motivate the adoption of practices and technologies that can reduce medication errors, and to ensure that professionals have the competencies required to deliver medications safely.

REFERENCES

Berwick DM. 2002. A user's manual for the IOM's "Quality Chasm" report. *Health Affairs (Millwood)* 21(3):80–90.

Christopherson G. 2004. *Person-Centered Health*. Notes: Draft document provided to IOM staff.

CIHSP (California Institute for Health System Performance). 2001. *A Compendium of Suggested Practices for Preventing and Reducing Medication Errors*. Sacramento, CA: CIHSP.

IOM (Institute of Medicine). 2001. *Crossing the Quality Chasm: A New Health System for the 21st Century*. Washington, DC: National Academy Press.

Leape LL, Kabcenell A, Berwick DM, Roessner J. 1998. *Breakthrough Series Guide: Reducing Adverse Drug Events*. Boston, MA: Institute for Healthcare Improvement.

4

Action Agenda to Support the Consumer–Provider Partnership

CHAPTER SUMMARY

A key step in improving the safety of the medication-use process is establishing a consumer–provider partnership. The consumer of health care—the patient—is the person with the greatest stake in identifying and preventing medication errors. The chapter addresses ways in which both consumers and providers (including physicians, nurses, and pharmacists) can strengthen the consumer–patient partnership. There are also many areas for improvement in consumer-oriented drug information.

According to a 2004 survey by the Kaiser Family Foundation, 48 percent of Americans are concerned about the safety of the medical care they and their families receive, and 55 percent are dissatisfied with the quality of the nation's health care—up from 44 percent who expressed this view in a survey conducted 4 years ago (KFF, 2004). Results of other national and international surveys indicate that 34 to 40 percent of individuals have experienced a medical error themselves or know of a family member or friend who has (CMWF 2005; NPSF, 1997). A National Patient Safety Foundation survey found that among those who had personally experienced an error, 40 percent of the errors were due to mistakes in diagnosis and wrong treatments. Medication errors accounted for 28 percent of the errors, while 22 percent were the result of mistakes during surgery. In a six-country survey by the Commonwealth Fund, 28 to 32 percent of patients in each country said treatment risks had not been completely explained during their hospital stay. In addition, 55 to 64 percent of patients said physicians had not always reviewed all their medications during the past year, and 47 to 69 percent stated that physicians did not always explain the side effects of medications (CMWF, 2005).

Usually, people are not told about an error unless injury or death occurs. In a nationally representative survey of hospital risk managers, the vast majority reported that their hospital's practice was to disclose harm at least some of the time, although only one-third of hospitals actually had board-approved policies for doing so in place (Lamb et al., 2003). More than half of respondents stated that they would always disclose a death or serious injury; when presented with actual clinical scenarios, however, respondents revealed they were much less likely to disclose preventable harm than to disclose nonpreventable harm of comparable severity. In a 2004 survey by the Premier Safety Institute, no respondents indicated that disclosures of errors causing serious or short-term harm were never given; 57 percent said such errors were frequently disclosed to patients or families, while 37 percent said such disclosures were always made (PSI, 2004).

The following is an example of a medication error that resulted in a fatality:

> Eighteen-month-old Josie King was admitted to the hospital for first- and second-degree burns received when she climbed into a hot tub. She spent 10 days in the pediatric intensive care unit, with her mother being vigilant as to the details of her care. Josie was recovering and was transferred to an intermediate care floor for a few more days. After her central line was removed, however, her condition worsened. Although her mother expressed concern about Josie's new symptoms, which at one point included sucking avidly on a wet washcloth, those concerns were not addressed by the shift nurses. Moreover, despite a doctor's order that no narcotics be administered to the child, and over the objections of her mother, Josie received a narcotic pain medication 2 days before she was to go home. She then experienced cardiac arrest. In retrospect, the child's symptoms reflected progressive dehydration. Josie's mother is among the many individuals, parents, and surrogates whose voices are often ignored by providers (JKF, 2002).

The following are examples of medication errors with the potential to result in death or serious harm:

> A child with leukemia was discharged from the hospital with a nasogastric tube in place for intermittent enteral feeding. While readmitted for chemotherapy, he developed an infection and had a peripherally inserted central catheter (PICC) emplaced for the administration of antibiotics. He recovered from the infection and was discharged. Shortly thereafter, the

PICC line clotted. His mother called the home care nurse. When the nurse arrived, she found that the mother was about to use a syringe of ginger ale to clear the PICC line and prevented a serious error. Having been taught to clear the child's feeding tube with ginger ale, the mother thought the same could be done with the PICC line. She is just one example of the many caretakers who do not receive adequate discharge counseling (Cohen, 2000).

A middle-aged man with newly developed asthma was prescribed an inhaler, but was not responding to treatment. During a follow-up visit, he described how he was using the inhaler. He would squirt two puffs in the air and breathe deeply for 15 minutes. He said he'd been instructed to do this by his doctor, who had picked up an inhaler, held it in the air, and released two puffs to demonstrate its use. The doctor had given the man no further instructions. The man had not read the instructions on the package because he was functionally illiterate. He is an example of the millions of Americans who do not receive adequate medication instructions and have difficulty with basic reading and writing (Cohen, 2000).

Each of the above cases illustrates the potentially lethal consequences of inadequate and ineffective interactions between consumers (patients or surrogates) and providers. The cases underscore the most common complaint about providers—they fail to take the time to listen and to explain. Some communication problems have been attributed to the fact that many health care providers focus on diseases and their management rather than on people, their lives, and their health issues (Lewin at al., 2005). Other issues concern the lack of understanding and respect for patients' rights to be informed and to play an active role in their and their family members' care. Unfortunately, such circumstances are commonplace (Annas, 2004; KFF, 2004; CMWF, 2005). Care delivered without good communication and follow-through on patient rights is provider-centric when in truth, consumers want and increasingly expect care that is patient-centered (Cleary, 1993). The Institute for Healthcare Improvement's program on Patient and Family Voices has identified key aspects of patient-centered care desired by consumers (see Box 4-1).

FOUNDATION FOR IMPROVEMENT

Improving safety and quality in the medication-use system requires a shift from the conventional approach to care toward a patient-centered model based on consumer–provider partnership and communication. The foundation for this change has several elements discussed in this chapter. First, all participants in the health care delivery system need to acquire a thorough understanding of what patient-centered care really entails in terms of both the consumer–provider relationship and the culture of the health

---

BOX 4-1
Patients' Expectations of Their Providers

- To be listened to, taken seriously, and respected as a care partner.
  - To have family/caregivers treated the same.
  - To participate in decision making at the level they choose.
- To always be told the truth.
  - To have things explained fully and clearly.
  - To receive an explanation and apology if things go wrong.
- To have information communicated to the entire care team.
  - To have care promptly and impeccably documented.
  - To have these records made available if requested.
- For care to be coordinated among all members of the health care team across settings.
  - To be supported emotionally as well as physically.
  - To receive high-quality, safe care.

SOURCE: IHI, 2005.

---

care organization. Second, consumers need to be empowered to play an active role in their care through the establishment of patient rights that are ensured at all points along the medication-use continuum, enhancing the presence, power, and participation of consumers in their relationships with providers. Third, certain basic, definitive actions can be taken to minimize and prevent medication errors and other safety issues; for example, the consumer can carry a medication list, and the provider can regularly practice medication reconcilation. Fourth, participants in the health care delivery system should seek to understand and address barriers to patient-centered care, patient–provider communication, and consumer medication self-management. Finally, resources need to be developed to support partnership, communication, and self-management. The first two of these elements are discussed below; the others are addressed in the remainder of the chapter.

Understanding Patient-Centered Care

Understanding patient-centered care is critical to quality and safety in medication use. Patient-centered care is an approach that adopts perspective of patients—what matters to them, what affects them either positively or negatively, and their experience of illness (Gerteis et al., 1993). The aim is to see people in their biopsychosocial entirety, understanding the whole person, sharing power and responsibility, and drawing attention to patients' individual identities (Armstrong, 1982; Stewart, 1995; Stewart et al., 1995; Mead and Bower, 2000). The approach recognizes that important aspects of the patient's experience have just as much to do with the quality of care delivery during interactions with medical staff as the actual medical care itself (Frampton et al., 2003). It focuses attention on the heart of the patient–provider relationship—communication during each clinical encounter, whether a consultation, intervention, or simple exchange. Patient-centered care that embodies both effective communication and technical skill is necessary to achieve safety and quality of care (Griffin et al., 2004).

Although a number of definitions have been presented in the academic and clinical literature (Frampton et al., 2003; Lewin et al., 2005), the Committee on Identifying and Preventing Medication Errors uses the multifaceted definition developed by Gerteis and colleagues (1993) and espoused in previous Institute of Medicine (IOM) reports. This definition encompasses seven primary dimensions of patient-centered care, as described in Box 4-2: (1) respect for patients' values, preferences, and expressed needs; (2) coordination and integration of care; (3) information, communication, and education; (4) physical comfort; (5) emotional support and alleviation of fear and anxiety; (6) involvement of family and friends; and (7) transition and continuity. Effective, patient-centered communication along these dimensions supports a more collaborative consumer–provider relationship whereby the joint definition of problems, treatment goals, and management strategies can be accomplished (Von Korff et al., 1997; Wolpert and Anderson, 2001). This collaboration, in turn, can lead to improved patient satisfaction, engagement in decision making, participation in prevention activities (Flach et al., 2004), better self-management of chronic conditions (Heisler et al., 2002), and adherence to medication regimens (Safran et al., 1998).

Even though the benefits of patient-centered communication are well understood, they have not been well implemented across health care settings, institutions, and practices (IOM, 2001). In today's health care system, such communication is sometimes sacrificed as a result of the intrusion of business into clinical practice, the pressures of limited time for office visits, the culture of medicalization, and the often all-consuming focus on technology (Teutsch, 2003). There is a misconception that supportive interactions require more staff or more time and are therefore more costly (Frampton et al., 2003). This is not necessarily the case. Rather, it could be argued that negative interactions (e.g., alienating patients, being unresponsive to their needs, or limiting their sense of control) can be very costly in terms of lost patient revenues, poor health outcomes, and, in some cases, increased likelihood of litigation (Frampton et al., 2003). For example, insufficient communication about medications can lead to nonadherence

BOX 4-2
Dimensions of Patient-Centered Care

1. *Respect for patients' values, preferences, and expressed needs.* Respecting patients' individuality and restoring their autonomy entails: paying attention to the impact that their condition or treatment has on their quality of life or subjective sense of well-being; involvement in decision making; being treated with dignity and respect, and sensitivity to their cultural values; and meeting their expectations and needs for autonomy.

2. *Coordination and integration of care.* Understanding patients' feeling of vulnerability and powerlessness in the face of illness and their need for competent and caring staff to coordinate and integrate clinical care effectively, including ancillary and support services, and "front-line" patient care.

3. *Information, communication, and education.* Respecting patients' need for information on clinical status, progress, and prognosis delivered accurately in a manner they understand; information on processes of care, how alternative treatments might affect their subjective well-being and clinical status, and information about the reasoning behind clinical decisions.

4. *Physical comfort.* Providing the most basic elements of physical comfort includes staff who listen and are attentive to patients' complaints about pain, help them with activities of daily living, and keep them clean and comfortable in an environment that is reasonably pleasant.

5. *Emotional support and alleviation of fear and anxiety.* Understanding that the emotions experienced in relation to illness may be as debilitating as the physical effects, and attending to and alleviating their fear and anxiety over clinical status, treatment, and prognosis; over the impact of the illness on self and family; and over the financial impact of the illness.

6. *Involvement of family and friends.* Accommodating patients' wishes for involvement or noninvolvement of family and friends relative to emotional support and decision making, and providing support and resources to family or friends who are caregiving in both immediate and extended term.

7. *Transition and continuity.* Addressing patients' concerns about their ability to care for themselves away from the clinical setting, their need to receive adequate information about their medications, dietary or other treatment regimens, and danger signals to look out for; their need for information about the plans made and services coordinated for continuing care and treatment; and their need for information to access clinical, social, physical, and financial support on a continuing basis if needed.

SOURCE: Gerteis et al., 1993.

and increased hospitalization (DiMatteo, 2004). Conversely, good communication can obviate the need for extensive discussions about the medication regimen with every patient during every visit.

Methods for incorporating patient-centered communication about medications into day-to-day clinical practice can be drawn from the Chronic Care Model (as well as others employed to develop consumers' self-management skills). The Chronic Illness Care Breakthrough Series Collaboratives established by the Institute for Healthcare Improvement and Associates in Process Improvement developed a five-component model of key steps to patient-centered self-management support (Glasgow et al., 2002) (see Figure 4-1). It is designed to organize evidence-based intervention components into an integrated and understandable iterative process appropriate for incorporation into busy primary care practices. The five components are as follows: (1) current self-management beliefs and behaviors are assessed, with feedback for both providers and patients; (2) the feedback prompts collaborative goal setting between patients and provider(s); (3) a personal action plan for self-management is developed; (4) initial self-management goals are refined and informed through the identification of anticipated barriers to and supports for the achievement

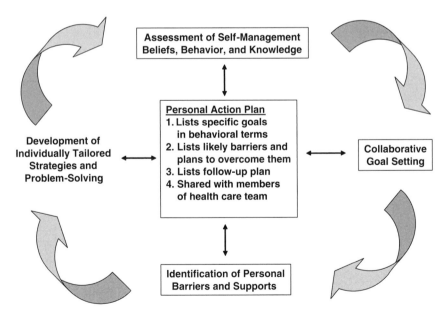

FIGURE 4-1 The Chronic Care Model: Key steps to patient-centered, self-management support.
SOURCE: Glasgow et al., 2002.

of those goals and a better understanding of the patient's perspective and the social environment in which self-management must be conducted; and (5) individually tailored strategies and problem-solving approaches are developed to enhance self-efficacy and provide patients with strategies for overcoming the barriers identified (Glasgow et al., 2002). These steps are repeated in an iterative, ongoing, flexible way at future encounters. Glasgow and colleagues (2002) believe this model is different from that used in most health care settings in that it is patient-centered, individualized, and self-correcting, and encompasses the overall care of a patient's health conditions rather than being an isolated activity.

Self-management education programs have been found to improve patient health outcomes (IOM, 2003). For example, a study that investigated the effects of self-management education and regular practitioner review for adults with asthma demonstrated a statistically significant reduction in the proportion of subjects reporting hospitalizations and emergency room visits, unscheduled physician visits, days lost from work, and episodes of nocturnal asthma (Gibson et al., 2000).

The above steps outlined for chronic care could easily be adapted to patient-centered care for improved medication self-management. In fact, Svarstad and colleagues (1999) developed a brief medication questionnaire for patients as a means of identifying those who need assistance with their medications, assessing their concerns, evaluating new ways to assist them, and monitoring their progress (including adherence). Additional research could be undertaken to develop methods for adapting the components of the Chronic Care Model to general medication self-management and the resources required to support patients and providers in a patient-centered, collaborative partnership.

Empowering Consumers in Their Health Care

The second critical element of the foundation for improving the safety and quality of the medication-use process through an emphasis on patient-centered care is the empowerment of consumers as equal partners in their health care. Equalizing and empowering consumers in their relationship with their providers requires assurance of their rights as patients in all health care settings. Embracing a set of basic patient rights that are endorsed and enforced by health care provider, accreditation, and regulatory organizations to support patient-centered medication management, informed decision making, and prevention of errors is necessary to improve the safety of medication use and the quality of care overall. As seen in the examples quoted earlier, patient rights are not important only in the abstract; they can literally save lives (Annas, 2004).

Many rights that empower consumers and protect them from harm have been instituted through codes, regulations, and laws governing informed consent prior to receipt of a medication, treatment, or procedure during an experimental clinical study or during clinical care. Informed consent is the fundamental ethical and legal doctrine that protects patients' rights to personal autonomy and bodily self-determination (Ridley, 2001). Where informed consent is relevant, the physician is required to discuss and disclose the following (AMA, 1998):

- Patient's diagnosis, if known
- Nature and purpose of a proposed medication, treatment, or procedure
- Risks and benefits of a proposed medication, treatment, or procedure
- Alternatives (including medication options), regardless of their cost or the extent to which they are covered by health insurance
- Risks and benefits of an alternative medication, treatment, or procedure
- Risks and benefits of not receiving or undergoing a treatment or procedure

Patients are also entitled to the opportunity to ask questions so they can elicit a better understanding of their treatment plan (medication or procedure) before proceeding with or refusing a proposed medical intervention.

Regulations of the U.S. Food and Drug Administration (FDA) govern informed consent requirements for participation in clinical trials. Vulnerable populations—children, pregnant women, those with mental illnesses, those of reduced competency, and prisoners—are given special consideration and, in some cases, extra protection by the federal government (Getz and Borfitz, 2002). As part of licensing, certification, and regulatory authority, state medical boards govern informed consent requirements in hospitals and ambulatory practice. Informed consent provisions are based on the American Medical Association's Code of Medical Ethics and standards set by the Joint Commission on Accreditation of Healthcare Organizations (JCAHO). While most state laws regarding informed consent are written for hospital care, precedent set by extensive case law applies these provisions equally to ambulatory care. In the realities of clinical practice, however, consumers are often not adequately informed to participate as partners in their care. For example, many aspects of medication therapy that should be discussed as fully as in an informed consent discussion are not. Often lacking is discussion of contraindications, side effects, adverse reactions, how to distinguish side effects and adverse reactions from the symptoms of disease, and what to do about them (Kerzman et al., 2005; Safran, 2003). Not all patients need a full discussion at every clinical encounter, especially if they are familiar with their medication(s), but such discussion should be recognized as a patient's fundamental right. This raises another core issue: a formal set of patient rights applicable in all health care settings has never been instituted at the federal or state level. Federal legislative attempts in the 1990s to pass a comprehensive patient bill of rights that would apply to health care services did not succeed, with the exception of consumers' right to sue their insurance payer for denial of benefits.

Health care provider and accreditation organizations have, however, been leaders in promulgating statements of patient rights. For example, the American Hospital Association recently recrafted its 1992 Patient's Bill of Rights to include principles of the patient care partnership, a model that represents a shift to patient-centered care. Those principles state what patients can expect during a hospital stay in terms of the hospital environment, participation in their care, protection of privacy, discharge preparation, and help with billing. JCAHO evaluates compliance with standards for ethics, rights, and responsibilities in hospital and ambulatory care settings. The purpose of these standards is to ensure that care, treatment, and services are provided in a way that respects and fosters patient dignity, autonomy, positive self-regard, civil rights, and involvement (JCAHO, 2005). Consideration is given to patients' abilities and resources; their cultural, psychosocial, and spiritual values; the relevant demands of their environment; and their wishes regarding the involvement of family members in their care. Other efforts to raise awareness of patient rights include those of the Tavistock Group—a group of experts representing health care stakeholders that developed a set of shared ethical principles to guide decision making in an integrated health care delivery system (Smith et al., 1999). Certain states have instituted a patient bill of rights, but provisions are not comprehensive, nor do they cover all health care settings (see Table 4-1 for examples).

While these efforts are steps in the direction of patient-centered care and patient rights, they do not go far enough. The committee believes that establishment of a basic set of patient rights—presented in Box 4-3—is essential to achieve patient-centered care, consumer activation and partnership, and improvements in safety and quality. Many but not all of these rights are established broadly in the U.S. Constitution (Amendments I and XIV[1]) and have been articulated by the courts through common law. Nonetheless, they remain difficult to enforce for patients and providers alike, especially for sick individuals (Annas, 2004). One important point listed in Box 4-3 that is not specifically provided for in the law is the right to be told

---

[1]Freedom of religion under the First Amendment allows citizens to make decisions according to their religious beliefs, including medical decisions regarding treatment. Due process under the Fourteenth Amendment as applied to health care ensures that citizens retain their right to life, liberty, and equal protection; meaning self determination and civil rights (patient rights).

TABLE 4-1 Examples of State Patient Rights Statutes

State	Provision	Providers/Facilities Covered
Alaska	Patient Medical Rights Alaska Stat. § 47.30.825 (2006)	Mental health facilities
California	Patients' Bill of Rights Cal. Health & Safety Code § 1599 (2006)	Nursing homes
Florida	Patient's Bill of Rights and Responsibilities Fla. Stat. § 381.026	Medical doctors, osteopaths, podiatrists, hospitals, and other health care facilities
Maryland	Patient Bill of Rights Md. HEALTH-GENERAL Code Ann. § 19-342	Hospitals
Massachusetts	Patients' Bill of Rights Annotated Laws of Michigan, ch. 111, § 70E (2005)	Hospitals, clinics, nursing homes
Mississippi	Patients Rights Miss. Code Ann. § 41-21-102	Mental health facilities

---

BOX 4-3
Improving Medication Safety: Actions for Nurses

• Establish safe work environments for medication preparation, administration, and documentation; for instance, reduce distractions and provide appropriate lighting.
• Maintain a culture of rigorous commitment to principles of safety in medication administration (for instance, the five rights of medication safety and cross-checks with colleagues, where appropriate).
• Remove barriers to and facilitate the involvement of patient surrogates in checking the administration and monitoring the effects of medications wherever and whenever they are administered.
• Foster a commitment to patients' rights as coproducers of their care.
• Develop aids for patient (or surrogate) self-management support.
• Enhance communication skills and team training so as to be prepared and confident in questioning medication orders and evaluating patient responses to drugs.
• Actively advocate for the development, testing, and safe implementation of electronic health records.
• Work to improve systems that address the most common near misses in the work environment.
• Realize they are part of a system and do their part to evaluate the efficacy of new safety systems and technology.
• Contribute to the development and implementation of error reporting systems, and support a culture that values accurate reporting of medication errors.

when an adverse event occurs. For example, if a patient is administered the wrong drug but is not injured, he or she should be told that the error occurred and what is being done to correct it. Thus, the committee believes disclosure of clinically significant errors should be included as an essential patient right. Enumerating patients' essential rights in one document would facilitate consumers' and providers' understanding and exercise of these rights and thereby improve the safety and quality of medication use. It also would clarify how the rights are to be applied day-to-day in clinical practice and ensure equality in application of the rights across health care settings.

COMPONENTS OF THE PATIENT–PROVIDER PARTNERSHIP FOR MEDICATION SAFETY

This section outlines components of the consumer–provider partnership that can contribute to the safety and quality of medication use. Components for consumers include activation and partnership, carrying a medication list, safety practices for self-care, and knowing where to find quality health and medication information. Components for providers include regular practice of medication reconciliation, patient education about medications, increased opportunities for consultation, respect for designated surrogates, and disclosure of errors.

Recommendation 1: To improve the quality and safety of the medication-use process, specific measures should be instituted to strengthen patients' capacities for sound medication self-management. Specifically:

• Patients' rights regarding safety and quality in health care and medication use should be formalized at the state and/or federal levels and ensured at every point of care.
• Patients (or their surrogates) should maintain an active list of all prescription drugs, over-the-counter (OTC) drugs, and dietary supplements they are taking; the reasons for taking them; and any known drug allergies. Every provider involved in the medication-use process for a patient should have access to this list.
• Providers should take definitive action to educate patients (or their surrogates) about the safe and effective use of medications. They should provide information about side effects, contraindications, and how to handle adverse reactions, as well as where to obtain additional objective, high-quality information.
• Consultation on their medications should be available to patients at key points in the medication-use process (during clinical

decision making in ambulatory and inpatient care, at hospital discharge, and at the pharmacy).

Components for Consumers

Consumers' awareness of health care quality and safety issues is growing, but fundamental principles related to the consumer's roles in addressing these issues are not widely known or implemented (NPSF, 2000). Several organizations, such as the Institute for Healthcare Improvement, Planetree, and the former Foundation for Accountability are developing strategies designed to advance patient-centered care (FACCT, 2001b; Frampton et al., 2003; IHI, 2005; Markle Foundation, 2005). One key element of these strategies is the empowerment and activation of consumers. Consumers who have already been activated with regard to medication safety generally gained this knowledge as the result of personal experience with an adverse event in either their own care or that of a family member or friend. Thus a sizable portion of the population does not know what constitutes appropriate and safe medication use, quality health care, and patient safety, or what practical steps consumers can take to protect themselves and their loved ones (NPSF, 2000).

Interventions that promote consumer empowerment and the acquisition of self-management skills emphasize the crucial role of patients in setting goals, establishing action plans, and identifying and overcoming barriers to effective self-management.

Consumer Activation and Partnership

Engagement of consumers in activities and behaviors that promote their health, well-being, and safety is an important component of current initiatives to redesign the health care system (Hibbard, 2004). Ideally, as informed and engaged partners in their health care, consumers contribute to efforts that improve the safety and quality of care while reducing costs to the system (IOM, 2001). In this role, they help produce desired health outcomes to the best of their ability. They make informed decisions about when to seek care; how to work with providers in selecting among treatment options on the basis of their own values and needs; how to work with providers in managing their conditions; what information to provide about their health and functioning to aid in diagnosis and treatment; and how to follow through on agreed-upon treatment plans, recommended lifestyle changes, and preventive actions (Hibbard, 2003).

Research has revealed that being an engaged and active participant in one's own care is linked to better health outcomes (Safran et al., 1998; Ansell, 1999; Lorig et al., 1999; Sawicki, 1999; Bodenheimer et al., 2002; Heisler et al., 2003; Flach et al., 2004). Some of the best research on patients' capability for self-management given adequate support and education stems from models developed for chronic conditions such as heart disease, stroke, lung disease, arthritis, and diabetes (see the earlier discussion of the Chronic Care Model). In these studies, providers educated patients about managing the symptoms and problems associated with their conditions and taught good medication self-management practices and healthful behaviors. For example, patients with vascular disease demonstrated high self-efficacy in medication use, exercise, and weight control when interventions emphasized the importance of self-management, supplied information on visible physiological changes and performance accomplishments, and used nursing staff for patient support and communications (Sol et al., 2006). Hartigan (2003) studied cancer patients receiving oral chemotherapy agents and noted their success with medication safety, optimal dosing, and adherence to the treatment plan when instructed by an oncology nurse in self-assessment, management of symptoms and medication side effects, and use of compliance aids (e.g., diaries, calendars, pillboxes with alarms). Nurses also provided telephone follow-up and triage to patients, reinforcing this support (Hartigan, 2003).

However, the ability and willingness of patients to assume this partnership role can vary depending on their health status. Many patients trust their health care providers and prefer that providers make appropriate decisions for them (Kravitz et al., 2003). In one study, for example, up to 34 percent of women recently diagnosed with breast cancer wanted to delegate all decision making to their provider (Degner et al., 1997). Another study found that 69 percent of patients with chronic conditions preferred such delegation of medical decisions (Arora and McHorney, 2000). The likelihood of preferring an active role increases with level of education and decreases significantly with age and severity of illness (Ende et al., 1989; Stiggelbout and Kiebert, 1997; Mansell et al., 2000).

Thus, consumer engagement should be viewed on a continuum from those who prefer a highly active role to those who prefer a more passive role (RWJF, 2000). For some individuals, their level of activation will change over time. Nevertheless, respect for patients' decisions about their care and level of partnership is paramount. No less important is respect for the level of participation desired by patient surrogates when patients themselves are unable to participate.

Carrying a Medication List

The single most important contribution consumers can make to medication safety and good medication self-management is maintaining an up-to-date medication list that includes prescription medications, OTC drugs, and dietary supplements; the reasons for taking these products; and all known drug and/or food allergies. Information about each drug should include its name, strength, dose, and frequency of administration. Patients should bring this list with them each time they visit their provider and have the provider verify the list with them. Ideally, they should carry it with them at all times in the event emergency care is needed. Indeed, patients have a responsibility to provide this information to their providers and designated surrogates to help prevent adverse drug events (ADEs) such as drug–drug interactions (Cohen, 2000). The medication list is especially important for those who have chronic conditions; see multiple providers; or take multiple medications, OTCs, and dietary supplements. Consumers should exercise their right to ask their prescriber questions if they do not understand their drug treatment regimen, especially side effects and contraindications, and communicate with their caregivers about any adverse changes in the way they feel after initiating a new medication. Providers should be sure that their patients understand the regimen and whom to contact if they have any further questions once they are at home.[2]

Many consumers do not know that their providers are supposed to reconcile their medications as they transition between different health care settings and patient care units. Carrying a medication list can help greatly in the reconciliation process. In particular, providers should reconcile patients' medications at each ambulatory encounter, at each admission to a hospital or readmission to long-term care, at each point of transfer between hospital units, and at hospital discharge.

Medication Safety Practices for Self-Care

When consumers become informed and engaged partners, they can decrease the probability that they will experience a medication error (Cohen, 2000). Actions range from the simple and routine, such as double-checking their prescription when dropping it off and picking it up from the pharmacy, to the more involved, such as maintaining an accurate personal medication record and a partnership with their provider in health care. The following are examples of actions consumers can take as empowered partners in their care:

---

[2]Examples of medication lists can be found at: (1) The Joint Commission for the Accreditation of Health Care Organizations (http://www.jcaho. org/general+public/gp+speak+up/speak up_brochure_meds.pdf and http://www.jcaho.org/general+public/gp+speak+up/speakup_card_meds.pdf); and (2) Institute for Healthcare Improvement (http://www.ihi.org/IHI/Topics/PatientSafety/MedicationSystems/Tools/MedicationReconciliationGuidelinesAndHome MedicationListLutherMidelfort.htm, http://www.ihi.org/IHI/Topics/PatientSafety/Medication Systems/Tools/Tools/WhatYouNeedtoKnowAboutMedicationSafety.htm, and http://www. ihi.org/IHI/Topics/PatientSafety/MedicationSystems/Tools/TheMedForm.htm).

• Ask questions and insist on answers from providers to guide their decision making on medication and nonmedication treatment options based on their personal values and needs.

• Insist that providers clarify specific aspects of the medication regimen (e.g., purpose, drug name, dosage, strength), identify possible side effects and what actions to take should they occur, and understand possible interactions with other medications and/or foods.

• Ensure that providers give them or direct them to written information about the drug appropriate to their level of health literacy, age, and language, and that they know where to obtain additional information about their medication(s) and health condition(s).

• Understand and retain their right to disagree and to say no—no to taking on a more active role, no to a particular provider's counsel, and no to medication therapy.

• Seek information and counseling to make informed self-care decisions when self-prescribing and administering OTC medications, herbal remedies, and dietary supplements.

Along with knowing their rights as patients and maintaining a medication list, understanding a basic set of practices for each step in the medication-use system can help consumers contribute to medication safety. These practices are outlined in Box 4-4 and discussed further later in the chapter.

Finding Quality Health and Medication Information

Consumers should become knowledgeable about where to find quality health and medication information to support them in self-care. They should know where and how to find this information at the public library, if these resources exist, and where to find the best information on the Internet (e.g., the National Library of Medicine's [NLM] MedlinePlus program) (see the section on actions for government and other stakeholders later in the chapter). In addition, they should keep a list of these references that they can refer to quickly and easily.

Components for Providers

Patient-centered care in the medication-use system requires improvement in many of the dynamics affecting the provider–patient relationship. Provider responsibilities in this regard include medication reconciliation, patient education, availability of counseling, respect for surrogates, and disclosure of errors. Just as important, consumers and surrogates can develop their understanding of the appropriate expectations they should have

---

BOX 4-4
Consumer Actions to Improve Medication Safety

Personal/Home Care

Consumers should:

- Maintain a list of the prescription drugs, nonprescription drugs, and other products, such as vitamins and minerals, they are taking.
- Take this list with them whenever they visit a provider, and have him or her review it.
- Be aware of where to find educational material related to their medication(s) in the local community and at reliable Internet sites.

Ambulatory Care/Outpatient Clinic

Consumers should:

- Have the prescriber write down the name of the drug (brand and generic, if available), what it is for, its dosage, and how often to take it, or provide other written material with this information.
- Have the prescriber explain how to use the drug properly.
- Ask about the drug's side effects and what to do if they experience a side effect.

Pharmacy

Consumers should:

- Make sure the name of the drug (brand or generic) and the directions for use received at the pharmacy are the same as what is written down by the prescriber.
- Know that they can review their list of medications with the pharmacist for additional safety.
- Know that they have the right to counseling by the pharmacist if they have any questions; they can ask the pharmacist to explain how to take the drug properly, what side effects it has, and what to do if they experience a side effect (just as they did with the prescriber).
- Ask for written information about the medication.

Hospital Inpatient Care

Consumers (or their surrogates) should:

- Ask the doctor or nurse what drugs are being given in the hospital.
- Not take a drug without being told the purpose for doing so.
- Exercise the right to have a surrogate present whenever they are receiving medication and are unable to monitor the medication-use process themselves.
- Prior to surgery, ask whether there are medications, especially prescription antibiotics, that they should take or any they should stop taking preoperatively.
- Prior to discharge, ask for a list of the medications they should be taking at home, have a provider review them, and be sure they understand how these medications should be taken.

---

of their providers for engaging in activities that promote quality and safety, and hold them accountable for meeting those expectations.

Medication Reconciliation

Medication reconciliation is a process designed to prevent medication errors at patient transition points. It is a multistep process that entails obtaining a complete and accurate list of the medications a patient is taking (including nonprescription and alternative medications) and comparing this list with both documentation in the patient's medical record during ambulatory care visits and the physician's admission, transfer, and/or discharge orders in inpatient settings (IHI, 2004). The purpose of the reconciliation process is to avoid or minimize errors of transcription, omission, duplication of therapy, and drug–drug and drug–disease interactions. Discrepancies are brought to the attention of the provider, and if appropriate, changes are made to the record or orders. The overarching goal is to facilitate continuity of care (Nickerson et al., 2005).

Several studies have shown that a significantly high number of discrepancies can be detected through the medication reconciliation process (Pronovost et al., 2003). Nickerson and colleagues (2005) found that of 481 drug therapy problems detected, 83.8 percent had a potentially significant or somewhat significant clinical impact. Another study of inpatient medical records found that the details of current medication use were either nonexistent or incorrect 85 percent of the time (Rozich and Resar, 2001). Bikowski and colleagues (2001) also demonstrated high rates of discrepancies in family practice. In 74 percent of cases studied, the patient was taking at least one medication that the physician was unaware of, or that the physician was aware of but was not actually part of the treatment regimen. Along with these statistics on medication incongruence, about 60 percent of medication errors in patient records occurred when patients were admitted, discharged, or transferred (Rozich and Resar, 2001).

Medication reconciliation has proven to be an effective means of achieving significant reductions in such discrepancies. The introduction of a series of reconciliation interventions in one hospital during a 7-month period decreased the rate of errors by 70 percent and that of adverse drug events by 15 percent (Rogers et al., 2006; Rozich et al., 2004). Pharmacy technicians in another hospital reduced the potential for medication errors by 80 percent within 3 months by obtaining a medication history from patients scheduled for surgery (Haig, 2003).

The Institute for Healthcare Improvement has simplified medication reconciliation into three steps applicable in all health care settings (IHI, 2004):

- Verification (collection of medication history/list)
- Clarification (ensuring that the medications and doses are appropriate)
- Reconciliation (documentation of changes)

The medication reconciliation process can be implemented in several ways. One method, especially when multiple providers are involved in a patient's care, is for health care organizations to maintain a system that allows each member of the care team (e.g., physician, nurse, pharmacist) access to the patient's medication list and medication administration record. Electronic health information systems (as discussed in Chapter 5) may be an efficient means to this end. During handoffs between sites of care (e.g., hospital to home) or between professionals (e.g., change in medical services or rotation of residents or attending physicians), the clinician receiving the patient should review and reconcile the patient's medication plan to ensure its completeness and accuracy. The Institute for Healthcare Improvement's *Getting Started Kit: Prevent Adverse Drug Events (Medication Reconciliation)—How-to-Guide* provides several strategies for implementing medication reconciliation processes within health care organizations (IHI, 2004).

Even though medication reconciliation is recognized as an effective means of preventing medication errors (Gleason et al., 2004; Ketchum et al., 2005), often it is overlooked and not performed (IHI, 2004: Rogers et al., 2006). Several barriers to implementing medication reconciliation were identified by Rodehaver (2005), who proposed actions that could be taken to overcome these barriers (see Table 4-2). Rather than continuing to leave reconciliation as a voluntary process, in 2003 JCAHO incorporated medication reconciliation as a key expectation for compliance with its National Patient Safety Goals (JCAHO, 2004). The intent is that by 2006, hospitals will implement reconciliation activities at all transition points, including transitions from the intensive care unit to medical or surgical units. The patient's updated medication regimen and list should be communicated to the "next provider of service" at all interfaces of care, and upon admission to and discharge from the facility. At admission and discharge, reconciliation activities should involve discussions with the patient or designated person (e.g., family member, significant other, surrogate decision maker). Implementing comprehensive medication reconciliation activities at all points of care as requested by JCAHO is a complex undertaking that may require remodeling of inpatient flow, provider workflow, and organizational information management. Studies should be undertaken to determine the most efficient and effective means of implementing the JCAHO requirements.

TABLE 4-2 Overcoming Barriers to the Implementation of Medication Reconciliation

Barrier	Actions to Overcome Barriers
Medical staff acceptance	• Increase the number and types of physicians on the team; include obstetricians, cardiologists, psychiatrists, and surgeons. • Review department-specific medical forms and physician discharge practices prior to implementation of standardized forms and practices. • Involve the medical staff executive committee as much as possible. • Initiate early discussions with physicians, such as obstetricians and cardiologists.
Concerns related to the accuracy of the solicited medication list	• Be aware that the information obtained from the patient and/or significant other is only as accurate as the informant. Knowing that the information is provided by a layperson, tolerate incomplete information related to dosage or frequency. Nursing and pharmacy personnel and physicians can assist in ensuring the accuracy of the list.
Ownership for medication oversight	• Shift the emphasis in organizational structure from delineation by discipline to patient care. • Focus on a team approach to medication reconciliation, which includes ownership on the part of the medical, nursing, and pharmacy staff.
Attitude that "my patient type is unique" and "you just don't understand"	• Take time to understand the process used by individual practitioners. • Help individuals assimilate "old" practices into the reconciliation process. • Have one-on-one conversations with resisters. Enable the process by assisting them at the point of patient admission or discharge. • Audit particular physician practices and compare them with those of their peers. • Allow time to enforce compliance. • Solicit the help of senior medical leadership. • Allow diffusion to occur gradually.
Inconsistency among residents and physician extenders	• Plan for continual rotation of residents, and plan appropriate education as needed. • Obtain buy-in of physician extenders.
Organizational climate versus small test of change	• Maintain the course of a small test of change regardless of internal pressures. • Implement the process unit by unit. Delay organizationwide implementation until medical, nursing, and pharmacy staff are ready.

SOURCE: Rodehaver, 2005.

Patient Education

Consumers should expect to be adequately educated by their providers about their medications and about appropriate medication self-management. Enhancing individuals' knowledge of and capacity for medication self-management requires, above all, high-quality communications with providers. Providers must be able and willing to understand and respond to the patient's implicit and explicit messages (Sundin and Jansson, 2003). They should attempt to elicit the patient's ideas, feelings, and preferences regarding health problems and possible treatments, daily routines, and the information needed to support self-management. Providers should understand that patients need different kinds of information at different times and for different purposes (Raynor et al., 2004). Moreover, they should understand that some points may be easily understood, while others may need to be reiterated, especially when the patient's receptivity is limited by physical debility or psychological/emotional states (Scott and Thompson, 2003). The information relayed should be accurate and complete relative to the patient's level of understanding (Reiser, 1980).

Part of the problem has been physician training—until recently, undergraduate and postgraduate training paid little attention to ensuring that doctors acquire the skills necessary to communicate well with patients (Maguire and Pitceathly, 2002). In the 1990s, medical schools sharpened their focus on communication skills (AAMC, 1999). The Association of American Medical Colleges (AAMC) initiated the Medical Schools Objectives Project to facilitate the process of enhancing teaching and assessment of communication skills. As a result of this and other efforts,[3] interpersonal skills and communication are one of six core competencies of graduate medical education required as part of the United States Medical Licensing Examination (Batalden et al., 2002; FSMB and NBME, 2005). However, there is significant variation among medical schools in the way and the extent to which communication skills are taught and assessed (AAMC, 1999; Makoul, 2003). Regardless of what method is used,[4] the reliability and effectiveness of observation and feedback can be compromised unless grounded in a coherent structured framework (Makoul, 2003).

---

[3]Revisions to the competencies of medical education were instituted by the Accreditation Council for Graduate Medical Education, the National Board of Medical Examiners, the Federation of State Medical Boards, and the Educational Commission for Foreign Medical Graduates.

[4]The primary teaching methods are small-group discussions and seminars (91 percent), lectures and presentations (82 percent), student interviews with simulated patients (79 percent), student observation of faculty with real patients (74 percent), and student interviews with real patients (72 percent) (AAMC, 1999).

The development of competency in communication has been a focus of nursing education for over 50 years. Nursing education programs are required to demonstrate attention to this core competency as part of the accreditation process (AACN, 1998). On many health care teams with excellent patient outcomes, nurses and nurse practitioners are used as the primary providers who listen, communicate with and educate patients and families, and coordinate care.

Even though some communication training has been incorporated in medical school curricula, most patient complaints about providers are related to problems with communication rather than clinical competency—specifically, that doctors do not listen to them (Richards, 1990). A study of the literature on patients' priorities for general practitioners found the most highly rated aspect of care to be "humanness," followed by competence/accuracy (Wensing et al., 1998). For some patients, the humanness element means the physician really listens and does not hurry them (Carroll et al., 1998). Patients' ratings of physicians' communication skills are strongly related to trust, but trust does not equate to unquestioning faith (Coulter, 2002). Patients need empathy, support, and reassurance, all essential features of the therapeutic relationship, but they also need honest information about their condition, options for treatment, and clinicians who listen to their concerns and preferences (Mechanic and Meyer, 2000).

It is widely recognized that provider–patient communications, including those regarding medications, typically are provider-oriented (e.g., the provider talking more than listening and asking few open-ended questions) (Berry et al., 2003). As a result, patients fail to receive all the information they need and desire about their medications, especially that related to risks, adverse side effects, and contraindications (Caress et al., 2002; Scott and Thompson, 2003; Garfield et al., 2004). Patients increasingly want more and better information about their condition and the expected outcome, more openness about medication side effects, and advice on what they can do for themselves (Meryn, 1998). Recognizing that some patients find it difficult to articulate their information needs or are reluctant to ask questions during medical visits, practitioners (physicians, nurse practitioners, physician assistants, pharmacists, nurses) should have the requisite training in communication to elicit their patients' understanding of the medication regimen and educational needs (Sleath et al., 1999). Box 4-5 outlines the core information that research indicates patients should receive about their medications (Sleath et al., 1999; Caress et al., 2002; Scott and Thompson, 2003; Garfield et al., 2004; Morrow et al., 2005).

The ability of providers to communicate medication information in an understandable manner is critical to adequately informing, educating, and empowering patients. In particular, both discussions and written information about medications should be appropriate to the patient's level of literacy, age, language, and culture. Providers must have resources available to manage the knowledge, practical, and attitudinal barriers that affect provider–patient communication. Information should be easy for patients to understand and follow when they are at home self-managing their regimen. For example, providers should be aware that the majority of individuals with literacy problems have difficulty following prescription directions and will require communication consistent with their literacy level (Safeer and Keenan, 2005). Patients may misunderstand the instruction to "take a tablet X times a day" but understand "take a tablet every X hours." When necessary, providers should have resources available to facilitate the patient's understanding of medication information orally and in writing. Such resources may include translation services for patients. Ambulatory care providers can have a nurse or technician on staff with the language skills necessary to support the needs of the practice's patient population, develop a partnership with a local pharmacist that can assist certain patients in confirming details of their medication regimen in their native language, or utilize centrally located telephone translation services.

Opportunities for Consultation

Successful medication self-management requires that consumers have multiple opportunities to gain knowledge about safe and effective medication use. Such consultations with providers should be readily available to consumers in all health care settings and at key points along the medication-use continuum. Specifically, consultations should take place during clinical decision making in ambulatory and hospital care, at hospital discharge, and at the time of dispensing by the local community pharmacy. Telephone consultations may be used to provide additional support to patients as they manage problems with and the effects of their medications. Access to consultation at these critical points in the medication-use continuum creates, in effect, a chain of communication that serves as the medication self-management support system. Conversely, poor communication at any of these points can lead to medication errors due to misunderstanding, inaccurate or incomplete information, or nonadherence (Morrow et al., 1988).

Because most health care is provided in community settings, the chain of communication begins with provider–patient consultations during ambulatory care. As discussed earlier, primary care providers play a crucial role in educating patients about the safe and effective use of prescription and nonprescription medications. Thus during ambulatory care consultations, providers must allow sufficient time for consultations with patients or surrogates about medication management (Raynor et al., 2004). Providers should be able to adapt to information needs that shift over time and

---

BOX 4-5
Core Information for Educating Patients
About Their Medications

• *Routine evaluation of all medications.* Providers should routinely evaluate the need for and effectiveness of all medications a patient is taking, and ensure that the patient understands critical information about the medications.

• *Different treatment options.* Providers should discuss with the patient all medication and other treatment options, including the expected benefits and risks of each option, in an objective manner (without overselling treatment benefits).

• *Name and purpose of each prescribed medication.* Most patients know the name of a medication they are taking, but fewer know why they are taking it, what type of drug it is (its class), how it works in their body, or how regular and long-term use differ (Raynor et al., 2004).

• *When and how to take the medication.* The patient needs to understand the regimen—how much of a medication they should take (dosage), how often (frequency), and with what special instructions (e.g., with food or on an empty stomach). When reviewing the regimen, providers should also review general medication safety practices.

• *Side effects and what to do about them.* Patients need to know:

   – About short- and long-term side effects of taking a medication (including the risk of dependency) and how to rely on self-observation to assess these effects.

   – About both minor and more severe effects, how they will affect day-to-day functioning, what to do about them, whom to contact, and when (Caress et al., 2002; Garfield et al., 2004; Raynor et al., 2004).

   – About the rate of occurrence of a side effect (e.g., X percent of patients experience it).

---

with changes in patients' health status. They should follow up closely on their patients' success or difficulties with a medication regimen so as to overcome the barriers to self-management discussed above and facilitate desired health outcomes. And it is essential that primary care providers function as the chief coordinator and record keeper of their patients' medication regimens from multiple providers.

Hospital providers also serve as important sources of patient education both during inpatient care and at discharge. Research shows that many patients desire more information about their health conditions, treatments, and procedures than they currently receive (Wilson et al., 2002; Scott and Thompson, 2003). During an inpatient stay, however, the extent to which patients want to be educated about their medications may vary according to individual preferences, severity of illness, or other factors. Patients or their surrogates should have access to regular consultations with physicians, nurses, and pharmacists to gain knowledge about the medications involved in the treatment plan. Evidence supports a team approach among these providers as a successful means of improving patient safety, quality of

- *Problems with other medications.* Patients receive information about drug–drug, drug–food, and drug–disease interactions mainly from pharmacy leaflets, but they express strong interest in receiving information from the provider who is prescribing a medication as well. This information should be included in the initial dialogue when medications are selected. Also, providers should educate patients about complementary and alternative medications that may be marketed for their condition, and any potential effects and interactions that may occur between these products and the prescribed medication (Ernst, 2001; IOM, 2005).
- *Adherence.* Providers should discuss with patients potential barriers to adherence and determine with the patient how best to handle them. Providers should discuss the short- and long-term effects of nonadherence. If it becomes obvious that there is a strong likelihood of intentional nonadherence for attitudinal reasons, providers should make the patient comfortable about disclosing that possibility so the best alternative treatments can be explored.
- *Role of medication.* Patients want information about the role of a medication in the healing, management, and recovery processes for their condition. They want to know the length of the treatment and how to tell whether the medication is working. They also need information about risk factors associated with their health conditions and how to minimize them.
- *Additional information.* Although the major focus of medication communications should be face-to-face discussions between patient and provider, printed materials can be a useful supplement (Johnson et al., 1986). Providers can offer written materials to their patients, as well as direct them to specific high-quality sources for information about their health condition, medications, and medication safety (e.g., clinical pharmacists, National Library of Medicine's MedlinePlus).

care, and health outcomes (Connor et al., 2002; Kaissi et al., 2003; Reiling et al., 2004). Providers should be particularly vigilant about educating patients at discharge, as many providers tend to overestimate patients' understanding of the medication regimen and its potential side effects (Kerzman et al., 2005). Discharge from the hospital is also a prime time for problems with medication reconciliation. Providers may overlook the need to resume medications that were suspended during hospitalization, and providers inside and outside of the hospital may inadvertently prescribe different medications for the same condition.

The quality of discharge planning and communication is an important determinant of patients' capacity for self-management and of overall health outcomes (Calkins et al., 1997). Registered nurses spend a large amount of time integrating patient care as part of planning for patients' discharge from hospitals or other health care facilities to enable continued care in the home, school, or long-term care facility; educating the patient and family about the patient's disease, course of therapy, medications, self-care activities, and other areas of concern to the patient; and preventing discontinuities in care (IOM, 2004d). Discharge communication is also an important factor affecting coordination of care during transitions from inpatient care to another setting. Hospital providers must ensure that both patients and their primary ambulatory care providers receive comprehensive information about the discharge plan, including the prescribed medication regimen, disease management if a chronic condition is present, and self-care activities to improve health status.

Another critical link in the chain of communication to support medication self-management is the local community pharmacist. Pharmacists have expertise in many aspects of medication use, yet are often underutilized in both hospital and community settings. Pharmacists are required by state law to provide consumers with medication consultation unless an individual waives his or her right. Because many consumers do not know that they have the right to utilize pharmacists in this capacity, they may unknowingly sign documents waiving consultation services. Pharmacists generally provide consultation upon request, but few serve as active facilitators of medication self-management. A daily workload characterized by a high volume of prescriptions to fill, large percentages of time (up to 85 percent) dedicated to claims adjudication, and staffing shortages inhibit pharmacists' ability to do so (Knowlton and Penna, 2003; Manasse and Thompson, 2005). Training pharmacy technicians to take over claims adjudication and bottle filling, as well as implementing robotics and other automated pharmacy systems, would allow pharmacists more time for counseling patients. Reducing costs in the above manner would generate some of the resources necessary to support medication management services for the general population, although additional resources may also be needed. Initial efforts to this end are included in the provisions of Part D of the Medicare Prescription Drug Improvement and Modernization Act of 2003, which requires pharmaceutical benefit plans to make available medication therapy management programs and pay pharmacists for these services. These medication therapy management programs are available only for certain beneficiaries—those using multiple medications, with multiple chronic conditions, and with expected drug expenditures of $4,000 annually. Pharmaceutical benefit plans provide the services through their own in-house staff and a toll-free 800 telephone number, rather than under fee-for-service contracts with community pharmacists. Medication therapy management is addressed further in Chapter 8.

Respect for Patient Surrogates

In compliance with existing laws, including those established through living wills, power of medical attorney, and other state and federal laws (Annas, 2004), providers should be aware of and strictly follow patients' arrangements for designated surrogates. If patients are unable or unwilling to make decisions on their own, providers must adhere to their alternative arrangements for health care decision making (PCSEPMBBR, 1982). Capacity for decision making is specific to a particular situation or episode and best understood from a functional perspective: the presence or absence of capacity does not depend on a person's health status or on the decision made, but on the individual's actual functioning in the decision-making process. Clearly, incoherent, unconscious, or otherwise incapacitated patients cannot make informed treatment decisions because they cannot receive a full and current explanation of their health problems and treatment options (Johnstone, 2000). Some patients may be technically capable of decision making but choose to defer to others, and this choice should be respected. Even if patients possess no decision-making capacity, ethical principles for protecting vulnerable populations dictate that providers speak to and inform them out of respect, beneficence, and justice (PCSEPMBBR, 1982; Getz and Borfitz, 2002). For example, someone with Parkinson's disease may be fully alert but unable to speak understandably or function physically. Nonetheless, providers should inform such a patient of decisions made by surrogates as care proceeds.

Patients should have the right to have someone of their choosing present whenever medications are being prescribed, administered, or monitored. Family members, friends, and significant others can have a far greater impact on patients' experiences with their illness, their safety, and their long-term health and happiness than any clinician (Gerteis et al., 1993). Relatives and friends take care of patients, offer love and support, remind patients to take medications, and monitor doctors' orders and nursing care. Patients may choose to have a family member, friend, or other person present for any number of other reasons important to them, such as assistance with health decision making, language translation, and emotional support. They may choose to have that person participate actively or passively. For example, at the patient's request, the designated person might be asked to double-check the dosage of a chemotherapy agent prepared for administration by a hospital nurse or to hold the patient's hand in prayer during the cycle of administration. Health care providers must expand their thinking about family from including only next of kin to encompassing other family members, friends, or designated others; recognize that involvement of these individuals is critical to patient-centered care; and be knowledgeable about laws that support such involvement (Gerteis et al., 1993).

Disclosure of Errors

Disclosure of medical errors signifies respect for both patient autonomy and ethical standards (Gerteis et al., 1993; Gallagher et al., 2003) and should be required of any medical practice. The majority (90 percent) of patients want and expect to be told about errors, particularly those that cause them harm (Wu et al., 1997; Brazeau, 1999; Blendon et al., 2002; Millenson, 2003; Mazor et al., 2004a; Gallagher and Levinson, 2005). However, rates of disclosure by providers have been quite low (about 30 percent)—this despite general agreement among providers that patients should be told about errors, as well as disclosure requirements outlined in hospital accreditation standards and some state laws (Sweet and Bernat, 1997; Blendon et al., 2002). The primary reasons for nondisclosure are fear of a malpractice suit, damage to the provider's or hospital's reputation, and the negative effect on provider–patient relationships. In reality, lack of disclosure is associated with lower levels of patient satisfaction, less trust of physicians, a more negative emotional response to care, and greater likelihood of a malpractice suit (Gallagher et al., 2003; Lamb, 2004; Mazor et al., 2004b).

Results of a number of studies confirm that patients want detailed explanations—they want to know what happened, what implications the error has for their health, why it happened, how the resulting problem will be corrected, and how future errors will be prevented (Gallagher et al., 2003; Mazor et al., 2004b; Manser and Staender, 2005). Just as important is the way an error is disclosed. Honesty and compassion in disclosure, along with a sincere apology, result in a more positive emotional response from the patient (Mazor et al., 2004b; Gallagher and Levinson, 2005). Health care providers must understand that disclosure of errors is part of a patient's fundamental rights and quality of care. Moreover, all providers should be trained in good communication skills related to error disclosure. Materials and programs to help accomplish this are starting to become available in the form of courses and educational videos (see, e.g., http://www. jhsph.edu/removinginsult/from/injury). Some organizations, such as the Veterans Health Administration (VHA), already are implementing policies for the disclosure of errors to patients or their representatives. The VHA published a directive in October 2005 stating that VHA facilities and individual VHA providers have an obligation to disclose adverse events to patients who have been harmed in the course of their care, including cases in which the harm may not be obvious or severe, or may be evident only in the future (VHA, 2005). The Harvard Medical School teaching institutions also have implemented guidelines for responding to adverse events (Harvard, 2006). The patient is free to involve family members in the disclosure process. Likewise, the University of Michigan Health System has instituted a disclosure program and has since seen reductions in legal costs (Wu, 2005). The "Sorry Works" Coalition also aims to promote error disclosure as an ethical imperative (SWC, 2005). However, these initiatives are not enough. Because there is no formal statute that dictates the seriousness of errors warranting disclosure, each health care organization defines this independently. To resolve these differences and respect the intent of patient rights, the committee believes patients have the right to know about any clinically significant error.

UNDERSTANDING AND OVERCOMING BARRIERS EXPERIENCED BY CONSUMERS AND PROVIDERS

In the current health care system, a number of barriers affect the ability of consumers to engage in safe and effective self-management of their medications and the ability of health care practitioners to change their day-to-day practices to support new consumer-oriented activities. These barriers can be classified into three main areas: knowledge deficits, practical barriers, and attitudinal factors (Cohen, 2000).

According to the Institute of Safe Medication Practices (ISMP), many of these barriers are the root cause of nonadherence (Baird et al., 1984; Ansell, 1999; Sawicki, 1999; Tamada et al., 1999; Cummings et al., 2000). Nonadherence to a recommended treatment regimen, both intentional and unintentional, is defined as not filling a prescription initially, not having a prescription refilled, omitting doses, taking the wrong dose, stopping a medication without the provider's consultation or advice, taking a medication incorrectly, taking a medication at the wrong time, or taking someone else's medication (Cohen, 2000). Box 4-6 summarizes statistics on nonadherence among patients in the U.S. population.

For providers, barriers can present themselves as factors contributing to errors in all phases of the medication-use system (many of which were summarized in Chapter 2). Factors that directly impact the consumer–provider relationship and consumers' capacity for medication self-management include the following:

- Inadequate continuing education programs and overreliance on marketing materials for new knowledge about medications
- Lack of patient educational materials and resources to support providers in this capacity
- Use of free samples without appropriate documentation or in lieu of other, more appropriate treatment options (medication and nonmedication) for a particular patient
- Complex, burdensome, time-consuming, and changing requirements associated with multiple payers and regulators
- Poor workflow design, inadequate continuity of care, and lack of systems approaches and information technologies, which compromise efficiency, effectiveness, and safety
- Lack of the support and leadership required to change from the current system to a patient-centered delivery system and a culture of safety

BOX 4-6
Rates of Inaccurate Medication Use by Consumers

Problems with adherence exist in all populations but tend to be somewhat more prevalent among vulnerable groups, such as those with low literacy, low English proficiency, or cognitive impairment; the uninsured; those over age 70; and those with polypharmaceutial regimens (NQF, 2005). The effects of nonadherence are substantial both for patients and in terms of costs to the health care system. A recent meta-analysis of 569 studies found that the average nonadherence rate was 25 percent, resulting in as many as 188 million visits to health care providers (including hospitalizations). Analysis by disease estimates nonadherence at 8.4 million for hypertension, 7.6 million for diabetes, and 4.5 million for cancer. Analysis by regimen suggests 112.2 million for medication, 49.4 million for diet, and 22.6 for exercise recommendations. Based on these rates, the costs of nonadherence could be very high (billions of dollars per year) (DiMatteo, 2004).

Individual studies have estimated significantly higher nonadherence rates. The University of Pennsylvania reported that about 50 percent of older adults have problems adhering to their prescribed regimen, and more than 10 percent of these cases result in hospital admissions (Schlenk et al., 2004). Other estimates of hospital admissions due to adverse drug events (ADEs) resulting from nonadherence are much higher: 23.5 percent for seniors (Michalsen et al., 1998) and 33 percent for all groups (McDonnell and Jacobs, 2002). Gurwitz and colleagues (2003) cite problems with patient adherence as a contributing factor in more than 20 percent of preventable ADEs that occurred at the prescribing and monitoring stages. A study of patients with hypertension and dyslipidemia who were prescribed a medication for each condition found that only 44.7 percent were adhering to their regimen 3 months after starting treatment, with a drop to 36 percent at 6 months and 1 year—a 64 percent nonadherence rate (Chapman et al., 2005). Other studies found that 20 to 71 percent of patients failed to take the prescribed dose, while 29 percent omitted taking the medication altogether (Bedell et al., 2000; Barat et al., 2001).

Some interventions designed to address adherence have been evaluated (e.g., interventions specific to a disease, dose simplification, reminders); these evaluations have not found consistent outcomes among patient groups. Part of the reason for this is that the issue of patient adherence has received very little attention in the literature on patient safety relevant to preventing ADEs.

A recent report of the National Quality Forum recommends the development of a set of standardized steps designed to improve adherence that could be implemented by providers as part of quality and safety improvement efforts (NQF, 2005). Where nonadherence is intentional and the result of informed patient preference, providers (and health care systems) need to understand these preferences and pursue other treatment options.

This section provides an overview of key issues underlying knowledge deficits, practical barriers, and attitudinal factors that constitute barriers for consumers and providers. Resources and strategies for adequately addressing these issues are necessary to achieve patient-centered care and the consumer–provider partnership envisioned in this report.

Knowledge Deficits

The single greatest barrier to patient education and good medication self-management is insufficient knowledge about the safe and effective use of medications. Both providers and patients often are forced to make decisions in spite of knowledge deficits and take calculated risks as they weigh the pros and cons of medication regimens.

At the most global level, there may be insufficient knowledge available about the risks, benefits, and use of a drug, particularly in certain patient populations. Issues that affect the development of an adequate knowledge base for providers and patients are discussed in Chapters 2 and 6. Providers themselves may lack up-to-date pharmacologic facts, especially given the volume of products on the market and frequently changing safety information (IOM, 2004c; Schultz and Perrier, 1976). As cited by Woolsey (2000), for example, a two-page package insert for cisapride, when printed in a 12-point font on 8.5 × 11 paper, is more than 10 pages long and contains more than 470 facts about the drug (PDR, 2000). Prescribers would have difficulty mastering all of this information for even a single drug, much less the 40 to 100 medications that they regularly prescribe (Woolsey, 2000). Most can manage simply the basic facts, including when to prescribe a drug; in which quantity, dose, and frequency; how to counsel patients about taking the drug; what to look for when monitoring for effects; and how to handle patient abuse of a drug (Horvatich and Schnoll, 1991). In addition, drug information may not be presented in a way that accommodates the needs of different providers (physicians, nurses, pharmacists) within the scope of different time-sensitive uses (e.g., emergency care, surgery, clinical practice, home care) or decision-support systems (IOM, 2004c).

Systems to assist physicians, nurses, pharmacists, and the public in dealing with the overwhelming volume of information on drugs have not been identified or are not being implemented (Woolsey, 2000). Poorly developed continuing education programs and methods of incorporating new information into day-to-day clinical practice are major factors contributing to providers' limited knowledge of medications (Balas et al., 1996; Blumenthal, 2004; Brennan et al., 2006). For example, physicians have little specific training or continuing education in prescribing medications for the elderly even though there is clear scientific evidence that these patients' physiological differences affect drug metabolism and safety (Avorn, 1990; Pereles and Russell, 1996; Peterson et al., 2005). Further lacking are specific methods for teaching older adults how to self-manage medications, as well as prevent such common errors as mixing OTC and prescription medications, discontinuing prescriptions, taking wrong doses, using incorrect techniques, and consuming inappropriate foods with specific medications (Curry et al., 2005). Another obstacle to better patient education and self-management is the tendency of the medical establishment to organize medical training and chronic disease management programs around single diseases and conditions despite the need for care that addresses those with multiple conditions taking multiple medications (Schroeder et al., 1986; Mullan, 1998). Lastly, use of complementary and alternative medications by consumers has increased dramatically, with a growing proportion requesting that these products be integrated into their treatment regimens (IOM, 2005). Except for selected hospitals, educational programs and licensure and credentialing requirements for integrated treatment with these products remain insufficient for the average practitioner (Cohen et al., 2005; IOM, 2005).

At the patient level, knowledge deficits are usually due to misunderstanding or the receipt of faulty or incomplete information about the medication regimen. Often such deficits are the product of limited provider–patient communications, low levels of literacy or English proficiency on the part of the patient, or inadequate educational materials and resources. The unfortunate result is that consumers' actual knowledge about illness, illness prevention, and the function of medications is generally quite low (Haugbolle et al., 2002). For example, in as many as 62 percent of patients, misunderstanding or forgetting instructions from health care providers or printed medication materials is an important reason for nonadherence and poor health outcomes (Jenkins et al., 2003; Skoglund et al., 2003). A study of medication misadventures resulting in emergency room visits found that 30 percent of patients had no understanding and another 30 percent only some understanding of proper medication use (Schneitman-McIntire et al., 1996). Another study demonstrated that 73 percent of patients discharged from the hospital were aware of the course and purpose of their medication, but were unaware of side effects, needed lifestyle changes, and correct medication schedules (Kerzman et al., 2005). Clearly, when consumers do not understand information about their medications, safety may be compromised (Cohen, 2000).

In other instances, misunderstandings in provider–patient communications are attributable to the patient's own lack of participation in the consultation, which can lead to inaccurate guesses and assumptions on the part of both provider and patient. Patients can also be confused by conflicting advice from their providers and other sources of information, such as pharmacy leaflets and the Internet (Bitten et al., 2000). One study of asthma patients found multiple examples of partial or total failure to understand drug information, even though patients had actively sought such information from a variety of professional and lay sources (Raynor et al., 2004).

Issues related to consumers' health literacy, in terms of low levels of both general literacy and English proficiency, and providers' cultural competence contribute further to deficits in knowledge about medications. According to the National Adult Literacy Survey, nearly half of all American adults (90 million people) have difficulty understanding and acting upon health information (IOM, 2004a). Health literacy is the degree to which individuals have the capacity to obtain, process, and understand basic health information and services as necessary to make appropriate health decisions (Ratzan and Parker, 2000). Functional literacy is the ability to use literacy to perform a task. It includes speech and speech comprehension (e.g., communicating symptoms to a doctor, discussing medication use), reading and writing (e.g., reading and understanding a prescription label, completing a medical history questionnaire), and basic math skills (e.g., calibrating a home care medical device, calculating the proper dose of a medicine). Even those with high general literacy skills may find health information difficult to obtain, understand, or use (IOM, 2004a); those Americans (40 million) with limited literacy and/or English proficiency, many of whom are poor, members of ethnic or cultural minorities, or with less than a high school education, are at a severe disadvantage in their ability to understand and act upon such information. For example, a Spanish-speaking patient may have an English-speaking physician who prescribes a heart medication to be taken once per day. Without an interpreter available, this patient, whose prescription has been filled in English, may translate the English words "once per day" as meaning "eleven times per day" in Spanish.

Another major factor contributing to the gap in knowledge, awareness, and understanding of medications among both high- and low-literacy groups is the inadequacy of drug information materials that are intended to supplement provider–patient communications and self-management. Few materials and resources are available to support providers in educating patients about their medications. Generally, educational exchanges with the provider are verbal; the provision of literature is relegated to the pharmacy, yet pharmacy leaflets vary in comprehensibility, utility, and design quality (Krass et al., 2002). The average pharmacy leaflet is written at a college reading level, four grade levels above the average reading comprehension level (grades 11–12) (Rolland, 2000), and lacks important information about precautions, drug–drug interactions, and symptoms of certain adverse reactions (Svarstad and Mount, 2001). Moreover, most pharmacies do not provide leaflets in commonly spoken languages to accommodate consumers with low English proficiency (Svarstad and Mount, 2001; Krass et al., 2002; IOM, 2004a). Knowledge deficits can be overcome by providing patients with more information or providing them with information in a more understandable forms, tailored to their level of education and their cultural/ethnic background (FACCT, 2001a; IOM, 2004a; AMA, 2005; AskMe3, 2005).

Practical Barriers

Practical barriers for providers generally can be classified as problems stemming from the health system itself, such as limited time for interactions with patients, prescribing requirements associated with multiple formularies, and lack of systems approaches and health information technology to improve workflow.

Providers are constrained in the amount of time they can spend with each patient for a number of reasons. Most visits to the doctor end with a prescription being written in the last 30 seconds, with limited discussion about the medication and the scope of important facts necessary for safe and effective medication use (George and Rabin, 1993; Gallagher et al., 2003; IOM, 2000). In a busy office practice, physicians often find it difficult to engage in lengthy discussions with patients about self-management, including medication use (Debusk et al., 1999; Ditmyer et al., 2003; Trude, 2003). Increased time pressures associated with clinical practice have been observed—patients waiting longer for appointments and more physicians reporting having inadequate time with patients (Trude, 2003). Constrained capacity also is the result of changes in the nature and prevalence of diseases in the population. Medical advances mean more treatment options are available to patients (Trude, 2003). People are living longer with chronic conditions that require more time to discuss treatment options and disease management, more complex coordination with other caregivers, and greater emphasis on preventive services (Trude, 2003). Some physician practices have employed physician assistants, nurse practitioners, nurse midwives, and clinical nurse specialists to counter the pressures of time and capacity. However, most ambulatory physicians cannot afford to hire additional office staff to assist them with patient education and counseling (Woolsey, 2000).

Prescribing requirements associated with multiple payers and formularies are another practical barrier affecting providers in their day-to-day practice activities. Some aspects of managing multiple different formulary requirements can be alleviated with the use of information technology.

For consumers, practical barriers to medication self-management inhibit an individual's ability to follow through on a prescribed medication regimen because of physiological, functional, or financial constraints. Such barriers include visual, hearing, and cognitive impairment; the inability to act on one's own behalf; complex medication regimens and adverse drug side effects; medication labeling and packaging that are difficult to read or use; and a lack of health insurance and the cost of drugs (Cohen, 2000). Seniors are particularly vulnerable as many of them are challenged by several of these barriers (NCHS, 1995).

Estimates of the number of people in the United States with visual difficulty (even wearing their usual eyeglasses) range from 7 to 20 million for all ages; 1.5 to 2.0 million are estimated to have severe visual impairment (i.e., near-total or total blindness) (AFB, 2004). Of particular concern is that four of the five major causes of vision impairment and blindness are associated with aging,[5] and the population of seniors is expected to double by 2030. Compromised ability to read instructions printed on drug containers or pharmacy leaflets creates a high potential for errors in self-managing medications. Consumers use a range of solutions, based generally on the severity of their impairment. For example, they may rely on friends or family members to read information on bottles or in leaflets, memorize the shape of a pill as it feels in their hand, use extra lighting and magnifiers, use a technological device (e.g., talking pill bottles, glucose meters with alerts) or a computer program that can convert printed information to Braille, or rely on their memory of oral communications (AFB, 2004). Nonetheless, methods for meeting the medication safety needs of individuals with various levels of visual impairment need to be more fully developed and widely distributed. Moreover, manufacturers need to make the printed information on prescription bottles easier to read for consumers in general.

Hearing-impaired individuals are compromised in their verbal communications with providers and pharmacists, which can lead to misunderstandings in the execution of the prescribed medication regimen. Since they are able to obtain and read written medication information, however, errors can be prevented more easily than for those with visual impairment.

Medication management requires not only a defined set of mental and physical skills, but also higher-level cortical processing and integration (Edelberg et al., 1999). With cognitive impairment, certain areas of the brain involved in thinking and higher-level executive functions (e.g., memory, language, reasoning, judgment, perception, attention, learning) are compromised to the point of interfering with the conduct of daily activities (NIMH, 2000; IOM, 2006). Even mild impairment, such as memory changes associated with the normal aging process, or fluctuating impairment, such as that associated with type II diabetes, can be a barrier to safe and effective medication self-management, especially when the ability to generate problem-solving strategies is required (Asimakopoulou and Hampson, 2002). Various interventions—psychosocial (e.g., caregivers, behavioral modification), technological (e.g., weekly pill organizers, electronic pagers), and others—can be effective in enhancing cognition and support for those with such impairment (Albert et al., 2003; Andrade et al., 2005).

---

[5]The major causes of visual impairment and blindness related to age are macular degeneration, cataracts, glaucoma, and diabetic retinopathy (NCHS, 1995).

The inability to perform self-care is another barrier to medication management when the impairment is high, when individuals are too sick to care for themselves, or when they are rendered unconscious. In such cases, individuals must rely completely on providers and other caregivers (e.g., family members, friends, surrogates) for medication management, safety, and error prevention. In these circumstances, informal caregivers require adequate training, education, and emotional support to carry out this role, whether for a short period, such as when a patient is postoperative, or for chronic conditions that require long-term care. Such caregivers can experience a significant burden that affects their quality of life and mental and physical health (McCullagh et al., 2005; Schrag et al., 2005; Vanderwerker et al., 2005), which in turn can result in medication errors.

It must be stressed that any policy or provider action that prevents a patient from having a designated surrogate present whenever the patient is receiving medication can be considered a barrier to safe and effective medication management. Given the amount of evidence for the occurrence of medication errors in hospitals, surrogates should be encouraged to question any professional about medications, routes of administration, and doses, and should be partners in reporting side effects patients may not be able to report themselves.

Another practical barrier to medication self-management can be the difficulty of opening a pill bottle or container, especially if an individual's manual dexterity has been compromised by his or her condition (e.g., arthritis, broken arm, disability). Such individuals may give up trying to open the bottle and simply not take the medicine.

Undesirable drug side effects (expected or not) distress patients, add to the burden of their illness, and increase the costs of care (Barsky et al., 2002). They may result in nonadherence or discontinuation of an otherwise appropriate therapy, or they may increase the complexity of the regimen as drug(s) are added to treat the side effects. Polypharmacy contributes significantly to the likelihood of adverse drug reactions and drug–drug interactions. Difficulties with side effects are exacerbated in those that have impaired renal and hepatic function as a result of either age (e.g., seniors) or illness (e.g., HIV) (Cohen, 2000; Murray and Kroenke, 2001). Drug toxicity can manifest as a decline in functional status (e.g., problems in performing activities of daily living, confusion, drowsiness, and depression) or a more pronounced acute or long-term reaction (e.g., vomiting, heart arrhythmia) (LeSage, 1991).

The inability to pay for medications (or for health care in general) is one of the most frequently cited practical barriers to medication adherence, as well as to overall self-management of health conditions (Safran et al., 2005; Piette et al., 2006). To minimize out-of-pocket costs for drugs, individuals who are uninsured or underinsured may not fill a prescriptions at all, skip doses, or take smaller doses to make the medication last longer (Cohen, 2000). Problems related to the cost of drugs are widespread; a recent poll showed that one of every three families has difficulty paying for prescriptions (AP, 2004). The elderly and those in lower income brackets are particularly affected by drug prices (Prutting et al., 1998), as are those subject to formularies that require high copayments even if no generic equivalent is available (Kamal-Bahl and Briesacher, 2004). Growing numbers of consumers are using the Internet to purchase lower-priced drugs, which may raise safety concerns (see Chapter 2).

Overcoming practical barriers requires a concerted effort to assist patients on the part of providers and other stakeholders. Providers should develop an understanding of how a medication regimen fits into the patient's life, including the practical barriers likely to arise. Providers should be able to direct patients and their surrogates to the appropriate resources for further assistance with medication management. They also should follow up with patients to see how they are handling the effects of their medication and whether they are encountering any barriers that could interfere with adherence. Pharmacists, drug manufacturers, and regulators should redesign product labels and instructions to make them easier to read and understand, and should redesign product containers so they are easier to use.

Attitudinal Factors

At the provider level, attitudinal factors that influence caregiving range from organizational leadership, culture, and priorities to individual providers' personal values. Improvements in patient safety (including medication safety and error prevention) are best achieved when health care organizations adopt a culture of safety (IOM, 2004c). A culture of safety[6] can be defined as an integrated pattern of individual and organizational behavior, based upon shared beliefs and values, that continuously seeks to minimize patient harm that may result from the processes of care delivery (Kizer, 1999). Several studies have documented that the existing health care culture is likely the greatest barrier to improving patient safety (Leape, 1998; O'Leary, 1998; Cohen et al., 2003; Manasse and Thompson, 2005). Patient safety and patient-centered care have not been made a priority (Gerteis et al., 1993; Manasse et al., 2002). Most events are handled within the con-

---

[6]A culture of safety encompasses several elements: shared beliefs and values about the health care delivery system; recruitment and training with patient safety as a priority; organizational commitment to detecting and analyzing patient safety events, including near misses; open communication about patient safety events (especially patient injury) within and outside the organization; and the establishment of a just culture (Kizer, 1999: IOM, 2004c).

text of a bureaucratic culture where errors are dealt with on an isolated, local basis, and lessons from failures are not integrated throughout the organization for purposes of improvement (Manasse and Thompson, 2005). The attitudes embodied in a culture of safety are not widely present within the majority of current health care organizations. To bring a culture of safety and quality to health care, fundamental change is required at both the organizational and individual practitioner levels (Bodenheimer, 1999). A core element of culture change is the patient-centered approach to care (Gerteis et al., 1993).

Patient-centeredness is an expression of organizational culture. While every health care organization's and practitioner's purpose is to serve patients, those that have successfully implemented a patient-centered approach to care have done so through a clear articulation of this mission of service, specific definition of the components of such service, and espousal of the approach by top management (Gerteis et al., 1993). Patient-centered care, then, permeates every facet of institutional life and practitoners' interactions with patients. Some organizational environments are more conducive to patient-centered care than others.[7] Chief attitudinal barriers to the adoption of patient-centered care from the organizational perspective are the failure to make patient-centered care a priority and redesign processes to support its multiple dimensions, lax or ineffective managerial intervention when such intervention can shape the quality of patient-centered care (e.g., efforts to attract, retain, and motivate the right people and socialize them into the institutional culture), and a lack of methods for measuring patients' perceptions (Gerteis et al., 1993). At the level of the individual provider, attitudinal barriers to patient-centered care are associated with a belief that the care being given *is* patient-centered, whereas the provider in fact may not fully understand the components of such interaction; external factors that negatively impact the provider–patient relationship;[8] preferences for formal sources of information (e.g., randomized controlled trials) for clinical decision making rather than patient preferences; frustration with poor

---

[7]It is more challenging to implement patient-centered care in large urban academic health centers. These centers must balance the myriad interests of clinical specialists; medical educators; academic researchers; politicians or government officials; and a community that may be deeply divided by class, race, and ethnicity. Complex lines of authority and governance typically connect the administration of a hospital with the medical school and the parent university, and in public institutions extend to involve civil service systems, government bureaucracy, and even local legislative processes (Gerteis et al., 1993).

[8]Examples include limited time to establish a bond with patients, technology encroaching on and replacing personal interactions, the litigiousness of medical practice, the comparison shopping approach to seeking services that increasingly characterizes consumers, and economic constraints that require uncomfortable discussions with the patient.

patient adherence to medical regimens rather than taking an empathetic approach to understand patient challenges; and challenges of the provider's own work environment (e.g., long hours).

Consumer-related attitudinal factors that affect medication self-management are rooted in the individual's belief system, culture, ethnicity, family, personal values, and previous experience with the health system (Cohen, 2000). Such factors affect everything from health beliefs to preferences regarding treatment, advance directives, organ donation, and disclosure, as well as truth telling (Berger, 1998). For example, cultural and religious beliefs can determine an individual's role preference in decision making. African Americans place greater emphasis on security, survival, and community than do white Americans, who place greater value on personal autonomy, empowerment, and control (Murray, 1992). Asian and Hispanic cultures emphasize family support and involvement in decision making, as well as high regard for and deference to the physician (Blackhall et al., 1995). Euthanasia is broadly accepted in the Netherlands, and nondisclosure of a cancer diagnosis is common practice in Italy and Japan (Berger, 1998).

According to Berger (1998), assessment of both good and harm is culturally mediated, and acceptance of medication varies by ethnic group. In fact, the influence of attitudinal factors is so strong that some health care interventions are unsuccessful because of the provider's failure to account for these factors. For instance, Afro-Caribbeans are less than half as likely as whites to take an antihypertensive medication (Morgan, 1995). White Americans are more likely to accept narcotic analgesics even if life is unintentionally shortened (Caralis et al., 1993). Herbal remedies are used commonly by Puerto Ricans to treat asthma and by Hispanics to treat diabetes (Zaldivar and Smolowitz, 1994; Pachter et al., 1995). Providers' recognition of the cultural and religious contexts of their patients' illnesses can thus be essential to a successful therapeutic relationship (Berger, 1998).

Culture and ethnicity aside, patients' personal experiences related to their health condition can influence their attitudes toward treatment and self-management. A growing portion of the population—36 percent in a recent survey (NCCAM, 2004)—uses complementary and alternative medications as part of the treatment plan or as a first step prior to the use of conventional medications. (Some organizations, such as the Dana Farber Cancer Institute, refer to these as integrative therapies.) Patients' preferences for these medications may engender a conflict between medical paternalism (the desire to do what is best for patients and protect them from foolish decisions) and patient autonomy (IOM, 2005). Moreover, individuals with serious and terminal illnesses may feel they are unable to tolerate any further traditional medicines with significant noxious side effects and prefer to seek relief with complementary and alternative therapies. Practitioners should demonstrate willingness, at the very least, to maintain a professional knowledge base on such medications, including results of the latest research studies, from which they can counsel their patients, guide decision making, and protect patient autonomy.

Individuals may have negative attitudes about prescription medicines and/or health care providers in general that may affect their willingness to follow a treatment regimen (Getz and Borfitz, 2002). Educated consumers may be cautious because providers have prescribed drugs in the past that turned out to be dangerous to people's health or have failed to prevent an ADE. They may also be aware that new drugs are not tested sufficiently to ensure that there will be no negative sequelae once the drugs are used outside of tightly controlled clinical trials in relatively healthy populations. Negative attitudes may be shaped as well by dislike of a medication's side effects or delivery method, concern about the perceived risk of using a particular medication, or a general reluctance to take any medication (Osman, 1997).

Conversely, people may overvalue the potential benefits of medications while ignoring or minimizing their risks. A recent article in the *New York Times* highlighted young people's sharing of psychiatric prescription medicines obtained from providers, their parents' medicine cabinets, and the Internet (Harmon, 2005). Youths are trading unused drugs with each other not to get high, but to feel more focused, better rested, less stressed, and less depressed. They also believe that general practitioners are too pressed for time to be familiar with the increasing inventory of psychiatric drugs and are happy to take suggestions from their friends. While they understand the risks of illegal drugs, such as cocaine and heroin, they have no grasp of the potential danger of misusing or overusing prescription drugs (Harmon, 2005). Additionally, older individuals struggling to pay for prescription drugs will often trade drugs with their friends to save money (Schommer et al., 2003).

The IOM's recent report on mental health and substance-use health care (IOM, 2006) expounds on the negative effects of stigma and discrimination on providers' recognition of the capacity of individuals with these conditions for self-efficacy in making decisions about and managing their illness and its care. In fact, stigma and discrimination act as direct impediments to patient-centered care. Those with mental health or substance-use conditions can experience stigma (negative attitudes about members of a group) and discrimination (behaviors that result from these attitudes) from society at large or from unenlightened clinicians. Such stereotypes (1) lessen patients' ability to participate in the management of their illness and achieve the desired outcomes; (2) encourage pessimistic and nontherapeutic attitudes and behaviors among clinicians, making them less likely to foster and support patients' self-management efforts;

and (3) promote discriminatory public policies that create barriers to patient-centered care and recovery. In the present context, because mental health care in America is highly medication-dependent, stigma and discrimination may affect deliberations about medication choice, administration modality, and who will monitor for side effects and determine the level of satisfaction with treatment outcomes.

Religious beliefs can affect medical treatment in such areas as prenatal and end-of-life decision making, as well as in more common decisions about medication use. In these situations, conflicts with medical recommendations are less about the clinical facts than about the meaning of the facts and their implications for further action (Curlin et al., 2005). Individuals who decline treatment for religious reasons do so more often in situations of relative uncertainty and under conditions in which treatment modalities offer modest benefit over faith in God for healing. However, some religions require that all medical interventions be declined, while others preclude the use of only certain treatments or medications (e.g., antidepressants). Regardless of the individual's reasons, courts have long held that patients have the right to refuse both medical treatment (*Schloendorff v. Society of N.Y. Hospital*, 211 N.Y. 125, 105 N.E. 92, 93 [1914]; *Cobbs v. Grant*, 502 P.2d 1, 12 [Cal 1972]), and mental health treatment or psychiatric medications (*Cruzan v. Director, Missouri Department of Health*, 497 U.S. 261 [1990]). For the majority of states, this includes the right of parents or guardians to refuse medical treatment for a child in their care based on religious beliefs without prosecution under federal laws governing abuse and neglect.[9] In life-or-death situations, however, a physician or hospital can obtain a court order to proceed with treatment for the child (Annas, 2004).

Attitudinal factors are more difficult to address than the other barriers discussed above as they embody an individual's personal beliefs and values, protected by the U.S. Constitution. Unless safety is seriously compromised (e.g., by youngsters trading drugs), most attitudinal factors should be taken into consideration when a medication regimen is being designed.

---

[9]Federal laws governing children and health care generally fall into two categories: (1) protection from abuse and neglect, in which the failure to provide adequate medical care is considered neglect (ACF, 2005), and (2) protection in clinical research through additional measures appropriate to the children's stage of development (IOM, 2004f). These laws rely on state statutes to provide relevant definitions or other elements essential to interpretation and application of the regulations. As a result, interpretations vary widely among the states. In 45 states, reliance of parents or guardians on spiritual healing is exempt from child abuse and neglect laws. The exceptions are Colorado, Hawaii, Massachusetts, Nebraska, and North Carolina, which repealed their religious exemption clauses.

RESOURCES TO SUPPORT THE
CONSUMER–PROVIDER PARTNERSHIP

Activating consumers on a national scale will require the development and refinement of resources to provide support at all stages of the medication-use process across all health care settings. Specifically, health and medication information and educational tools must be revised to have consumer-friendly formats; a variety of supportive interventions for medication safety and self-management education should be developed and tested; systems that provide around-the-clock access to clinical support should be developed; information technology tools should incorporate programs that support medication management and general self-care; and regulatory councils should expand consumer participation. All stakeholders in the health system (e.g., government regulators, payers, employers, industry) should make contributions to the development and implementation of these means of support for consumers and providers.

Recommendation 2: Government agencies (i.e., the Agency for Healthcare Research and Quality [AHRQ], the Centers for Medicare and Medicaid Services [CMS], the Food and Drug Administration [FDA], and the National Library of Medicine [NLM]) should enhance the resource base for consumer-oriented drug information and medication self-management support. Such efforts require standardization of pharmacy medication information leaflets, improvement of online medication resources, establishment of a national drug information telephone helpline, the development of personal health records, and the formulation of a national plan for the dissemination of medication safety information.

• Pharmacy medication information leaflets should be standardized to a format designed for readability, comprehensibility, and usefulness to consumers. The leaflets should be made available to consumers in a manner that accommodates their individual needs, such as those associated with variations in literacy, language, age, and visual acuity.
• The NLM should be designated as the chief agency responsible for Internet health information resources for consumers. Drug information should be provided through a consumers' version of the DailyMed program, with links to the NLM's Medline Plus program for general health and additional drug information.
• CMS, the FDA, and the NLM, working together, should undertake a full evaluation of various methods for building and funding a national network of drug information helplines.

- CMS, the FDA, and the NLM should collaborate to confirm a minimum dataset for personal health records and develop requirements for vendor self-certification of compliance. Vendors should take the initiative to improve the use and functionality of personal health records by incorporating basic tools to support consumers' medication self-management.
- A national plan should be developed for widespread distribution and promotion of medication safety information. Health care provider, community-based, consumer, and government organizations should serve as the foundation for such efforts.

Pharmacy Leaflets

Written information about prescription drugs for consumers is available in various forms (e.g., medication guides, pharmacy leaflets, patient package inserts,[10] websites). Consumers rely primarily on pharmacy-distributed documents (i.e., medication guides and leaflets) for basic information and instructions about their medications. Medication guides (as defined in Chapter 2) are pharmaceutical company–produced and FDA-approved labels that are required to be provided to consumers for drugs that pose a serious and significant public health concern if certain circumstances exist.[11] While the law (21 Code of Federal Regulations Part 208) requiring distribution of medication guides was not formally passed until 1999 (NARA, 1999), the FDA began requiring additional warnings and consumer-oriented information for certain high-risk drugs, such as isoproterenol products, in the late 1960s and for oral contraceptives (by means of patient package inserts) in the 1970s (DHHS, 1996). Through these early initiatives, the FDA recognized the benefit of such information to safe, effective medication use. At several points in subsequent decades, the FDA sought to pass formal regulations requiring the provision of consumer-oriented information for all prescription drugs; each time, however, the

---

[10]Patient package inserts are labels written for consumers based on FDA and drug company discussions. The inserts provide basic information about the drug, including its major and common risks and efficacy, and pertinent disease-specific information in consumer-friendly language. Unlike professional product labels, patient package inserts are generally not included in the product container, and they are not required for most drugs. Pharmacies are not required to dispense them, except for oral contraceptives and estrogen-containing products.

[11]Medication guides are to be handed out if (1) patient labeling could help prevent serious adverse effects; (2) supplemental information about the seriousness of the drug's risks (relative to its benefits) is warranted because such information could affect patients' decision to use or continue to use the drug; or (3) supplemental information on adherence to directions for use is crucial to the drug's effectiveness (FDA, 2005).

legislation failed.[12] Instead, Public Law 104-180 was passed in 1996, establishing a process for voluntary development and distribution of medication information for consumers in the form of pharmacy leaflets.

Pharmacy leaflets (also known as consumer medication information or CMI)—the computerized printouts that are attached to or placed in the prescription bag at the pharmacy—are now the most common form of medication information received by consumers. Neither the FDA nor state boards of pharmacy regulate the content of the leaflets, although the FDA did produce the Keystone report (DHHS, 1996), which provides guidance on leaflet design and content. If written in a clear, understandable manner, leaflets can be an important supplement to provider–patient communications. They can help bridge information gaps, clarify specific instructions, reinforce safety precautions, and increase adherence (Bernardini et al., 2000). For such results to occur, however, the leaflets must be easy to read, understand, and act upon (Gustafsson et al., 2003).

Unfortunately, a number of studies have confirmed that the quality of pharmacy leaflets remains inadequate, and varies widely from one pharmacy vendor to another and from one drug to another (Morrow et al., 1988; Svarstad and Mount, 2001; USP, 1999). Primary problems include a lack of standardized consumer-friendly nomenclature, incomplete or inaccurate information, inadequate layout and design for readability, and a lack of regulatory review and approval prior to use. A U.S. Pharmacopeia (USP) study found that these and various cognitive features can affect consumers' ability to find, understand, remember, and use the information provided (USP, 1999). Many types of health information, ranging from informed consent forms and public health information to prescription instructions and health education materials, are provided in written form characterized by jargon and technical language that make them unnecessarily difficult for consumers to use (Rudd et al., 2000). Cultural, language, and age differences exacerbate problems with comprehension, particularly since leaflets cannot be adjusted to accommodate individual needs (Gustafsson et al., 2003). There have been exceptions (such as the USP MedCoach leaflets with gender-specific and easy-to-read versions), but they have proved difficult to maintain. Research has found that key information deemed by consumers to be most important to them but missing or deficient in the leaflets is that related to risks (i.e., contraindications and drug interactions), followed by administration (i.e., directions and precautions) (Meryn, 1998; Svarstad and Mount, 2001; Garfield et al., 2004; Raynor et al., 2004).

---

[12]Refer to the *Action Plan for the Provision of Useful Prescription Medicine Information* (DHHS, 1996), also known as the Keystone report, for a historical review of the efforts of the FDA and others in this regard.

A major part of the problem has been follow-through on the processes established by Public Law 104-180. Specifically, the law set basic standards for content and design, and there are plans to study the extent of leaflet distribution at two specific target dates (2001/2002 and 2006/2007). However, the standards were never fully developed or implemented, and the most extensive studies on content and design have been undertaken by other organizations, such as USP, and individuals. As a result, most pharmacies distribute leaflets, but the only standard is a de facto one set by the market. To move forward with leaflet design, the FDA published a draft guidance document in May 2005 describing how vendors should implement the Keystone criteria. However, those criteria need further improvement to address critical barriers experienced by consumers when trying to read, understand, and act on medication information in the leaflets. Remaining concerns about leaflet readability, comprehensibility, and usefulness to the consumer must be resolved to support safe and effective medication use.

Additional work on human and cognitive factors engineering aspects of content and design should be undertaken for the various consumer information sources (i.e., pharmacy leaflets, medication guides). Expanded studies should be based on well-known cognitive principles identified in the USP (1999) study, including the following:

- Information load (i.e., the amount of information presented)
- Study time (i.e., the limited amount of time someone will actually spend reading the information)
- Depth of processing (i.e., the way information can be processed to increase memory and understanding)
- Chunking (i.e., breaking up items into smaller, more manageable pieces)
- Linguistic coding (i.e., internal ways of naming or coding information to increase memory and understanding)
- Prior knowledge and knowledge structures from previous experiences that may make it easier to learn and recall new information
- Cognitive task scenarios that test the ability to utilize the information in problem solving situations (USP, 1999).

Along with work on human and cognitive factors, studies should be undertaken to develop and evaluate pictograms that could be used in leaflets to accommodate certain populations. Some studies have evaluated the use of pictograms to improve readability and comprehensibility, but their findings do not support major improvements in the comprehensibility of leaflet information (TGA, 2002; Hameen-Anttila et al., 2004; USP, 1999). In one study, reasons for neutral results included disconnects between pictograms and leaflet information, nonuse of text within pictograms to reinforce the message, and too many visual elements (USP, 1999). For example, pictograms meant to convey "ask/tell your doctor if you are pregnant" were interpreted as "don't use this drug if you are pregnant;" other pictograms meant to convey "don't drive" and "don't share medicines" did not translate at all. Researchers agree, however, that standardized, well-designed, and comprehensively tested pictograms would be valuable and safe to use for intended patient populations, particularly those in vulnerable groups (e.g., children, the elderly, those with poor sight or low literacy skills) (Hameen-Anttila et al., 2004).

Implementation of the leaflets designs can be relatively simple. Pharmacy database vendors can develop software programs that allow the pharmacist to generate a leaflet according to selected characteristics to accommodate the individual needs of consumers.

Lastly, the lack of an established regulatory review prior to distribution has compromised the effectiveness of leaflets. The committee believes FDA leadership is necessary to ensure that leaflet content and design promote safe and effective medication use and accommodate the needs of all consumer populations. The FDA could establish an advisory council for this purpose. Box 4-7 outlines specific tasks for leaflet improvement that encompass but go beyond those identified in the Keystone report (DHHS, 1996).

Pharmacy Container Labels

Along with pharmacy leaflets, the labels applied to medication containers dispensed at the pharmacy warrant significant improvement. Container labels that are difficult to read or easy to confuse with those for other medications increase the likelihood that an error will occur (Cohen, 2000). (Issues concerning the external packaging and labeling generated by drug manufacturers, which affect health care providers, are discussed in Chapter 6; the discussion here focuses on bottle labels generated at the pharmacy, which affect consumers.)

At the community pharmacy, almost all medications are dispensed in similar-looking brown, bottle-shaped containers with white labels providing basic drug information. Warnings (e.g., may cause drowsiness, take with food) are placed horizontally on the containers on yellow stickers that may include a pictogram. Typically for drug information and warnings, the point size is quite small (i.e., 10 or smaller), and the labels may contain abbreviations, acronyms, or other terms that are difficult for consumers to read and understand. Moreover, the readability of label information is compromised when the label is placed horizontally so that it can be read only by turning the bottle around, and when characters are compressed to fit the small space of the label (Wogalter and Vigilante, 2003).

BOX 4-7
Principles for Improving Pharmacy Medication
Information Sheets (Leaflets)

The FDA and the National Library of Medicine should:
- Develop a consumer-friendly set of terms and concepts (nomenclature) that can be applied to all printed materials, including leaflets. This nomenclature should be flexible enough to accommodate differences among patient populations, such as age, health status, ability to understand, and language. It should be transferable to data standards associated with consumer-oriented information technologies.
- Produce leaflets in multiple languages that can be printed from pharmacy database systems on demand to meet the needs of consumers with low or no English proficiency. Additionally, the FDA should work with the appropriate organizations to make leaflet medication information available for the visually impaired and the blind.
- Provide information in a format that progresses into greater detail.

The FDA should:
- Establish a visual standard for the layout of leaflets as a model for pharmacies to follow. The layout should place information in order of importance to and use by the consumer. Specifically, information should be presented in the following order:
  - Name of medication and brief description of regimen
  - Instructions for use (per clinician's orders)
  - Contraindications
  - Precautions and warnings
  - Other use information (e.g., how it works, monitoring of effects)
  - Side effects (occurrence rate and what to do about them)
  - Contacts for emergencies and patient safety information
  - Additional information sources (e.g., MedlinePlus)
- Ensure that leaflet content is presented in 12-point type at a minimum. Along with other criteria from the Keystone report (DHHS, 1996) study, descriptions should be in active, short phrases or sentences.
- Review and approve all medication leaflets to be distributed by pharmacies. Regulators should create a medication safety council with consumer representatives to review and approve materials.
- Develop measures for regularly evaluating the readability, comprehensibility, and usefulness of leaflets.

Sometimes warning labels are stuck on the bottles over other important information or each other. These problems of readability and comprehensibility are compounded for those individuals with visual or hearing impairment, memory problems, or language or literacy difficulties (Drummond et al., 2004). Moreover, opening containers with safety caps can be problematic for older individuals, exacerbating their difficulties in taking their medications (Beckman et al., 2005).

Several studies of all types of labeling have demonstrated the importance of label format—point size, font type, font compression, design/layout, and terminology (including acronyms)—for readability, comprehensibility, and usefulness to consumers (Cramer, 1998; Cohen, 2000; Wogalter and Vigilante, 2003). For example, Drummond and colleagues (2004) noted significant improvements in comprehension and adherence among older adults when the label font was Arial 22 or the equivalent—almost three times the point size normally used on medication labels. Adjusting the format of pharmacy bottle labels is one of the simplest, lowest-cost means of improving consumer understanding of the information presented (Wogalter and Vigilante, 2003).

Some pharmacies are experimenting with new designs for the shape of medication containers and for labels. For example, the new bottle and label design implemented by pharmacies at Target™ retail stores, called Clear Rx™, is an upside-down bottle made from red clear plastic with flat front/back surfaces for printed information, including up to five warnings (Hafferty, 2005). Removable colored rings can be added around the bottle opening to differentiate family members' medications or an individual's different medications. On the label, light blue bands separate each item of labeling information. The name of the prescription is in bold and all capital letters, highlighted by a light gray background. Below the drug name are the instructions for use, followed by a colored band, then secondary information, such as the number of tablets/capsules, date, number of refills, prescriber's name, drug routing information, and pharmacy phone numbers (Hafferty, 2005). Additional information about side effects and warnings are printed on a small card that slips under the back portion of the label.

The FDA is now exploring the development of a general set of requirements for redesigning pharmacy containers and labels to improve their safety and quality. Comparative studies of different designs should be undertaken to determine those optimally useful to consumers. Such efforts should incorporate the principles of human factors engineering and include thorough testing in the general population. As with pharmacy leaflets, attention should be given to the needs of various consumer groups; different designs may be necessary to accommodate these varying needs.

Drug Information on the Internet

The proliferation of Internet-based health information over the last decade has given consumers immediate access to valuable resources such as medical journals and libraries, disease management guidelines, medication information, and treatment alternatives, and consumers are increasing their use of the Internet to obtain this information. The proportion of adults who have sought health information online grew from 27 percent (54 million) in 1998 to 53 percent (117 million) in 2005 (HI, 2005). Many consumers believe that Internet health information is highly reliable (37 percent) or somewhat reliable (53 percent). In reality, however, the quality of health and drug information on the Internet remains quite variable (Griffiths and Christensen, 2000; Berendt et al., 2001; Eysenbach et al., 2002; Risk and Petersen, 2002). This variability stems from the multitude of sources of information and differing standards (or the lack thereof) for developing content (Silberg et al., 1997; Berland et al., 2001; Eysenbach et al., 2002).

Most drug information on the Internet is not peer reviewed, but is developed from lay or commercial sources. Those sources may include other Internet sites that attempt to provide medical information for all needs (e.g., http://www.drkoop.com, webmd.com), that target specific health and medication information needs (e.g., American Cancer Society [http://www. cancer.org], http://www.hopkins-aids.edu), or that are maintained by health care providers and pharmaceutical companies (Gawande and Bates, 2000). Much drug information from nonpeer-reviewed sources tends to be poor and on occasion can even be harmful (Doupi and van der Lei, 1999; Boyer et al., 2001; Crocco et al., 2002). Many Internet pharmacies that sell prescription drugs, OTCs, dietary supplements, and complementary and alternative medications are particularly known for presenting inadequate, inaccurate, misleading, or fraudulent information (Eysenbach et al., 2002; Bessell et al., 2003; Molassiotis, 2004; Oakley, 2005). Yet in many cases, these sources are the first retrieved from Internet search engines (Peterson et al., 2003). The commercial website of a drug's pharmaceutical manufacturer, which highlights the drug's benefits and downplays its risks, tends to be one of the first retrieved as well. Because most consumers do not go beyond the first page of search results, they are not easily or automatically accessing the highest-quality or most objective drug information from the most respected sources, such as the National Library of Medicine (NLM). They may not know exactly where to find the best information or how to evaluate the quality of information from various sites. Moreover, the most respected sources of drug information— the NLM, the FDA, other government sources, peer-reviewed journals, health care provider organizations, consumer organizations, and pharmaceutical companies—are available online in multiple formats, at various levels of detail, and often with data that conflict with each other, further confusing consumers (Eysenbach et al., 2002).

Government agencies are collaborating to develop reliable, high-quality, consumer-friendly health and medication information available to the general public online through the NLM. In particular, NLM's MedlinePlus program provides information online in English that is easy to read, with interactive tutorials and voice recordings to facilitate learning (Personal communication, E. Humphreys, 2003). The tutorials, available for more than 150 health topics, are a popular feature in part because they are suitable for those with low levels of literacy. In addition to providing standardized health information, the NLM has a leadership role in the development of standardized electronic drug information for providers through the DailyMed program. The DailyMed database, as its name suggests, is intended to provide updates of medication information to the public on a daily basis (Brown et al., 2003). The NLM's MedlinePlus program does provide consumer-oriented drug information developed by several sources. However, greater standardization is needed. On MedlinePlus, consumers should have access to the electronic versions of standardized pharmacy leaflets and consumer-oriented versions of product package inserts (or patient information sheets). The FDA has been working with pharmaceutical companies to standardize the latter inserts (see Chapter 6), but more work is needed on current versions to employ more consumer-friendly nomenclature.

An important aspect of raising public awareness of quality information available at the NLM website is ensuring that this information is placed as the first to be retrieved when consumers search the Internet for health and medication information. Such placement of the NLM's resources and peer-reviewed literature is critical to improving consumer education and access to information resources. The NLM, search engine developers, and Internet service providers should collaborate to develop mechanisms that support the NLM's placement as a top resource for Internet health information.

The committee believes continued leadership by the NLM and the FDA is necessary to make health and medication information widely available to the public in standardized form and everyday language. The NLM should receive funding for several specific tasks aimed at advancing the online availability of quality health and medication information (see Box 4-8).

Telephone Helpline

Telephone intervention and helpline support programs in several countries have proven to be a successful resource for consumers seeking medical advice and information. Consumers can receive advice around the clock about general self-care and self-management of symptoms related to their health condition, medication, or drug side effects, as well as information about their health and prescription drug benefits. Helplines are an important supplement to provider services, giving consumers immediate access to effective care when they are unsure how best to care for themselves or for another as a designated surrogate. Such interventions have resulted in im-

---

BOX 4-8
Tasks the National Library of Medicine Should Undertake to Develop Quality Internet Resources for Drug Information

- Expand the language offerings of MedlinePlus health information and interactive tutorials to accommodate those who do not possess proficiency in English.
- Develop interactive tutorials for medication information (i.e., pharmacy leaflets). Such tutorials should be available to consumers in a number of different languages.
- Develop and maintain a standardized glossary of medication-related terms to help consumers understand the differences between particular medical concepts or terms. A link to the glossary should be available on each MedlinePlus medication information webpage.
- Maintain a patient safety library for consumers, containing general information on medication safety practices and where to report problems.
- Work with other government agencies or private groups to develop criteria for evaluating the quality of health information for consumers on the Internet. A "seal of approval" or a "trusted site" designation (similar to the "Good Housekeeping seal of approval") should be developed that is easily recognizable to consumers.
- Work with Internet service providers and search engine developers to establish mechanisms for making the NLM-based health and medication information and top-quality peer-reviewed literature first results of consumers' online information searches.

---

proved health outcomes, decreased provider and emergency room visits, and ultimately reduced health care expenditures (Reigel et al., 2002; Bosworth et al., 2005; Caithain et al., 2005). Self-confidence and self-efficacy in handling one's own health problems are also noted benefits of telephone interventions (Brooks et al., 2004).

Currently, most telephone helplines are available through health care providers and target certain health conditions, such as cancer (Jefford et al., 2005), chronic heart failure (Reigel et al., 2002), rheumatoid arthritis (Hughes et al., 2002), hypertension (Bosworth et al., 2005), and mental health problems (De Leo et al., 2002). Some address the needs of specific patient populations (e.g., pediatric patients) and are manned by physicians who share resources (Poole et al., 1993). For providers, the *Physicians' Desk Reference* (PDR, 2005) provides lists of toll-free numbers for pharmaceutical companies staffed by nurses and pharmacists well qualified to provide drug information.

In Western Australia, nurses provide health information associated with general practice by telephone statewide (Turner et al., 2002); similar services are offered nationally in Canada (Robb, 1996), Denmark (Christensen and Olesen, 1998), and the United Kingdom (Caithain et al., 2005). The National Health Service (NHS) in the United Kingdom has by far the most well-developed telephone intervention and helpline support system in the world—NHS Direct (Caithain et al., 2005). Individuals can call the service and receive advice for a per minute fee; the average call costs £18.00 or roughly US$31.00. In all cases, nurses are the primary health professionals providing telephone intervention and helpline support (Greatbatch et al., 2005). Strict protocols and standards for evaluating consumers' health needs, along with clinical decision-support software, guide the helpline consultations.

In the United States, consumers receive telephone assistance with questions about their prescription medications by directly contacting their health care provider, local pharmacist, or prescription benefit manager or going to the emergency room. This approach may not be able to meet the growing health demands and information needs and the changing demographics of the U.S. population. Use of all medications has increased tremendously in recent decades, now representing 11 percent of overall health care expenditures (NCHS, 2005). Of these expenditures, ADEs are the largest safety-related cost to the health system. Many of these events are the result of misunderstanding proper use of a drug. There are also enormous gaps in timely access to advice and information about medications, particularly for the 43 million Americans who are uninsured (IOM, 2004b) and those with literacy and language difficulties (IOM, 2004a).

Consumers need quick, easy access to drug information, advice about minor problems, and information on what to do about side effects and adverse reactions for the range of products on the market. The committee believes establishing a national drug information telephone helpline (a "drugline") could serve this purpose. The drugline would give consumers a third option for obtaining information about proper medication use, complementing paper and online sources they may not be able to access, read, or understand. In particular, establishing the drugline would accelerate the availability of medication assistance to consumers with health literacy, language, and other barriers. However, it will take significant time and funding to expand existing online resources. Building a national drugline similar to that in the United Kingdom would be expensive. In fiscal year 2002–2003, the cost of the NHS Direct program was £124 million (US$216.6 million). Thus, leveraging the existing health care and public health infrastructure may be the best option for developing the drugline and trimming the overall costs for doing so.

One possibility may be the expansion of poison control centers to include drug safety counseling. Several centers have collaborated with nearby universities and already initiated expansion in this capacity. For example, the Arizona Poison and Drug Information Center operates as part of the University of Arizona, Health Sciences Center, College of Pharmacy, providing accessible poison- and medication-related emergency treatment advice; referral assistance; and comprehensive information on poisons and toxins, poison prevention, and the safe and proper use of medications (APDIC, 2005). As another example, along with counseling on poison-related events, the Rocky Mountain Poison and Drug Center provides health and safety information on the safe and effective use of medications, adverse reactions, drug interactions, and drug use during pregnancy and lactation (RMPDC, 2006). Pharmaceutical companies contract with the center to provide their customers 24-hour access to medical information, to collect information on adverse drug events, and to meet other regulatory requirements. The Denver Health Nurse Line also is part of the Rocky Mountain Poison and Drug Center, providing 24-hour access to medical triage for health concerns. Potentially, a combination of existing funds from local, state, and private sources could be used, together with additional allocations from private and federal sources, to finance such expansion of poison control centers nationwide.

A drawback to this approach may be the question of whether most poison control centers are adequately funded and structured to handle drug information and counseling services. Currently most are not, but they can be. The 2004 IOM report *Forging a Poison Prevention and Control System* highlighted many of the issues involved, citing financial instability, lack of network or systems infrastructure (each operates independently), lack of effective links to the nation's public health system, and data collection that operates through a proprietary system (IOM, 2004e). The report made several recommendations for improvement, many of which have yet to be implemented. Policy makers should revisit the recommendations of this report in evaluating possibilities for development of the proposed drugline.

The federal government should undertake a full evaluation of various methods for building a national network of drug information helplines and develop strategies for their ongoing funding and financing. Knowledge gained from the successful telephone intervention and helpline support programs mentioned above can be incorporated into the strategy for developing these centers, along with other guidance outlined in Box 4-9. The druglines should include a mechanism for consumers to report ADEs and medication errors.

Personal Health Records

Emerging information and communications technologies have great potential to improve consumers' self-management of their health and health conditions (Markle Foundation, 2005). Over the last 5 years, several initiatives have been launched to develop and market computerized personal health records (PHRs) as a viable technology to support self-management. In general, PHRs were intended to function as an extension of electronic health

BOX 4-9
Guidelines for a National Drugline

The drugline should:

• Provide telephone access to medication information consistent with the standards for information available through the NLM's MedlinePlus.
• Provide medication information in multiple languages, accessible through touch- or voice-activated menus.
• Have qualified health care professionals (pharmacists, nurses) available to discuss medications with consumers as requested.
• Provide consumers with information about when, where, and how to report problems with their medications, through either the drugline or another system, such as MedWatch.
• Be accessible to consumers around the clock, 365 days a year.
• Include options for obtaining general information about medication safety and specific medications.
• Provide the opportunity to report an ADE or medication error.

records (EHRs) that would allow individuals to access certain portions of their health record (e.g., medication record, laboratory test results) through a secure portal. Individuals would also be able to enter information in the PHR/EHR system, such as that related to diet, exercise, adherence to treatment/medication plans, and OTC medications. However, slow adoption of EHRs by providers overall and some concerns about the privacy and security of health information on the part of consumers have resulted in several different types of web-based and stand-alone systems (Waegemann, 2002): (1) offline PHRs are composed of health-related documents carried in paper-based files or booklets, or electronically on a CD-ROM or smart card; (2) commercial PHRs store a consumer's health information on a secure webpage; (3) functional/purpose-based PHRs are web-based records accessible for a specific service, such as emergency care; (4) provider-based PHRs are those for which the provider or health plan makes portions of personal health information available through the provider's website/portal; and (5) partial PHRs allow an individual to keep an electronic file of health information and literature about diseases and conditions downloaded from the web, and also can be used by the web provider for marketing purposes.

Most PHRs function simply as a file of data; only a few have capabilities to support self-management. Yet even a holding file plus some modest upgrades can be useful to facilitate medication self-management. Specifically, the following functionality should be required for PHRs: information about safe medication use; printable medication record sheets with areas for listing drug allergies; patient safety reporting forms; and links to online drug libraries, drug interaction checkers, and medication adherence tools. The Markle Foundation Connecting for Health Initiative identified components of a minimum dataset for PHRs: (1) personal and emergency contact information, (2) physician and insurance information, (3) health condition information, (4) medications, (5) allergies, (6) immunization history, (7) certain test results, (8) surgical history, (9) health risks, (10) lifestyle information, and (11) advance directives (Markle Foundation, 2003).

Innovative tools designed for specific patient populations (e.g., seniors) to support medication adherence and self-monitoring of medication effects could prove highly useful to increase compliance. Eventually, PHRs and more comprehensive disease management programs can be integrated; at this time, however, they remain independent.

Information Dissemination

Important information and resources must be readily accessible to consumers to increase their awareness, knowledge, and active involvement with regard to medication safety on a national scale. Consumers should be able to obtain information not only from their providers, but also through community-based resources, consumer organizations, and public health networks. The information available should include general medication safety practices or tips, as well as guidelines for specific medications and polypharmacy regimens, medication self-management strategies, and methods for reporting ADEs and medication errors. Also, information should be available in both paper and electronic format, with variations to accommodate the consumer's individual needs and preferences. The lack of an overall strategy and resources for dissemination of information on medication use and safety has resulted in limited consumer knowledge and activation. Thus, the broad array of organizations already interacting with the medication-use system should develop strategic plans and leverage their resources to disseminate such information more broadly to consumers. Some examples of organizations that have developed consumer-friendly brochures or leaflets on general safe medication practices that providers can distribute to patients or consumers can print from the Internet are highlighted in Box 4-10.

Along with brochures, other means of disseminating information should be used, such as the development of health information resource centers. For example, retail pharmacies could set up medication kiosks for consumers[13] who would like to look up or print out additional information about

---

[13]This idea was proposed in the early 1990s and considered by retail pharmacies (Goldschmidt and Goodrich, 2004; Schuerenberg, 2005). The Baylor Sammons Breast Imaging Center in Dallas has set up several kiosks as part of a pilot project to facilitate patient registration and information retrieval (Fusco and Whiteside, 2005). A few small-scale studies could be undertaken to evaluate the best use of resources for such purposes and areas of greatest impact on consumers.

BOX 4-10
Examples of Consumer Medication Safety Materials

The National Council on Patient Information and Education (NCPIE) has developed several brochures describing what consumers can do to improve medication safety and prevent errors. Examples are *Be MedWise: Use Over-the-Counter Medicines Wisely* (http://www.bemedwise.org/brochure/bemedwise_english_brochure.pdf) and *Prescription Pain Medicines: What You Need to Know* (http://www.talkaboutrx.org/assocdocs/ TASK/18/pain_bro.pdf).

The Massachusetts Coalition for the Prevention of Medical Errors has published a guide for patients and families titled *Your Role in Safe Medication Use* (http://www.mhalink.org/public/prodserv/Docs/consumerguide.pdf).

The FDA collaborated with the Council on Family Health to produce such brochures as *Be an Active Member of Your Health Care Team* (http://www.fda.gov/cder/consumerinfo/Active12panel.pdf) and *Medicines and You: A Guide for Older Adults* (http://www.fda.gov/cder/consumerinfo/MedandYouEng.pdf).

The American Pharmacists Association has developed a brochure on *Avoiding Medication Errors* (http://www.pharmacyandyou.org/aboutmedicine/med.html).

The Institute for Safe Medication Practices has produced a pamphlet titled *Be an Informed Consumer* (http://www.ismp.org/Consumer/Brochure.html).

The above materials are a good start for information on safe medication use, but their dissemination is not as widespread as is needed. Moreover, the materials need to specify where to find additional information about health and medications, such as the NLM's MedlinePlus website (http://medlineplus.gov), and how to report problems or ADEs through the FDA's MedWatch Program (http://www.fda.gov/medwatch).

their medications. Public libraries could establish health resource areas for consumers interested in obtaining health and medication information or leaflets. School health programs and libraries could distribute child- or adolescent-oriented materials on safe medication use and what to do should a problem occur. Waiting areas in ambulatory care offices could serve as venues for patient education through videotapes, computers, and/or paper-based information on health conditions and on good medication self-management practices. The waiting area could display lively posters explaining the patient's rights and responsibilities with regard to medication safety (e.g., why it is important for the doctor to know if the patient is taking herbal or other dietary supplements).

Communication networks already in place, such as those associated with the public health infrastructure, should be utilized for medication safety initiatives. The Centers for Disease Control and Prevention recently completed the consolidation of its dissemination activities into one center—the National Center for Health Marketing (NCHM). The goal of NCHM is to help people actively use accessible, accurate, relevant, and timely health information and interventions to protect and promote their

---

BOX 4-11
Actions to Disseminate Medication Information and Resources

- Stakeholders should develop and disseminate materials that specifically address medication safety–related topics.
- Community-based health resource centers should be established in public and school libraries to facilitate consumer education.
- Providers should utilize ambulatory care, hospital, or pharmacy space and resources to make even limited medication information available.
- Government and consumer organizations should utilize their extensive communications networks to expand dissemination activities to include basic patient safety tips, medication safety information, and guidance on where to access quality health and medication information on the Internet.

NOTE: Medication information used for dissemination activities should be scientifically accurate, useful, and comprehensible to patients and their families, rather than the type of information used for commercial purposes.

---

health and that of their families and communities (CDC, 2005). The center has a number of divisions that could be employed for dissemination of medication safety information, including the divisions of Public and Private Partnerships, Consumer Services, and State and Local Public Health Systems. Other federal communication networks affiliated with the FDA, the NLM, and CMS could provide additional resources to broaden dissemination activities. Consumer organizations (e.g., Consumers Union, American Association of Retired Persons) could also serve as valuable resources. As membership-based organizations, they have extensive networks reaching out to millions of Americans and offering significant opportunities to expand communications about medication safety. Their members have access to information through online and paper publications that often include health and medication information. These organizations also provide telephone information helplines to assist their members in understanding important information, such as that on drug benefit plans. Actions the committee believes should be taken to better disseminate information and resources on medication safety are summarized in Box 4-11.

REFERENCES

AACN (American Association of Colleges of Nursing). 1998. *The Essentials of Baccalaureate Education for Professional Nursing Practice.* Washington, DC: AACN.

AAMC (Association of American Medical Colleges). 1999. *Report III: Contemporary Issues in Medicine: Communication in Medicine.* Washington, DC: AAMC.

ACF (Administration for Children and Families). 2005. *Overview of Abuse and Neglect.* [Online]. Available: http://nccanch.acf.hhs.gov/topics/overview/index.cfm [accessed March 27, 2006].

AFB (American Foundation for the Blind). 2004. *Submission to the FDA for the Medicare Prescription Drug Improvement and Modernization Act of 2003: Study on Making Prescription Pharmaceutical Information Accessible for Blind and Visually Impaired Individuals.* Docket 2004N-0221, June 25, 2004.

Albert SM, Flater SR, Clouse R, Todak G, Stern Y, Marder K. 2003. Medication management skill in HIVL I. Evidence for adaptation of medication management strategies in people for cognitive impairment. II. Evidence for a pervasive lay model of medication efficacy. *AIDS and Behavior* 7(3):329–338.

AMA (American Medical Association). 1998. *Informed Consent.* [Online]. Available: http://www.ama-assn.org/ama/pub/category/4608.html [accessed December 2005].

AMA. 2005. *Helping Your Patients Understand.* [Online]. Available: http://www.ama-assn.org/ama/pub/category/9913.html [accessed February 6, 2006].

Andrade AS, McGruder HF, Wu AW, Celano SA, Skolasky RL, Selnes OA, Huang IC, McArthur JC. 2005. A programmable prompting device improves adherence to highly active antiretroviral therapy in HIV-infected subjects with memory impairment. *Clinical and Infectious Diseases* 41(6):875–882.

Annas GJ. 2004. *The Rights of Patients: The Authoritative ACLU Guide to the Rights of Patients.* 3rd ed. New York: New York University Press.

Ansell JE. 1999. Empowering patients to monitor and manage oral anticoagulation therapy. *Journal of the American Medical Association* 281(2):182–183.

AP (Associated Press). 2004. *Almost a Third of Americans Say Paying for Drugs Is a Problem in Their Families.* [Online]. Available: http://www.ipsos-na.com/news/pressrelease.cfm?id=2064 [accessed November 15, 2005].

APDIC (Arizona Poison and Drug Information Center). 2005. *Arizona Poison and Drug Information Center.* [Online]. Available: http://uanews.org/cgi-bin/WebObjects/UAMaster Calendar.woa/2/wa/goPrint?EventID=1232 [accessed March 21, 2006].

Armstrong D. 1982. The doctor-patient relationship: 1930-1980. In: Wright P, Treacher A, eds. *The Problems of Medical Knowledge. Examining the Social Construction of Medicine.* Edinburgh, Scotland: Edinburgh University Press.

Arora NK, McHorney A. 2000. Patient preferences for medical decision making: Who really wants to participate? *Medical Care* 38(3):325–341.

Asimakopoulou K, Hampson SE. 2002. Cognitive functioning and self-management in older people with diabetes. *Diabetes Spectrum* 15(2):116–121.

AskMe3, Partnership for Clear Health Communication. 2005. *Information for Patients.* [Online]. Available: http://www.askme3.org [accessed February 6, 2006].

Avorn J. 1990. The elderly and drug policy: Coming of age. *Health Affairs* 9(3):6–19.

Baird MG, Bentley-Taylor MM, Carruthers SG, Dawson KG, Laplante LE, Larochelle P, MacCannell KL, Marquez-Julio A, Silverberg LR, Talbot P. 1984. A study of efficacy, tolerance and compliance of once-daily versus twice-daily metoprolol (Betaloc) in hypertension. Betaloc Compliance Canadian Cooperative Study Group. *Clinical and Investigative Medicine* 7(2):95–102.

Balas EA, Austin SM, Mitchell JA, Ewigman BG, Bopp KD, Brown GD. 1996. The clinical value of computerized information services. A review of 98 randomized clinical trials. *Archives of Family Medicine* 5(5):271–278.

Barat I, Andreasen F, Damsgaard EMS. 2001. Drug therapy in the elderly: What doctors believe and patients actually do. *British Journal of Clinical Pharmacology* 51:615–622.

Barsky AJ, Saintfort R, Rogers MP, Borus JF. 2002. Nonspecific medication side effects and the nocebo phenomenon. *Journal of the American Medical Association* 287(5):622–627.

Batalden P, Leach D, Swing S, Dreyfus H, Dreyfus S. 2002. General competencies and accreditation in graduate medical education. *Health Affairs* 21(5):103–111.

Beckman AGK, Parker MG, Thorslund M. 2005. Can elderly people take their medicine? *Patient Education and Counseling* 59:186–191.

Bedell SE, Jabbour S, Goldberg R, Glaser H, Gobble S, Young-Xu Y, Graboys TB, Ravid S. 2000. Discrepancies in the use of medications: Their extent and predictors in an outpatient practice. *Archives of Internal Medicine* 160(14):2129–2134.

Berendt M, Schaefer B, Heglund MJ, Bardin C. 2001. Telehealth for effective disease state management. *Home Care Provider* 6(2):67–72.

Berger J. 1998. Culture and ethnicity in clinical care. *Archives of Internal Medicine* 158:2085–2090.

Berland GK, Elliott MN, Morales LS, Algazy JI, Kravitz RL, Broder MS, Kanouse DE, Munoz JA, Puyol JA, Lara M, Watkins KE, Yang H, McGlynn EA. 2001. Health information on the Internet: Accessibility, quality, and readability in English and Spanish. *Journal of the American Medical Association* 285(20):2612–2621.

Bernardini C, Ambrogi V, Perioli L, Tiralti MC, Fardella G. 2000. Comprehensibility of the package leaflets of all medicinal products for human use: A questionnaire survey about the use of symbols and pictograms. *Pharmacological Research* 41(6):679–688.

Berry DL, Wilkie DL, Thomas CR, Fortner P. 2003. Clinicians communicating with patients experiencing cancer pain. *Cancer Investigation* 21(3):374–381.

Bessell TL, Anderson JN, Silagy CA, Sanson LN, Hiller JE. 2003. Surfing, self-medicating, and safety: Buying nonprescription and complimentary medicines via the Internet. *Quality and Safety in Health Care* 12:88–92.

Bikowski RM, Ripsin CM, Lorraine VL. 2001. Physician-patient congruence regarding medication regimens. *Journal of the American Geriatrics Society* 49(10):1353–1357.

Bitten N, Stevensen FA, Barry CA, Barber N, Bradley C. 2000. Misunderstandings in prescribing decisions in general practice: Qualitative study. *British Medical Journal* 320:484–488.

Blackhall LJ, Murphy ST, Frank G, Michel V, Azen S. 1995. Ethnicity and attitudes towards patient autonomy. *Journal of the American Medical Association* 274:820–825.

Blendon R, DesRochies C, Brodie M, Benson JM, Rosen AB, Schneider E, Altman DE, Zapert K, Herrmann M, Steffenson AE. 2002. Views of practicing physicians and the public on medical errors. *New England Journal of Medicine* 347(24):1933–1940.

Blumenthal D. 2004. Doctors and drug companies. *New England Journal of Medicine* 351(18):1885–1890.

Bodenheimer T. 1999. The American health care system: The movement for improved quality in health care. *New England Journal of Medicine* 340(6):488–492.

Bodenheimer T, Lorig K, Holman H, Gumbach K. 2002. Patient self-management of chronic disease in primary care. *Journal of the American Medical Association* 288(19):2469–2475.

Bosworth HB, Olsen MK, Gentry P, Orr M, Dudley T, McCant F, Oddone EZ. 2005. Nurse administered telephone intervention for blood pressure control: A patient-centered multifactoral intervention. *Patient Education and Counseling* 57(1):5–14.

Boyer EW, Shannon M, Hibberd PL. 2001. Web sites with misinformation about illicit drugs. *New England Journal of Medicine* 345(6):469–471.

Brazeau C. 1999. Disclosing the truth about a medical error. *American Family Physician* 60:1013–1014.

Brennan TA, Rothman DJ, Blank L, Blumenthal D, Chimonas SC, Cohen JJ, Goldman J, Kassirer JP, Kimball H, Naughton J, Smelser N. 2006. Health industry practices that create conflicts of interest: A policy proposal for academic medical centers. *Journal of the American Medical Association* 295(4):429–433.

Brooks D, Fancott CA, Falter LB, McFarlane A, Nonoyama ML. 2004. The development of a helpline for chronic obstructive pulmonary disease. *Patient Education and Counseling* 54:329–336.

Brown SH, Levin R, Lincoln MJ, Kolodner RM, Nelson SJ. 2003. *United States Government Progresses Toward a Common Information Infrastructure for Medications.* Bethesda, MD: National Library of Medicine.

Caithain AO, Goode J, Luff D, Strangleman T, Hanlon G, Greatbatch D. 2005. Does NHS Direct empower patients? *Social Science and Medicine* 61:1761–1771.

Calkins DR, Davis RB, Reiley P, Phillips RS, Pinco KLC, Delbance TL, Iezzoni LI. 1997. Patient-physician communication at hospital discharge and patients' understanding of the postdischarge treatment plan. *Archives of Internal Medicine* 157:1026–1030.

Caralis PV, Davis B, Wright K, Marcial E. 1993. The influence of ethnicity and race on attitudes toward advance directives, life prolonging treatments, and euthanasia. *Journal of Clinical Ethics* 4:155–165.

Caress AL, Luker K, Woodcock A, Beaver K. 2002. An exploratory study of priority information needs in adult asthma patients. *Patient Education and Counseling* 47:319–327.

Carroll L, Sullivan FM, Colledge M. 1998. Good health care: Patient and professional perspectives. *British Journal of General Practice* 48:1507–1508.

CDC (Centers for Disease Control and Prevention). 2005. *Health Marketing and Communication at the New CDC.* [Online]. Available http://cdc.confex.com/cdc/nic2006/techprogram/P11748.HTM [accessed May 8, 2006].

Chapman RH, Benner JS, Petrilla AA, Tierce JC, Collins SR, Battleman DS, Schwartz S. 2005. Predictors of adherence with antihypertensive and lipid-lowering therapy. *Archives of Internal Medicine* 165(10):1147–1152.

Christensen MB, Olesen F. 1998. Out of hours service in Denmark: Evaluation five years after reform. *British Medical Journal* 316:1502–1505.

Cleary PD, Edgman-Levitan S, Walker JD, Gerteis M, Delbanco TL. 1993. Using patient reports to improve medical care: A preliminary report from 10 hospitals. *Quality Management in Health Care* 2(1):31–38.

CMWF (The Commonwealth Fund). 2005. *Commonwealth International Survey on Sicker Adults.* New York: CMWF.

Cohen MH, Hrbek A, Davis RB, Schachter SC, Eisenberg DM. 2005. Emerging credentialing practices, malpractice liability policies, and guidelines governing complimentary and alternative medical practices and dietary supplement recommendations: A descriptive study of 19 integrative health care centers in the United States. *Archives of Internal Medicine* 165(3):289–295.

Cohen MM, Eustis MA, Gribbins RE. 2003. Changing the culture of patient safety: Leadership's role in health care quality improvement. *Joint Commission Journal on Quality and Safety* 29(7):329–335.

Cohen MR. 2000. *Medication Errors: Causes, Prevention, and Risk Management.* Sudbury, MA: Jones and Bartlett Publishers.

Connor M, Ponte PR, Conway J. 2002. Multidisciplinary approaches to reducing error and risk in a patient care setting. *Critical Care Nursing Clinics of North America* 14(4):359–367.

Coulter A. 2002. Patients' views of the good doctor: Doctors have to earn trust. *British Medical Journal* 325:668–669.

Cramer JA. 1998. Enhancing patient compliance in the elderly: Role of packaging aids and monitoring. *Drug Therapy* 12(1):7–15.

Crocco AG, Villasis-Keever M, Jadad AR. 2002. Two wrongs don't make a right: Harm aggravated by inaccurate information on the Internet. *Pediatrics* 109(3):522–523.

Cummings SR, Palermo L, Browner W, Marcus R, Wallace R, Pearson J, Blackwell T, Eckert S, Black D. 2000. Monitoring osteoporosis therapy with bone densitometry: Misleading changes and regression to the mean. *Journal of the American Medical Association* 283(10):1318–1321.

Curlin FA, Roach CJ, Gorawara-Bhat R, Lantos JD, Chin MH. 2005. When patients choose faith over medicine: Physician perspectives on religiously related conflicts in the medical encounter. *Archives of Internal Medicine* 165:88–91.

Curry LC, Walker C, Hogstel MO, Burns P. 2005. Teaching older adults to self-manage medications: Preventing adverse drug reactions. *Journal of Gerontological Nursing* 31 (4):32–42.

De Leo D, Buono MD, Dwyer J. 2002. Suicide among the elderly: The long-term impact of a telephone support and assessment intervention in northern Italy. *British Journal of Psychiatry* 181:226–229.

Debusk RF, West JA, Miller NH, Taylor CB. 1999. Chronic disease management: Treating the patient with disease(s) vs treating disease(s) in the patient. *Archives of Internal Medicine* 159(22):2739–2742.

Degner LF, Kristjanson LJ, Bowman D, Sloan A, Carriere KC, O'Neil J, Bilodeau B, Watson P, Mueller B. 1997. Information needs and decisional preferences in women with breast cancer. *Journal of the American Medical Association* 277(18):1485–1492.

DHHS (U.S. Department of Health and Human Services). 1996. *Action Plan for the Provision of Useful Prescription Medicine Information: Steering Committee for the Collaborative Development of a Long-Range Action Plan for the Provision of Useful Prescription Medicine Information.* Washington, DC: DHHS.

DiMatteo MR. 2004. Variations in patients' adherence to medication recommendations: A qualitative review of 50 years of research. *Medical Care* 42(3):200–209.

Ditmyer MM, Price JH, Telljohann SK, Rogalski F. 2003. Pediatricians' perceptions and practices regarding prevention and treatment of Type 2 diabetes mellitus in children and adolescents. *Archives of Pediatric and Adolescent Medicine* 157(9):913–918.

Doupi P, van der Lei J. 1999. Rx medication information for the public and the WWW: Quality issues. *Medical Informatics and the Internet Medicine* 24(3):171–179.

Drummond SR, Drummond RS, Dutton GN. 2004. Visual acuity and the ability of the visually impaired to read medication instructions. *British Journal of Othamology* 88:1541–1542.

Edelberg HK, Shallenberger E, Wei JY. 1999. Medication management capacity in highly functioning community-living older adults: Detection of early deficits. *Journal of the American Geriatrics Society* 47(5):592–596.

Ende J, Kazis L, Ash A, Moskowitz MA. 1989. Measuring patients' desire for autonomy: Decision making and information-seeking preferences among medical patients. *Journal of General Internal Medicine* 4:23–30.

Ernst E. 2001. Informed consent in complimentary and alternative medicine. *Archives of Internal Medicine* 161:2288–2292.

Eysenbach G, Powell J, Kuss O, Sa ER. 2002. Empirical studies assessing the quality of health information for consumers on the World Wide Web. *Journal of the American Medical Association* 287(20):2691–2700.

FACCT (Foundation for Accountability). 2001a. *Consumers and Quality. What Do They Know? What Do They Want? Results from FACCT Consumer Research 1996–2000.* Portland, OR: FAACT and New York: Markle Foundation.

FACCT. 2001b. *Development of a Consumer Communications Toolkit: Report and Findings from the Leapfrog Group's 2001 Focus Groups.* Portland, OR: FAACT and New York: Markle Foundation.

FDA (U.S. Food and Drug Administration). 2005. *Patient Labeling and Risk Communication*. [Online] Available: http://www.fda.gov/cder/Offices/ODS/labeling.htm [accessed January 2, 2006].

Flach SD, McCoy KD, Vaughn TE, Ward MM, Bootsmiller BJ, Doebbeling BN. 2004. Does patient-centered care improve provision of preventive services? *Journal of General Internal Medicine* 19:1019–1026.

Frampton SB, Gilpin L, Charmel PA. 2003. *Putting Patients First: Designing and Practicing Patient-Centered Care*. San Francisco, CA: Jossey-Bass.

FSMB (Federation of State Boards of Medicine) and NBME (National Board of Medical Examiners). 2005. *United States Medical Licensing Examination*. [Online]. Available: http://www.usmle.org [accessed March 23, 2006].

Fusco R, Whiteside J. 2005. Kiosks win patient kudos and speed registration. *Healthcare Benchmarks and Quality Improvement* 12(2):20–21.

Gallagher TH, Levinson W. 2005. Disclosing harmful medical errors to patients. *Archives of Internal Medicine* 165:1819–1824.

Gallagher TH, Waterman AD, Ebers AG, Fraser VJ, Levinson W. 2003. Patients' and physicians' attitudes regarding the disclosure of medical errors. *Journal of the American Medical Association* 289(8):1001–1007.

Garfield S, Francis SA, Smith FJ. 2004. Building concordant relationships with patients starting antidepressant medication. *Patient Education and Counseling* 55:241–246.

Gawande AA, Bates DW. 2000. *The Use of Information Technology in Improving Medical Performance: Part III. Patient-Support Tools*. [Online]. Available: http://www.medscape.com/viewarticle/408035 [accessed November 7, 2005].

George CF, Rabin KH. 1993. *Improving Patient Information and Education on Medicines*. Geneva, Switzerland: International Medical Benefit/Risk Foundation-RAD-AR.

Gerteis M, Edgman-Levitan S, Daley J, Delbanco T. 1993. *Through the Patient's Eyes: Understanding and Promoting Patient-Centered Care*. San Francisco, CA: Jossey-Bass.

Getz K, Borfitz D. 2002. *Informed Consent: A Guide to the Risks and Benefits of Volunteering for Clinical Trials*. Boston, MA: Thomson CenterWatch.

Gibson PG, Coughlan J, Wilson AJ, Abramson M, Bauman A, Hensley MJ, Walters EH. 2000. Self-management education and regular practitioner review for adults with asthma. *Cochrane Database Systematic Review* (2):CD001005.

Glasgow RE, Funnell MM, Bonomi AE, Davis C, Beckham V, Wagner EH. 2002. Self-management aspects of the improving chronic illness care breakthrough series: Implementation with diabetes and heart failure teams. *Annals of Behavioral Medicine* 24(2): 80–87.

Gleason KM, Groszek JM, Sullivan C, Rooney D, Barnard C, Noskin GA. 2004. Reconciliation of discrepancies in medication histories and admission orders of newly hospitalized patients. *American Journal of Health System Pharmacists* 61(16):1689–1695.

Goldschmidt L, Goodrich GL. 2004. Development and evaluation of a point-of-care interactive patient education kiosk. *Journal of Telemedicine and Telecare* 10(Supplement 1):30–32.

Greatbatch D, Hanlon G, Goode J, Caithain AO, Strangleman T, Luff D. 2005. Telephone triage, expert systems, and clinical expertise. *Sociology of Health and Illness* 27(6): 802–830.

Griffin SJ, Kinmonth AL, Veltman MWM, Gillard S, Grant J, Stewart M. 2004. Effect on health-related outcomes of interventions to alter the interaction between patients and practitioners: A systematic review of trials. *Annals of Family Medicine* 2(6):595–608.

Griffiths KM, Christensen H. 2000. Quality of Web-based information on treatment of depression: Cross sectional survey. *British Medical Journal* 321(7275):1511–1515.

Gurwitz JH, Field TS, Harrold LR, Rothschild J, Debellis K, Seger AC, Cadoret C, Fish LS, Garber L, Kelleher M, Bates DW. 2003. Incidence and preventability of adverse drug events among older persons in the ambulatory setting. *Journal of the American Medical Association* 289(9):1107–1116.

Gustafsson J, Kalvemark S, Nilsson G, Nilsson JLG. 2003. A method to evaluate patient information leaflets. *Drug Information Journal* 37:115–125.

Hafferty E. 2005. *Clear Rx: Design on Drugs.* [Online]. Available: http://www.brand channel.com/print_page.asp?"ar_id=248&section=profile [accessed December 27, 2005].

Haig K. 2003. *One Hospital's Journey Toward Patient Safety–A Cultural Revolution. Medscape Money and Medicine* 4(2). [Online]. Available: http://www.medscape.com/view article/460721 [accessed May 8, 2006].

Hameen-Anttila K, Kemppainen K, Enlund H, Bush PJ, Marja A. 2004. Do pictograms improve children's understanding of medicine leaflet information? *Patient Education and Counseling* 55:371–378.

Harmon A. 2005. Young, assured and playing pharmacist to friends. *New York Times.* p. 16.

Hartigan K. 2003. Patient education: The cornerstone of successful oral chemotherapy treatment. *Clinical Journal of Oncology Nursing* 7(6):21–24.

Harvard. 2006. *When Things Go Wrong: Responding to Adverse Events. A Consensus Statement of the Harvard Hospitals.* [Online]. Available: http://macoalition.org/documents/respondingToAdverseEvents.pdf [accessed April 13, 2006].

Haugbolle LS, Sorensen EW, Henriksen HH. 2002. Medication- and illness-related factual knowledge, perceptions, and behavior in angina pectoris patients. *Patient Education and Counseling* 47:281–289.

Heisler M, Bouknight RR, Hayward RA, Smith DM, Kerr EA. 2002. The relative importance of physician communication, participatory decision making, and patient understanding in diabetes self management. *Journal of General Internal Medicine* 17(4):243–252.

Heisler M, Vijan S, Anderson RM, Ubel PA, Bernstein SJ, Hofer TP. 2003. When do patients and their physicians agree on diabetes treatment goals and strategies, and what difference does it make? *Journal of General Internal Medicine* 18:893–902.

HI (Harris Interactive). 2005. *Number of Cyberchondriacs: U.S. Adults Who Go Online for Health Information Increases to Estimated 117 Million.* [Online]. Available: http://harrisinteractive.com/news/newsletters/healthnews/HI_HealthCareNews2005Vol5_Iss08.pdf [accessed November 5, 2005].

Hibbard JH. 2003. Engaging health care consumers to improve the quality of care. *Medical Care* 41(1):I-61–I-70.

Hibbard JH. 2004. New roles for patients and consumers in assuring high quality care. *Virtual Mentor: Ethics Journal of the American Medical Association* 6(6). [Online]. Available: http://www.ama-assn.org/ama/pub/category/12500.html [accessed September 26, 2006].

Horvatich PK, Schnoll SH. 1991. Filling the knowledge gap: A continuing medical education course on prescribing drugs with abuse potential. *New York State Journal of Medicine* 91(11):40S–42S.

Hughes RA, Carr ME, Thwaites CEA. 2002. Review of the function of a telephone helpline in the treatment of outpatients with rheumatoid arthritis. *Annals of the Rheumatic Disease* 61:341–345.

IHI (Institute for Healthcare Improvement). 2004. *Getting Started Kit: Prevent Adverse Drug Events (Medication Reconciliation).* How-To-Guide. Boston MA: IHI.

IHI. 2005. *Consumer Involvement.* [Online]. Available: http://www.ihi.org/IHI/Topics/HIVAIDS/ConsumerInvolvement.htm [accessed February 8, 2006].

IOM (Institute of Medicine). 2000. *To Err Is Human: Building a Safer Health System.* Washington, DC: National Academy Press.

IOM. 2001. *Crossing the Quality Chasm: A New Health System for the 21st Century*. Washington, DC: National Academy Press.

IOM. 2003. *Priority Areas for National Action Transforming Health Care Quality*. Washington, DC: The National Academies Press.

IOM. 2004a. *Health Literacy: A Prescription to End Confusion*. Washington, DC: The National Academies Press.

IOM. 2004b. *Insuring America's Health*. Washington, DC: The National Academies Press.

IOM. 2004c. *Patient Safety: Achieving a New Standard for Care*. Washington, DC: The National Academies Press.

IOM. 2004d. *Keeping Patients Safe: Transforming the Work Environment of Nurses*. Washington, DC: The National Academies Press.

IOM. 2004e. *Forging a Poison Prevention and Control System*. Washington, DC: The National Academies Press.

IOM. 2004f. *Ethical Conduct of Clinical Research Involving Children*. Washington, DC: The National Academies Press.

IOM. 2005. *Complementary and Alternative Medicines in the United States*. Washington, DC: The National Academies Press.

IOM. 2006. *Improving the Quality of Health Care for Mental and Substance-Use Conditions*. Washington, DC: The National Academies Press.

JCAHO (Joint Commission on Accreditation of Healthcare Organizations). 2004. *2005 Joint Commission National Patient Safety Goals*. [Online]. Available at: http://www.jcipatient safety.org/show.asp?durki=9344&site=164&return=9335 [accessed May 26, 2005].

JCAHO. 2005. *Ethics, Rights, and Responsibilities. 2005 Hospital Accreditation Standards*. Chicago, IL: JCAHO.

Jefford M, Kirke B, Grogan S, Yeoman G, Boyes A. 2005. Australia's cancer helpline: An audit and caller profile. *Australian Family Physician* 34(5):393–394.

Jenkins L, Britten N, Stevenson F, Barber N, Bradley C. 2003. Developing and using quantitative instruments for measuring doctor-patient communication about drugs. *Patient Education and Counseling* 50:273–278.

JKF (Josie King Foundation). 2002. *Sorrel's Speech to IHI Conference*. [Online]. Available: http://www.josieking.org/speech.html [accessed February 1, 2006].

Johnson MW, Mitch WE, Sherwood J, Lopes L, Schmidt A, Hartley H. 1986. The impact of a drug information sheet on the understanding and attitude of patients about drugs. *Journal of the American Medical Association* 256(19):2722–2724.

Johnstone MJ. 2000. Informed consent and the betrayal of patient's rights. *Australian Nursing Journal* 8(2):1320–1385.

Kaissi A, Johnson T, Kirschbaum MS. 2003. Measuring teamwork and patient safety attitudes of high-risk areas. *Nursing Economics* 21(5):211–218.

Kamal-Bahl, S, Briesacher B. 2004. How do incentive-based formularies influence drug selection and spending for hypertension? *Health Affairs* 23(1):227–236.

Kerzman H, Baron-Epel O, Toren O. 2005. What do discharged patients know about their medication? *Patient Education and Counseling* 56:276–282.

Ketchum K, Grass CA, Padwojski A. 2005. Medication reconciliation: Verifying medication orders and clarifying discrepancies should be standard practice. *American Journal of Nursing* 105(11):78–79.

KFF (Kaiser Family Foundation). 2004. *National Survey on Consumers' Experiences with Patient Safety and Quality Information*. Menlo Park, CA: KFF.

Kizer KW. 1999. *Large System Change and a Culture of Safety. Enhancing Patient Safety and Reducing Errors in Health Care*. Chicago, IL: National Patient Safety Foundation.

Knowlton CH, Penna RP. 2003. *Pharmaceutical Care*. 2nd ed. Bethesda, MD: American Society of Health System Pharmacists.

Krass I, Svarstad BL, Bultman D. 2002. Using alternative methodologies for evaluating patient education leaflets. *Patient Education and Counseling* 47:29–35.

Kravitz RL, Bell RA, Azari R, Kelly-Reif S, Krupat E, Thom DH. 2003. Direct observation of requests for clinical services in office practice: What do patients want and do they get it? *Archives of Internal Medicine* 163(14):1673–1678.

Lamb RM. 2004. Open disclosure: The only approach to medical error. *Quality Health Care* 13:3–5.

Lamb RM, Studdert DM, Bohmer RMJ, Berwick DM, Brennan TA. 2003. Hospital disclosure practices: Results of a national survey. *Health Affairs* 22(2):73–83.

Leape LL. 1998. *Creating a Culture of Safety*. Paper presented at: Enhancing Patient Safety and Reducing Errors in Health Care, Rancho Mirage, CA.

LeSage J. 1991. Polypharmacy in geriatric patients. *Nursing Clinics of North America* 26(2): 273–290.

Lewin SA, Skea ZC, Entwistle V, Zwarenstein M, Dick J. 2005. Interventions for Providers to Promote a Patient-Centered Approach in Clinical Consultations (Review). The Cochrane Collaboration.

Lorig KR, Sobel DS, Stewart AL, Brown BW, Bandura A, Ritter P, Gonzalez VM, Laurent DD, Holman HR. 1999. Evidence suggesting that a chronic disease self-management program can improve health status while reducing hospitalization: A randomized trial. *Medical Care* 39(1):5–14.

Maguire P, Pitceathly C. 2002. Key communication skills and how to acquire them. *British Medical Journal* 325:697–700.

Makoul G. Communication skills education in medical school and beyond. 2003. *Journal of the American Medical Association* 289(1):93.

Manasse HR, Thompson KK. 2005. *Medication Safety: A Guide for Health Care Facilities*. Bethesda, MD: American Society of Health System Pharmacists.

Manasse HR, Turnbull JE, Diamond LH. 2002. Patient safety: A review of the contemporary American experience. *Singapore Medical Journal* 43(5):254–262.

Mansell D, Poses RM, Kazis L, Duefield CA. 2000. Clinical factors that influence patients' desire for participation in decisions about illness. *Archives of Internal Medicine* 160:2991–2996.

Manser T, Staender S. 2005. Aftermath of an adverse event: Supporting health care professionals to meet patient expectations through open disclosure. *Acta Anaesthesiologica Scandinavica* 49:728–734.

Markle Foundation. 2003. *The Personal Health Working Group: Final Report. Connecting for Health: A Public-Private Collaborative*. New York: Markle Foundation.

Markle Foundation. 2005. *Connecting Americans to Their Health Care: Empowered Consumers, Personal Health Records, and Emerging Technologies*. New York: Markle Foundation.

Mazor KM, Simon SR, Gurwitz JH. 2004a. Communicating with patients about medical errors. *Archives of Internal Medicine* 164:1690–1697.

Mazor KM, Simon SR, Yood RA, Martinson BC, Gunter MJ, Reed, GW, Gurwitz JH. 2004b. Health plan members' views about disclosure of medical errors. *Annals of Internal Medicine* 140(6):409–418.

McCullagh E, Brigstocke G, Donaldson N, Kalra L. 2005. Determinants of caregiving burden and quality of life in caregivers of stroke patients. *Stroke* 36(10):2181–2186.

McDonnell PJ, Jacobs MR. 2002. Hospital admissions resulting from preventable adverse drug reactions. *Annals of Pharmacotherapy* 36(9):1331–1336.

Mead N, Bower P. 2000. Patient-centeredness: A conceptual framework and review of empirical literature. *Social Science and Medicine* 51(7):1087–1110.

Mechanic D, Meyer S. 2000. Concepts of trust among patients with serious illness. *Social Science and Medicine* 51:657–658.

Meryn S. 1998. Improving doctor-patient communication. *British Medical Journal* 316:1922–1930.

Michalsen A, Konig G, Thimme W. 1998. Preventable causative factors leading to hospital admission with decompensated heart failure. *Heart* 80:437–441.

Millenson M. 2003. The silence. *Health Affairs* 22(3):103–112.

Molassiotis A. 2004. Quality and safety issues of web-based information about herbal medicines in the treatment of cancer. *Complementary Therapies in Medicine* 12(4):217–227.

Morgan M. 1995. The significance of ethnicity for health promotion: Patients' use of antihypertensive drugs in inner London. *International Journal of Epidemiology* 24:S79–S84.

Morrow DG, Leirer V, Sheikh J. 1988. Adherence and medication instructions: Review and recommendations. *Journal of the American Geriatrics Society* 36:1147–1160.

Morrow DG, Weiner M, Young J, Steinley D, Deer M, Murray MD. 2005. Improving medication knowledge among older adults with heart failure: A patient-centered approach to instruction design. *The Gerontologist* 45(4):545–552.

Mullan F. 1998. Eugene McGregor, MD: A legacy of general practice. *Journal of the American Medical Association* 279(14):1117–1120.

Murray MD, Kroenke K. 2001. Polypharmacy and medication adherence: Small steps on a long road. *Journal of General Internal Medicine* 16(2):137–139.

Murray RF. 1992. Minority perspectives on biomedical ethics. In: Pellegrino E, Mazzarella P, Corsi P, eds. *Transcultural Dimensions in Medical Ethics*. Frederick, MD: University Publishing Group.

NARA (National Archives and Records Administration). 1999. *Title 21–Food and Drugs: Chapter I–Food and Drug Administration, Department of Health And Human Services. Part 208–Medication Guides for Prescription Drug Product*s (Effective 6-1-99). [Online]. Available: http://www.access.gpo.gov/nara/cfr/waisidx_99/21cfr208_99.html. Notes: 21 CFR 208 [accessed March 23, 2006].

NCCAM (National Center for Complimentary and Alternative Medicine). 2004. *The Use of Complementary and Alternative Medicine in the United States*. [Online]. Available: http://nccam.nih.gov/news/camsurvey_fs1.htm#use [accessed February 6, 2006].

NCHS (National Center for Health Statistics). 1995. *National Health Interview Survey on Disability*. [Online]. Available: http://www.cdc.gov/nchs/about/major/nhis_dis/nhis_dis.htm [accessed November 15, 2005].

NCHS. 2005. *Health, United States, 2005*. Hyattsville, MD: NCHS.

Nickerson A, MacKinnon NJ, Roberts N, Saulnier L. 2005. Drug-therapy problems, inconsistencies, and omissions identified during a medication reconciliation and seamless care service. *Healthcare Quarterly* 8:65–72.

NIMH (National Institute of Mental Health). 2000. *Cognitive Research*. Bethesda, MD: NIMH.

NPSF (National Patient Safety Foundation). 1997. *National Patient Safety Foundation at the AMA*. North Adams, MA: NPSF.

NPSF. 2000. *National Agenda for Action: Patients and Families in Patient Safety*. Chicago, IL: NPSF.

NQF (National Quality Forum). 2005. *Improving Use of Prescription Medications: A National Action Plan*. Wu HW, Nishimi RY, Kizer KW, eds. Washington, DC: NQF.

O'Leary DS. 1998. Organization, Evaluation, and a Culture of Safety. Paper presented at: Enhancing Patient Safety and Reducing Errors in Health Care, Rancho Mirage, CA.

Oakley A. 2005. Focus on: Information technology. Online drug information for dermatology patients. *Journal of Drugs and Dermatology* 4(1):108–113.

Osman LM. 1997. How do patients' views about medication affect their self management in asthma? *Patient Education and Counseling* 32:S43–S49.

Pachter LM, Cloutier MM, Bernstein BA. 1995. Ethnomedical (folk) remedies for childhood asthma in a mainland Puerto Rican community. *Archives of Pediatric and Adolescent Medicine* 149:982–988.

PCSEPMBBR (President's Commission for the Study of Ethical Problems in Medicine and Biomedical and Behavioral Research). 1982. *Making Health Care Decisions: The Ethical and Legal Implications of Informed Consent in the Patient-Practitioner Relationship.* New York: U.S. Government Printing Office.

PDR (Physicians' Desk Reference). 2000. *Physicians' Desk Reference.* Montvale, NJ: Medical Economics Co.

PDR. 2005. *Physicians' Desk Reference*, edition 2006. Montvale, NJ: Thomson PDR.

Pereles I, Russell ML. 1996. Needs for CME in geriatrics. Part 2: Physician priorities and perceptions of community representatives. *Canadian Family Physician* 42:632–640.

Peterson G, Aslani P, Williams KA. 2003. How do consumers search for and appraise information on medicines on the Internet? A qualitative study using focus groups. *Journal of Medical Internet Research* 5(4):e33.

Peterson JF, Kuperman GJ, Shek C, Patel M, Avorn J, Bates DW. 2005. Guided prescription of psychotropic medications for geriatric inpatients. *Archives of Internal Medicine* 165(7):802–807.

Piette JD, Heisler M, Horne R, Alexander GC. 2006. A conceptually based approach to understanding chronically ill patients' responses to medication cost pressures. *Social Science and Medicine* 62(4):846–857.

Poole SR, Schmitt BD, Carruth T, Peterson-Smith A, Slusarski M. 1993. After-hours telephone coverage: The application of an area-wide telephone triage and advice system for pediatric practices. *Pediatrics* 92:670–679.

Pronovost P, Weast B, Schwarz M, Wyskiel RM, Prow D, Milanovich SN, Berenholtz S, Dorman T, Lipsett P. 2003. Medication reconciliation: A practical tool to reduce the risk of medication errors. *Journal of Critical Care* 18(4):201–205.

Prutting SM, Cerveny JD, MacFarlane LI, Wiley MK. 1998. An interdisciplinary effort to help patients with limited prescription drug benefits afford their medication. *Prescription Drug Assistance* 91(9):815–820.

PSI (Premier Safety Institute). 2004. *Survey on Disclosure Practices.* Oak Brook, IL: PSI.

Ratzan SC, Parker RM. 2000. Introduction. In: Selden CR, Zorn M, Ratzan SC, Parker RM, eds. *National Library of Medicine Current Bibliographies in Medicine: Health Literacy.* NLM Pub. No. CBM2000-1. Bethesda, MD: National Institute of Health, U.S. Department of Health and Human Services.

Raynor DK, Savage I, Knapp P, Henley J. 2004. We are the experts: People with asthma talk about their medicine information needs. *Patient Education and Counseling* 53:167–174.

Reigel B, Carlson B, Kopp Z, LePetri B, Glaser D, Unger A. 2002. Effect of standardized nurse case-management telephone intervention on resource use in patients with chronic heart failure. *Archives of Internal Medicine* 162:705–712.

Reiling JG, Knutzen BL, Wallen TK, McCullough S, Miller R, Chernos S. 2004. Enhancing the traditional hospital design process: A focus on patient safety. *Joint Commission Journal on Quality and Safety* 30(5):233.

Reiser S. 1980. Words as scalpels: Transmitting evidence in the clinical dialogue. *Annals of Internal Medicine* 92:837–842.

Richards T. 1990. Chasms in communication. *British Medical Journal* 301:1407–1408.

Ridley DT. 2001. Informed consent, informed refusal, informed choice: What is it that makes a patient's medical treatment decisions informed? *Medical Law* 20(2):205–214.

Risk A, Petersen C. 2002. Health information on the Internet: Quality issues and international initiatives. *Journal of the American Medical Association* 287(20):2713–2715.

RMPDC (Rocky Mountain Poison and Drug Center). 2006. *Organization History.* [Online]. Available: http://www.rmpdc.org/history/index.cfm [accessed March 21, 2006].

Robb N. 1996. Telecare acting as an "electronic grandmother" for New Brunswickers. *Canadian Medical Association Journal* 154(6):903–904.

Rodehaver C. 2005. Medication reconciliation in acute care: Ensuring an accurate drug regimen on admission and discharge. *Joint Commission Journal on Quality and Patient Safety* 31(7):406–413.

Rogers G, Alper E, Brunelle D, Federico F, Fenn CA, Leape LL, Kirle L, Ridley N, Clarridge BR, Bolcic-Jankovic D, Griswold P, Hanna D, Annas CL. 2006. Reconciling medications at admission: Safe practice recommendations and implementation strategies. *Joint Commission Journal on Quality and Patient Safety* 32(1):37–50.

Rolland PD. 2000. Reading level of drug information printouts: A barrier to effective communication of patient medication information. *Drug Information Journal* 34:1329–1338.

Rozich JD, Resar RK. 2001. Medication safety: One organization's approach to the challenge. *Journal of Clinical Outcomes Management* 8:27–34.

Rozich JD, Howard RJ, Justeson JM, Macken PD, Lindsay ME, Resar RK. 2004. Standardization as a mechanism to improve safety in health care: Impact of sliding scale insulin protocol and reconciliation of medications initiatives. *Joint Commission Journal on Quality and Safety* 30(1):5–14.

Rudd RE, Colton T, Schact R. 2000. *An Overview of Medical and Public Health Literature Addressing Literacy Issues: An Annotated Bibliography. Report #14.* Cambridge, MA: National Center for the Study of Adult Learning and Literacy.

RWJF (Robert Wood Johnson Foundation). 2000. *Patient Education and Consumer Activation in Chronic Disease.* Princeton, NJ: RWJF.

Safeer RS, Keenan J. 2005. Health literacy: The gap between physicians and patients. *American Family Physician* 72(3).

Safran DG. 2003. Defining the future of primary care: What can we learn from patients? *Annals of Internal Medicine* 138(3):248–255.

Safran DG, Taira DA, Rogers WH, Kosinski M, Ware JE, Tarlov AR. 1998. Linking primary care performance to outcomes of care. *Journal of Family Practice* 47(3):213–220.

Safran DG, Neuman P, Schoen C, Kitchman MS, Wilson IB, Cooper B, Li A, Chang H, Rogers WH. 2005. Prescription drug coverage and seniors: Findings from a 2003 National Survey. *Health Affairs (Millwood)* W5-152–W5-166.

Sawicki PT. 1999. A structured teaching and self-management program for patients receiving oral anticoagulation: A randomized controlled trial. *Journal of the American Medical Association* 281(2):145–150.

Schlenk EA, Dunbar-Jacob J, Engberg S. 2004. Medication nonadherence among older adults: A review of strategies and interventions for improvement. *Journal of Gerontologic Nursing* 30(7):33–43.

Schneitman-McIntire O, Farnen TA, Gordon N, Chan J, Toy WA. 1996. Medication misadventures resulting in emergency department visits at an HMO medical center. *American Journal of Health-System Pharmacy* 53(12):1416–1422.

Schommer JC, Mott DA, Hansen RA, Cline RR. 2003. Selected characteristics of senior citizens prescription drug payment and procurement in 1998 and 2001. *Journal of Managed Care Pharmacy* 9(5):453–456.

Schrag A, Hovis A, Morley D, Quinn N, Jahanshahi M. 2005. Caregiver burden in Parkinson's disease is closely associated with psychiatric symptoms, falls, and disability. *Parkinsonism and Related Disorders* 12(1):35–41.

Schroeder SA, Showstack JA, Gerbert B. 1986. Residency training in internal medicine: Time for a change? *Annals of Internal Medicine* 104(4):554–561.

Schuerenberg BK. 2005. Kiosks serve up e-Rx convenience. *Health Data Management* 13(11): 56, 58.

Schultz PE, Perrier CV. 1976. Inadequacy of information about drugs. *International Journal of Clinical Pharmacology* 14(4):255–258.

Scott JT, Thompson DR. 2003. Assessing the information needs of post-myocardial infarction patients: A systemic review. *Patient Education and Counseling* 50:167–177.

Silberg WM, Lundberg GD, Musacchio RA. 1997. Assessing, controlling, and assuring the quality of medical information on the Internet. *Journal of the American Medical Association* 277(15):1244–1245.

Skoglund P, Isacson D, Kjellgren KI. 2003. Analgesic medication: Communication at pharmacies. *Patient Education and Counseling* 51:155–161.

Sleath B, Roter D, Chewning B, Svarstad B. 1999. Asking questions about medication: Analysis of physician-patient interactions and physician perceptions. *Medical Care* 37(11): 1169–1173.

Smith R, Hiatt H, Berwick D. 1999. Shared ethical principles for everyone in healthcare: A working draft from the Tavistock Group. *British Medical Journal* 318(7178):248–251.

Sol BG, van der Graaf Y, van der Bijl JJ, Goessens NB, Visseren FL. 2006. Self-efficacy in patients with clinical manifestations of vascular diseases. *Patient Education and Counseling* 61(3):443–448.

Stewart M. 1995. Effective physician-patient communication and health outcomes: A review. *Canadian Medical Association Journal* 152(9):1423–1433.

Stewart M, Brown JB, Weston WW, McWhinney IR, McWilliam CL, Freeman TR. 1995. *Patient-Centered Medicine: Transforming the Clinical Method.* Thousand Oaks, CA: Sage.

Stiggelbout AM, Kiebert GM. 1997. A role for the sick role. Patient preferences regarding information and participation in clinical decision-making. *Canadian Medical Association Journal* 157(4):383–389.

Sundin K, Jansson L. 2003. Understanding and being understood as a creative caring phenomenon in care of patients with stroke and aphasia. *Journal of Clinical Nursing* 12: 107–116.

Svarstad BL, Mount JK. 2001. *Evaluation of Written Prescription Information Provided in Community Pharmacies.* Rockville, MD: FDA.

Svarstad BL, Chewning BA, Sleath BL, Claesson C. 1999. The brief medication questionnaire: A tool for screening patient adherence and barriers to adherence. *Patient Education and Counseling* 37(2):113–124.

SWC (Sorry Works Coalition). 2005. *Homepage: Sorry Works Coalition.* [Online]. Available: http://www.sorryworks.net [accessed March 22, 2006].

Sweet MP, Bernat JL. 1997. A study of the ethical duty of physicians to disclose errors. *Journal of Clinical Ethics* 8:341–348.

Tamada JA, Garg S, Jovanovic L, Pitzer KR, Fermi S, Potts RO. 1999. Noninvasive glucose monitoring: Comprehensive clinical results. *Journal of the American Medical Association* 282(19):1839–1844.

Teutsch C. 2003. Patient-doctor communication. *The Medical Clinics of North America* 87(5):1115–1145.

TGA (Therapeutic Goods Administration). 2002. *Review of the Labelling Requirements for Medicines: Consumer-Focused Labelling—A Way Forward?* Australia: Commonwealth Department of Health and Ageing.

Trude S. 2003. *So Much to Do, So Little Time: Physician Capacity Constraints 1997-2001.* Tracking Report: Results from the Community Tracking Study. Washington, DC: Center for Studying Health System Change.

Turner VF, Bentley PJ, Hodgson SA, Collard PJ, Drimitis R, Rabune C, Wilson AJ. 2002. Telephone triage in Western Australia. *Medical Journal of Australia* 176:100–103.

USP (U.S. Pharmacopeia). 1999. *Optimizing Patient Comprehension Through Medicine Information Leaflets.* Rockville, MD: USP.

Vanderwerker LC, Laff RE, Kadan-Lottick NS, McColl S, Prigerson HG. 2005. Psychiatric disorders and mental health service use among caregivers of advanced cancer patients. *Journal of Clinical Oncology* 23(28):6899–6907.

VHA (Veterans Health Administration). 2005. *Disclosure of Adverse Events to Patients. VHA Directive 2005-049.* Washington, DC: VHA.

Von Korff M, Gruman J, Schaefer J, Curry SJ, Wagner EH. 1997. Collaborative management of chronic illness. *Annals of Internal Medicine* 127(12):1097–1102.

Waegemann CP. 2002. The vision of electronic health records. *Journal of Medical Practice Management* 18(2):63–65.

Wensing M, Jung HP, Mainz J, Olesen F, Grol R. 1998. A systematic review of the literature on patient priorities for general practice care. Part 1: Description of the research domain. *Social Science and Medicine* 47:1573–1588.

Wilson IB, Ding L, Hays RD, Shapiro MF, Bozette SA, Cleary PD. 2002. HIV patients' experiences with inpatient and outpatient care. *Medical Care* 40(12):1149–1160.

Wogalter MS, Vigilante WJ. 2003. Effects of label format on knowledge acquisition and perceived readability by younger and older adults. *Ergonomics* 46(4):327–344.

Wolpert HA, Anderson BJ. 2001. Management of diabetes: Are doctors framing the benefits from the wrong perspective? *British Medical Journal* 323(7319):994–996.

Woolsey RL. 2000. Drug labeling revisions—Guaranteed to fail? *Journal of the American Medical Association* 284(23):3047–3049.

Wu AW. 2005. *Removing Insult from Injury—Disclosing Adverse Events.* [Online]. Available: http://www.sorryworks.net/article28.phtml [accessed March 22, 2006].

Wu AW, Cavanaugh TA, McPhee SJ, Lo B, Micco GP. 1997. To tell the truth: Ethical and practical issues in disclosing medical mistakes to patients. *Journal of General Internal Medicine* 12:770–775.

Zaldivar A, Smolowitz J. 1994. Perceptions of the importance placed on religion and fold remedies by nonMexican American Hispanic adults with diabetes. *Diabetes Educator* 20:303–306.

5

Action Agenda for Health Care Organizations

CHAPTER SUMMARY

Health care providers need to develop safer medication-use systems. This chapter presents the committee's recommendation for systemic changes in three settings—inpatient, nursing home, and outpatient—and in care transitions. Recognizing that systemic change takes time, the committee proposes ways in which individual physicians, pharmacists, and nurses can improve medication safety in the short term. In addition, health care providers must acknowledge that the work of making medication use safer is never finished. Thus the chapter provides guidance on ways to monitor for medication errors.

This chapter presents the committee's recommendation for systemic changes aimed at improving the safety of medication use. These recommendations are directed at providers in three settings—inpatient, nursing home, and outpatient—as well as in care transitions, which can be especially problematic with respect to the risk of medication errors. In formulating its recommendations, the committee bore in mind the diversity of each of these settings; for example, the outpatient setting encompasses ambulatory care, home care, community pharmacies, care in schools, and assisted living. Overall, the committee believes patients should be involved in their medication-related care in all settings, with the extent of their autonomy being determined by their preferences and capacity.

The committee's recommendation is intended to apply to all of the above settings, although the way it is implemented will vary by setting, as will the medication-use systems and the errors and adverse drug events (ADEs) that may occur. In the inpatient setting, for example, major safety issues include medication selection and administration (Bates et al., 1995a). By contrast, in nursing homes and the outpatient setting, monitoring is especially important (Gandhi et al., 2003; Gurwitz et al., 2000, 2003). In all settings, access to patient-specific and reference information is central to delivering safe medication-related care.

Actions identified by the committee that can be taken to improve medication safety by individual prescribers are summarized in Box 5-1, by individual pharmacists in Box 5-2, and by individual nurses in Box 5-3. The committee's recommendation for systemic changes across health care settings is then presented. The remainder of the chapter provides a detailed discussion of the specifics of this recommendation.

Many of the actions for providers listed in Boxes 5-1 to 5-3 are recommended by the Joint Commission on Accreditation of Healthcare Organizations (JCAHO) and the National Quality Forum (NQF). Since 2003, JCAHO has set annual National Patient Safety Goals (JCAHO, 2005) and included a survey of compliance with the requirements as part of the accreditation process. Many of the National Patient Safety Goals relate to medications (see Box 5-4). The Agency for Healthcare Research and Quality (AHRQ) requested that the NQF use an expert consensus process to define a list of best safety practices. The resulting NQF report, *Safe Practices for Better Healthcare*, listed 30 practices that should be universally adopted in applicable care settings, 13 of which involve the use of medications (see Box 5-5), and another 27 practices (15 of which are medication-related) that should receive high priority for additional research (NQF, 2003).

A number of additional key points should be emphasized. First, having a safety culture is pivotal to improving medication safety. To institute a safety culture, senior management must devote adequate attention to safety and provide sufficient resources to quality improvement and safety teams. Senior management must also authorize resources to invest in technologies that have been demonstrated to be effective but are not yet widely implemented in most organizations, such as computerized provider order entry (CPOE) and electronic health records. It has become increasingly clear that the introduction of any of these technologies requires close attention to business processes and ongoing maintenance. A number of studies have shown that these tools can have unintended and adverse consequences, and that avoiding such consequences requires addressing business and cultural issues.

Improvements in the safe use of medications need to be implemented within the context of an overall quality improvement program, specifically

BOX 5-1
Improving Medication Safety: Actions for Prescribers

- Reconcile medications at transition points, e.g., admission, discharge, transfer. (All)
- Make routine the reconciliation of medication changes with the pharmacy record. (NH/AL, Out)
- Avoid verbal orders except in urgent situations and emergencies. (In)
- Be aware of other medications the patient is taking when prescribing. (NH/AL)
- Keep an accurate medication list (including over-the-counter and complementary and alternative medications). (Out)
- Ask patients to bring their medications in periodically. (Out)
- Ask about allergies when prescribing a new medication. (Out)
- Inform the patient of indications for all medications. (Out)
- Ask regularly whether patients are taking their medications, including as-needed drugs, as nonadherence may signal issues other than knowledge deficits, practical barriers, or attitudinal factors. (Out)
- Ask the primary pharmacy about the patient's refill history. (Out)
- Consider that new complaints may represent side effects of medications. (NH/AL)
- Explain common or significant side effects when prescribing. (Out)
- Ask regularly about side effects or adverse drug events (ADEs). (All)
- Prescribe electronically when possible. (All)
- Use readback with verbal orders when feasible. (All)
- Avoid abbreviations. (All)
- Include patient age and weight when applicable. (All)
- Work as a team with pharmacists and nurses. (In)
- Work as a team with consultant pharmacists and nurses. (NH/AL)
- Work as team with the primary pharmacist and nurses. (Out)
- Adhere to Class I clinical indications and guidelines. (All)
- Use special caution with high-risk medications (All), especially warfarin. (NH/AL)
- Exercise particular caution in high-risk situations—when stressed, sleep-deprived, angry, or supervising inexperienced personnel. (All)
- Consult electronic or other reference sources for questions. (All)
- Report errors and ADEs. (All)
- Include medications when transferring patients between providers. (In)
- Standardize and improve transfers between covering physicians and other providers. (NH/AL)
- Standardize communication about prescriptions within the practice; standardize and improve handoffs to the primary pharmacist. (Out)
- Actively monitor the patient for response to medication therapy, and use validated instruments when possible. (Out)
- Minimize the use of free samples; when dispensing free samples, apply standards similar to those a pharmacy would use. (Out)

NOTE: All = all prescribers; In = inpatient prescriber; NH/AL = nursing home/assisted living prescriber; Out = outpatient prescriber.

BOX 5-2
Improving Medication Safety:
Actions for Individual Pharmacists

- Monitor the medication safety literature and other resources regularly for information related to medication errors, and take action to ensure that similar errors will be avoided in the local practice setting. (Amb and Hosp)
- Develop, implement, and follow a medication error avoidance plan. (Amb)
- As part of this plan, establish a routine procedure for double-checking filled prescriptions waiting to be picked up and verifying the accurate entry of data on new prescriptions into computer systems. (Amb)
- Monitor error frequencies, and correct system problems associated with errors. (Amb and Hosp)
- Use the show-and-tell counseling method to detect and correct dispensing errors; this should include verification of patient identity. (Amb)
- Educate consumers regarding error prevention techniques and resources (e.g., websites such as http://www.ismp.org, http://www.safemedication.com, and http://www.ahrq. gov). (Amb)
- Pharmacy managers designate a medication safety officer with responsibility for improving the safety of prescription filling processes. (Amb)
- Advocate for a medication safety officer with responsibility for improving medication safety throughout the hospital. (Hosp)
- Create a safe work environment by optimizing lighting levels, using a magnifying lens or resizable scanned prescription for viewing prescription slips, minimizing distractions, and arranging drug storage areas to call attention to drugs with a high potential for errors leading to patient harm. (Amb)
- Create a safe work environment by optimizing lighting levels and minimizing distractions and interruptions. (Hosp)
- Advocate for a statewide medication safety coalition, to include the state board of pharmacy, pharmacy organizations, practitioners, and consumers. (Amb and Hosp)
- Report errors and near misses to both internal and external medication error reporting programs or systems to help others learn how to avoid similar problems. (Amb and Hosp)
- Request resources needed to promote accurate prescription dispensing (clinical decision support, bar code verification technology, time for counseling patients). (Amb)
- Be assertive in requesting resources needed to promote accurate medication processing and dispensing (clinical decision support, bar code verification technology). (Hosp)
- Actively pursue a tiered system of clinical alerts that can facilitate better response to serious medication safety issues (e.g., suppress trivial warnings and retain those with a high probability of patient risk). (Amb and Hosp)
- Evaluate and continuously monitor new technologies (e.g., automated prescription filling machines) regarding the risk of introducing medication errors. (Amb)
- Evaluate and continuously monitor new technologies (e.g., infusion pumps, automated medication dispensing machines) regarding the risk of introducing medication errors. (Hosp)

• Regularly make targeted follow-up calls to patients (e.g., those with asthma, chronic pain, hypertension) to assess how they are faring with new medications, learn about any side effects or potential ADEs, and ensure that medications are being taken properly. (Amb)

• Work with nurses to make regular targeted follow-up calls to discharged patients (e.g., those with asthma, chronic pain, hypertension) or use mailed questionnaires to assess how these patients are faring with prescribed medications, learn about any side effects or potential ADEs, ensure that medications are being taken properly, and answer any questions patients may have.

NOTE: Amb = ambulatory care pharmacist; Hosp = hospital pharmacist.

BOX 5-3
Improving Medication Safety: Actions for Nurses

• Establish safe work environments for medication preparation, administration, and documentation; for instance, reduce distractions and provide appropriate lighting.

• Maintain a culture of rigorous commitment to principles of safety in medication administration (for instance, the five rights of medication safety and cross-checks with colleagues, where appropriate).

• Remove barriers to and facilitate the involvement of patient surrogates in checking the administration and monitoring the effects of medications wherever and whenever they are administered.

• Foster a commitment to patients' rights as coproducers of their care.

• Develop aids for patient (or surrogate) self-management support.

• Enhance communication skills and team training so as to be prepared and confident in questioning medication orders and evaluating patient responses to drugs.

• Actively advocate for the development, testing, and safe implementation of electronic health records.

• Work to improve systems that address the most common near misses in the work environment.

• Actively participate in or lead evaluations of the efficacy of new safety systems and technology.

• Contribute to the development and implementation of error reporting systems, and support a culture that values accurate reporting of medication errors.

BOX 5-4
National Patient Safety Goals of the Joint
Commission on Accreditation of Healthcare
Organizations Relating to Medication Use

Goal 1: Improve the accuracy of patient identification

1A. Use at least two patient identifiers (neither to be the patient's room number) whenever administering medications or blood products, taking blood samples

continued

and other specimens for clinical testing, or providing any other treatments or procedures.

1B. Prior to the start of any invasive procedure, conduct a final verification process to confirm the correct patient, procedure, site, and availability of appropriate documents. This verification process uses active—not passive—communication techniques.

Goal 2: Improve the effectiveness of communication among caregivers

2A. For verbal or telephone orders or for telephonic reporting of critical test results, verify the complete order or test result by having the person receiving the order or test result "read-back" the complete order or test result.

2B. Standardize a list of abbreviations, acronyms, and symbols that are not to be used throughout the organization.

2C. Measure, assess and, if appropriate, take action to improve the timeliness of reporting, and the timeliness of receipt by the responsible licensed caregiver, of critical test results and values.

2E. Implement a standardized approach to "hand off" communications, including an opportunity to ask and respond to questions.

Goal 3: Improve the safety of using medications

3B. Standardize and limit the number of drug concentrations available in the organization.

3C. Identify and, at a minimum, annually review a list of look-alike/sound-alike drugs used in the organization, and take action to prevent errors involving the interchange of these drugs.

3D. Label all medications, medication containers (e.g., syringes, medicine cups, basins), or other solutions on and off the sterile field in perioperative and other procedural settings.

Goal 8: Accurately and completely reconcile medications across the continuum of care

8A. Implement a process for obtaining and documenting a complete list of the patient's current medications upon the patient's admission to the organization and with the involvement of the patient. This process includes a comparison of the medications the organization provides to those on the list.

8B. A complete list of the patient's medications is communicated to the next provider of service when it refers or transfers a patient to another setting, service, practitioner or level of care within or outside the organization.

Goal 13: Encourage the active involvement of patients and their families in the patient's care as a patient safety strategy

Define and communicate the means for patients to report concerns about safety and encourage them to do so.

SOURCE: JCAHO, 2005.

BOX 5-5
The National Quality Forum's Safe
Practices for Better Health Care

Among the 30 safe practices identified by the NQF consensus report, the following 13 relate to medication use:

1. Create a health care culture of safety.

3. Specify an explicit protocol to be used to ensure an adequate level of nursing based on the institution's usual patient mix and the experience and training of its nursing staff.

5. Pharmacists should actively participate in the medication-use process, including at a minimum, being available for consultation with prescribers on medication ordering, interpretation and review of medication orders, preparation of medications, dispensing of medications, and administration and monitoring of medications.

6. Verbal orders should be recorded whenever possible and read back to the prescriber—i.e., a health care provider receiving a verbal order should read or repeat back the information that the prescriber conveys in order to verify the accuracy of what was heard.

7. Use only standardized abbreviations and dose designations.

8. Patient care summaries or other similar records should not be prepared from memory.

9. Ensure that care information, especially changes in orders and new diagnostic information, is transmitted in a timely and clearly understandable form to all of the patient's current health care providers who need that information to provide care.

12. Implement a computerized prescriber order entry system.

25. Decontaminate hands with either a hygienic hand rub or by washing with disinfectant soap prior to and after direct contact with the patient or objects immediately around the patient.

27. Keep workspaces where medications are prepared clean, orderly, well lit, and free of clutter, distraction, and noise.

28. Standardize the methods for labeling, packaging, and storing medications.

29. Identify all "high alert" drugs (e.g., intravenous adrenergic agonists and antagonists, chemotherapy agents, anticoagulants and antithrombotics, concentrated parenteral electrolytes, general anesthetics, neuromuscular blockers, insulin and oral hypoglycemics, narcotics and opiates.

30. Dispense medications in unit-dose or, when appropriate, unit-of-use form, whenever possible.

SOURCE: NQF, 2003.

---

within the clinical unit—a small group of clinicians and staff working together with a shared clinical purpose to provide care for a defined set of patients (Mohr and Batalden, 2002). Research on highly effective clinical units has indicated that they share a number of characteristics (Mohr and Batalden, 2002). Such units (1) integrate information within the care delivery process (often with technology playing a key role); (2) monitor processes and outcomes routinely to assess the quality of care delivered; (3) provide care through multidisciplinary teams sharing information among providers and patients; (4) make resources available for quality improvement, including staff training; and (5) work within a larger management environment that is supportive of quality improvement. The application of these ideas at LDS Hospital, Salt Lake City, Utah, led to reduced ADE rates and postoperative deep wound and organ space infection rates (IOM, 2004). Similarly, application of these principles in intensive care units (ICUs) has led to reductions in medication errors in patient transfer orders using medication reconciliation (Pronovost et al., 2003a) and to reduced ICU lengths of stay using a one-page daily goals form to improve the effectiveness of communication among the care team (Pronovost et al., 2003b).

The committee also believes that all organizations in all settings need to monitor rates of medication errors and ADEs more effectively. Most organizations have focused solely on spontaneous reporting, which is necessary but not sufficient. While spontaneous reporting has and will continue to produce highly valuable information, especially at the regional and national levels, internal improvement at the organizational level requires ongoing measurement of meaningful rates. Observation is valuable for assessing administration. In addition, it will increasingly be possible to detect errors and ADEs through computerized monitoring, and such monitoring produces much more reliable information about rates of errors and ADEs in the patient population than does spontaneous reporting.

Recommendation 3: All health care organizations should immediately make complete patient-information and decision-support tools available to clinicians and patients. Health care systems should capture information on medication safety and use this information to improve the safety of their care delivery systems. Health care organizations should implement the appropriate systems to enable providers to:

- Have access to comprehensive reference information concerning medications and related health data.
- Communicate patient-specific medication-related information in an interoperable format.
- Assess the safety of medication use through active monitoring and use these monitoring data to inform the implementation of prevention strategies.
- Write prescriptions electronically by 2010. Also by 2010, all pharmacies should be able to receive prescriptions electronically.

By 2008, all prescribers should have plans in place to implement electronic prescribing.
* Subject prescriptions to evidence-based, current clinical decision support.
* Have the appropriate competencies for each step of the medication-use process.
* Make effective use of well-designed technologies, which will vary by setting.

ACCESS TO POINT-OF-CARE REFERENCE INFORMATION

Providers should have access to comprehensive reference information concerning medications and related health data.

A number of studies have examined the information needs of practicing clinicians (Covell et al., 1985; Gorman, 1995; Gorman and Helfand, 1995; Ely et al., 1999, 2005; Shablinsky et al., 1999). These studies have found that patient care generates a large number of clinical questions, regardless of the provider's specialty. Covell and colleagues (1985) found that internal medicine physicians, both generalists and primary care, generated approximately two clinical questions for every three patients seen. Gorman (1995) found that physicians asked slightly over one question per two patients (Gorman, 1995), while Barrie and Ward (1997) found they asked just over one question per five patients. Much less is known about the information needs of providers other than physicians, but it is reasonable to assume that nurses, pharmacists, and others have frequent needs for clinical information. It should be noted that research indicates nurses prefer to gain knowledge from personal experience and interactions with coworkers and patients rather than from journal articles, textbooks, or research resources (Thompson et al., 2001; Estabrooks et al., 2005).

Most investigators have found that the majority of the questions raised by clinicians during patient care go unanswered[1] (Covell et al., 1985; Gorman, 1995; Ely et al., 1999). Moreover, when clinicians do seek further information, they spend, on average, only 2 minutes doing so. By contrast, one study found that trained librarians took an average of more than 10 minutes to find answers to well-formulated clinical questions all focused on a single illness (Giuse et al., 1994). The clinical impacts of the decision not

---

[1]Examples related to medications are: "This patient is already on a maximal dose of the most potent statin. Which secondary drug—niacin, ezetimibe, or a fibrate—has the greatest impact on stroke and myocardial infarction?" and "This patient is not doing well on valproic acid for controlling bipolar symptoms. Would it be better to add an atypical antipsychotic or switch to another primary medication?"

to seek further information have not been rigorously evaluated, though it is reasonable to assume that such impacts do occur.

Remaining current, even in highly focused areas, has become extremely difficult for clinicians (Giuse et al., 1994). Thirty years ago, it was estimated that there were 1 million facts in the core body of general knowledge in internal medicine (Pauker et al., 1976). This number has likely increased significantly since that time. Nonetheless, most clinicians still rely primarily on memory and clinical experience. Despite the widespread availability of data through the World Wide Web, little improvement in knowledge management has been documented over the past decade (Covell et al., 1985; Gorman, 1995; Ely et al., 2005). Even when clinicians have access to electronic databases, the process of seeking information from these sources is typically so time-consuming as to be impractical in many patient care settings (Alper et al., 2001). With the continuing expansion of medical information, this situation is unlikely to improve without new approaches to knowledge management (Smith, 1996).

The decision to initiate a clinical intervention requires the synthesis of a wide array of data, resulting at a minimum in a probable diagnosis and logical therapeutic options. Medications are the most common options offered (Woodwell and Cherry, 2004). The continuing availability of new pharmacotherapeutic options creates an ongoing need for new knowledge to ensure safe prescribing. Appropriate and safe pharmacotherapy demands not only knowledge of the medication itself, but also appropriate decision making prior to the start of therapy, an understanding of how the medication may interact with coexisting illnesses and medications, and knowledge of requirements for monitoring for success and side effects. Dealing with all these variables requires an extraordinary degree of information synthesis (Smith, 1996). Not surprisingly, then, practicing clinicians indicate a need for highly synthesized and abridged information (Grandage et al., 2002).

Access to the Clinical Knowledge Base

Given that the knowledge base and decision processes are often unique to a particular care setting, clinicians require knowledge gathered from studies conducted in appropriate settings with appropriate patient populations and in a particular stage of the care process (Oxman et al., 1993). The concept of just-in-time information, a given in many businesses, has developed in medicine over the past decade in response to this challenge (Ebell, 1999; Ely, 2001). Practicing clinicians also require information that has been critically analyzed, typically combining the results of a number of studies and presented in clinically relevant form (Smith, 1996; Grandage et al., 2002). The past two decades have seen a shift from teaching individual clinicians how to evaluate the medical literature (Oxman et al., 1993) to answering clinical questions through larger, organized approaches, best exemplified by the Cochrane Collaboration (The Cochrane Library, 2004), national task forces on prevention (CTFPHC, 2005; DHHS, 2005), and the Family Physicians Inquiries Network (FPIN, 2005), as well as numerous commercial endeavors. Most of these approaches are focused on interpretation and analysis of the medical literature; far fewer focus as well on the ability to search for and deliver the knowledge in a rapid and reproducible fashion. Yet both of these aspects of the process are critical if improved care and safety are to be realized.

There are two methods of delivering information to practicing clinicians—the passive lookup of information and the proactive interactive search for information. The Cochrane Collaborative is an example of a passive lookup information source. The collaborative has established a quality standard for creating critically reviewed clinical answers. The reviews are available through several channels, including the Internet, local intranets, and programs available on handheld devices (CC, 2005). A number of organizations are now designing ways to produce answers for busy clinicians (Epocrates, 2005; FPIN, 2005; JFP, 2005), including databases with tags for rapid searches and multiple delivery methods. Applications of this type are typically available in both web versions and versions that can be run on personal digital assistants (PDAs) (Ebell et al., 2002; Beattie, 2003; Lu et al., 2003; Barrett et al., 2004; Taylor, 2005). The current lack of Internet access from the bedside or examination room of most care locations in the United States has helped fuel PDA-based approaches to clinical information management (Rothschild et al., 2002). The rapid growth of PDA computing capabilities has spurred major advances in health information programs (Galt et al., 2005). The ability to update information daily, offer robust search capabilities, and imbed clinical algorithms in these programs enhances their utility for clinicians who are facile and regular users. Nonetheless, the stand-alone nature of these systems renders them but an intermediate step in the quest for robust knowledge management systems for health care providers.

Even with the enhanced compilation of clinical information and the improved databases and search engines of current knowledge management systems, applications that require the active engagement of a clinician will not be used as often as they should be. Full clinical decision support requires systems that support hyperlinks from data within an electronic health record (EHR) to information repositories (Kamel Boulos et al., 2002; Maviglia et al., 2005). Existing systems provide primarily links to static data, such as greater information on a laboratory test or drug monograph information. With improved capabilities for structured data capture, EHRs could facilitate the review of diagnostic features and testing, as well as choices among therapeutic options during patient care, through embedded hyperlinks and queries based on real-time data (Kamel Boulos et al., 2002). The basic approach to data collection inherent in most EHRs in use today may need to be reconsidered if the power of such systems is to be fully realized. The power of appropriate structured clinical data linked to data repositories is illustrated by the Transhis project (Hofmans-Okkes and Lamberts, 1996; Okkes et al., 2001).

Pharmacotherapeutic Decision Support

As the complexity of medical care and medical treatments increases, appropriate and safe care requires that just-in-time information be routinely available to guide diagnostic, treatment, and monitoring activities. Linking of structured data in EHRs to clinical information repositories, together with continuous monitoring of decisions associated with selected activities, such as diagnosis, testing, and treatment, offers the best opportunity for rapidly improving the safety of care. Current working examples of this model are primarily in the pharmacotherapeutic arena, where monitoring of drug–allergy, drug–drug, and drug–disease interactions is common with computerized physician order entry (CPOE) packages. Unfortunately, the benefits of active alert systems have been offset in many cases by the high volume of clinically irrelevant messages, leading to frustration and alert fatigue among clinicians (Payne et al., 2002; Weingart et al., 2003), though this does not need to be the case (Shah et al., 2005). The poor concordance of the output of decision-support tools has also been noted (Abarca et al., 2004; Fernando et al., 2004). Indeed, low user acceptance of current active clinical decision-support systems may hinder the acceptance of EHRs overall, although reminder systems, typically based on patient gender and age (for prevention and screening activities) or diagnosis (for chronic disease care) are beginning to demonstrate the ability to improve care and gain user acceptability (McDonald et al., 1984; Shea et al., 1996; Burack and Gimotty, 1997; Hayes et al., 1999). Medication monitoring systems with carefully defined metrics (such as depression scales or bipolar screens) may become increasingly important as black box warnings become more common (Personal communication, Wilson Pace, February 8, 2006).

COMMUNICATION OF MEDICATION-RELATED INFORMATION

Providers should communicate patient-specific medication-related information in an interoperable format.

Lessons Learned from Hurricane Katrina:
The Importance of Interoperable Medication Data

In 2005, after the devastation of Hurricane Katrina, the country witnessed some of the consequences of the failure to have health care data in an interoperable format. Until this time, although some experts and high-level administrators had some appreciation of the potential role of a national infrastructure for health care information, other key stakeholders, such as payers, did not fully recognize that potential (Sung et al., 2003). After Katrina left hundreds of thousands homeless and forced them to relocate, the health care system was left scrambling to supply these people with lost medications and medical equipment (GAO, 2005). Fortunately, companies such as Walgreens were able to retrieve patients' medication lists, enabling providers to serve these individuals. States with immunization registries were able to retrieve these data so that children could enroll in new schools. Health care systems such as the Department of Veterans Affairs (VA) demonstrated the potential of national EHRs by having available all the information needed to piece together the pharmaceutical and other needs of their patients. Jonathan Perlin, undersecretary for health at the VA, perhaps stated the issue best when he said that after seeing how technology facilitated ongoing health care for Katrina victims, "you wonder why people use horse and buggy tools in the information age" (Bower, 2005).

The most significant event in terms of electronic access to Katrina victims' medical information was the creation of Katrinahealth.org, an electronic medical record accessible to authorized doctors or pharmacists managing Katrina evacuees. The information on the site was compiled and made accessible within 4 weeks of the disaster by a broad group of private companies, public agencies, and national organizations, including medical software companies; pharmacy benefit managers; chain pharmacies; local, state, and federal agencies; and a national foundation. Katrinahealth.org is now a utility that can be used in any disaster.

Katrinahealth.org was formed from data that were in a format that supported their sharing and reuse. Three lessons were reinforced by this effort. First, it is vital that a medication list be accurate and complete. Pharmaceuticals, durable medical equipment (such as eyeglass prescriptions and settings for sleep apnea assistance devices), and important patient data (including medical conditions) are all potential or standard components of such a list. In addition, for these data to be maximally useful, they must be in a structured format including such components as the medication name, dose, route, frequency, duration, and start date. The messaging standard National Council for Prescription Drug Programs script (NCPDP, 2005), which is supported under the Medicare Modernization Act, already specifies this level of detail in its medication segment. Finally, these data must be formatted in a way that unambiguously allows systems from different manufacturers to understand both their structure and content, so that, for example, all versions of a generic medication are identifiable by all systems required to review them. These last two principles are the essential characteristics of interoperability (James, 2005; Wallace, 2005).

Interoperability allows data to be easily aggregated, stored, retrieved into a single view, and shared. As emphasized in a recent report of the Commission for Systemic Interoperability (CoSI, 2005), interoperability allows national-level aggregation of data, making it possible to assess trends in emerging diseases or to recognize patterns of symptoms in cases of bioterrorism. Interoperability also has the potential to allow data access to be governed by a single set of rules, thereby providing patients with greater security and confidentiality.

Missing information is the rule rather than the exception in medicine (Smith et al., 2005). In a recent study of medical errors by Woolf and colleagues (2004), 80 percent of the errors were initiated by miscommunication, including a lack of communication between physicians, misinformation in medical records, mishandling of patient requests and messages, inaccessible records, mislabeled specimens, misfiled or missing charts, and inadequate reminder systems.

Almost all health care situations can benefit from interoperable medication lists. Emergency department clinicians typically see patients without prior knowledge of their medications, problems, or allergies (Benson and Westphal, 2005; Kobusingye et al., 2005; Lappa, 2005). Primary care providers often do not know which medications have been prescribed by other providers or are actually being taken by the patient. In most health care settings, the lack of an accurate list of medications, problems, and allergies places patients at risk for ADEs due to drug–drug interactions or allergies (Benson et al., 1988; Carpenter and Gorman, 2002; Weingart et al., 2004). Although pharmacy chains may have a reasonably accurate list of medications, they rarely have accurate information about risk factors for potential ADEs, and they have no information about alternative and complementary medications, food supplements, or dietary habits that may affect drug metabolism and drug interactions (Isetts et al., 2003). This lack of information provided to pharmacists is especially concerning given their established role as a safety net in detecting potential errors (Kuyper, 1993).

Those with the greatest stake in detecting potential errors are patients and their families. Having an understandable list of medications, problems, and allergies can give patients and their surrogates the information they need to scrutinize their medications (Sutcliffe et al., 2004; Porter et al., 2005).

Sharing of medication data offers the potential to mitigate overprescribing and underprescribing (Waldron, 1977; Tafreshi et al., 1999); improve the follow-up of patients taking medications, such as antidepressants (Simon et al., 2004, 2005); and address the rising problem of prescription drug abuse (Brushwood, 2003). In some cases, interoperable data on patient medications, problems, and allergies is already shared among pharmacy systems, but these data are accessible to few patients in their homes, physicians in the ambulatory setting, or emergency departments (Peth, 2003; Kaboli et al., 2004). These data could also provide important information for school nurses and chronic care facilities (Stupalski and Russell, 1999; Farris et al., 2003). The public health sector could benefit from such information as well. After Hurricane Katrina, for example, the Centers for Disease Control and Prevention was limited in its ability to conduct surveillance for illness and injury by such factors as misclassification of illnesses or injuries on the standardized form by participating facilities and the lack of aggregate baseline data, both of which would be improved by interoperability (CDC, 2005).

Role of Interoperability in the Transfer of Patients Between Sites of Care

The process of transferring patients and their information from one provider or site to another, also called "handoff," is fraught with errors due to poor communication (IOM, 2000; Volpp and Grande, 2003; Solet et al., 2005). Many of these errors could be mitigated by the provision of an accurate history of medications, problems, and allergies. For example, hospitals do not routinely seek a medication record from a patient's primary pharmacy. As a result, the admissions medication record is anecdotal and often omits or misrepresents medications that are being taken. Similarly, on discharge there is no communication back to the primary pharmacist of medication changes that have been ordered while the patient is in the hospital. Work conducted in the emergency departments of Indianapolis demonstrates the improvements that are possible when handoffs are supported by interoperable information systems (Overhage et al., 1995; McDonald et al., 2005). The improved safety associated with the provision of patient-specific medication information has been demonstrated for both emergency departments (Anglemyer et al., 2004; Croskerry et al., 2004) and the inpatient setting (Petersen et al., 1998). Indeed, interoperable medication data can improve the safety of care generally and of medication use in particular in handoffs involving all care settings.

Both paper and electronic formats can be used to improve patient care and patient safety (Tufo et al., 1977; Weed, 2004). However, electronic tools for data capture (order entry) and retrieval offer automated consolidation of data from multiple sources (Overhage et al., 1995; Finnell et al., 2003), remote access as needed (Torre, 2004), and automated decision support (Bates et al., 1995b, 1999, 2001; Abookire et al., 2000; Grasso et al., 2003; Kaushal et al., 2003; Field et al., 2004). CPOE systems for both ambulatory and inpatient care support faxing, messaging, and bidirectional communication of prescription information (eHI, 2004). Each of these tools improves access to original data and provides these data in a format that is legible and potentially interoperable.

In sum, the availability of interoperable data is a lynchpin of a safer health care system, as noted by the Institute of Medicine (IOM) in its report on patient safety (IOM, 2004). Systems provided with these data are uniquely able to provide health care providers with feedback on aspects of their medication prescribing practices about which they might otherwise be unaware (Meyer, 2000; Galloway et al., 2002). This information can also be used for continuing medical education (CME) and evaluation as a part of maintenance of certification, helping providers remain current with the best practices for safe health care delivery. Research suggests that when provided with information on how their behavior can be improved in a timely fashion, health care providers will make these changes (Neilson et al., 2004). Finally, it must be emphasized that as noted by the Commission for Systemic Interoperability, "Having an electronic medication record for every American is a critical step toward achieving true interoperability in healthcare, giving treating physicians the information they need when they need it, allowing more effective care for their patients. It will bring all the medications an individual is currently taking to the doctor's attention at the time important decisions about new prescriptions are being made" (CoSI, 2005).

In effect, interoperable medication data can facilitate more efficient medication reconciliation,[2] particularly at admission and discharge, when discrepancies are an important problem and a frequent cause of ADEs (Forster et al., 2005). Providing such data electronically is even more important now that JCAHO has established that by 2006, hospital organizations must institute a process for comprehensive medication reconciliation at admission, at transitions to and from internal patient care units, and at discharge with the "next provider of service." Interoperable medication data will be the most feasible approach to accomplishing this goal.

MONITORING AND SAFETY IMPROVEMENT

Providers should assess the safety of medication use through active monitoring and use these monitoring data to inform the implementation of prevention strategies.

---

[2]Reconciliation involves comparing what a person is taking in one setting with what is being provided in another setting to avoid errors of transcription, omission, duplication of therapy, and drug–drug and drug–disease interactions.

BOX 5-6
Detection Methods for Medication Errors and ADEs

- Attendance at medical rounds or review of nurse change-of-shift reports to look for clues that an error has occurred (Andrews et al., 1997; Baker, 1997)
- Chart review (Bates et al., 1995a,b)
- Comparison of drugs removed from an automated drug dispensing device with physician orders (Shuttleworth and Ruelle, 1996)
- Computerized analysis to identify patients receiving target drugs that may be used to treat a medication error or a search for serum drug concentration orders that may indicate an overdose (Bates et al., 1995b)
- Direct observation for detecting medication administration errors (Allan and Barker, 1990; Barker et al., 2002)
- Monitoring of doses returned to the pharmacy (indicating possible dose omissions) (Gift et al., 1996)
- Examination of death certificates (Phillips et al., 1998)
- Comparison of medication administration records with physician orders (Cunningham et al., 1996)
- Voluntary reports of medication errors (Phillips, 2002)
- Stimulated self-reports using interviews (Bates et al., 1995a,b)
- Urine testing as evidence of omitted drugs and unauthorized drug administration (Ballinger et al., 1974)

Accurate counting of medication errors and ADEs using appropriate detection methods is now possible and is critical for establishing the scope of the error problem. Accurate counts also enable providers to assess the impact of error prevention efforts. The discussion in this section focuses on what health care providers can do to improve medication safety through the use of error detection and monitoring techniques; the use of external reporting programs for safety improvement, introduced in Chapter 2, is discussed in Chapter 8.

Many health care systems monitor medication errors by tracking self-reported errors. Experts generally acknowledge that such reports detect a small percentage of the true number of errors and ADEs, but they believe this approach is the only feasible option. There are, however, better methods for counting errors. The goal of the committee's recommendation in this area is to assist health care providers in selecting improved methods for monitoring of medication errors and ADEs while maintaining the recognized benefits of current reporting mechanisms.

Numerous detection methods for medication errors and ADEs have been employed (see Box 5-6). The selection of a method for inpatient settings can be facilitated by answers to the following questions:

• Are we most interested in focusing on medication errors for inpatient settings that lead to patient injury (ADEs)? If yes, review the methods described in Table 5-1.

• Are we interested in detecting as many errors as possible for inpatient settings so that real system problems can be identified more quickly and prevention efforts prioritized? If yes, review the methods described in Table 5-2.

• ADE and error detection methods for outpatient settings are summarized in Table 5-3.

Some of the methods available for detecting errors and ADEs are described in greater detail below. These include reporting, chart review, computerized detection of ADEs (Classen et al., 1991; Evans et al., 1991; Bates et al., 2003), observation of medication administration (Barker et al., 2002),

TABLE 5-1 ADE Detection Methods: Inpatient Setting

Detection Method	Description	Source of Data
Chart review (see Morimoto et al., 2004)	Data sources are screened for evidence that an ADE occurred	Medical record (including electronic notes), orders
Computer-generated signals	Computer screens orders, laboratory values, and other data for indicators that an ADE may have occurred; reviewer follows up on results	Triggers from computerized data (e.g., laboratory results, order for antidote)
Electronic notes	Software screens chart for evidence of an ADE; reviewer follows up on results	Electronic health record, discharge summaries (Murff et al., 2003)
Self-report, voluntary	Providers submit data about events	Patients, medical record
Self-report, prompted	Providers are interviewed to see whether any incidents have occurred	Providers

and audits of prescriptions filled in community pharmacies to monitor dispensing errors (Flynn et al., 2003).

Reporting of Medication Errors and ADEs

Voluntary reports, while not appropriate for measuring the actual frequency of errors, are useful as a basis for root-cause analysis and for identification of error trends involving certain medications, doses, forms, and routes. Trend analyses and data mining benefit from having very large databases—hence the efforts being made to increase error reporting and to combine databases (see Chapter 8).

Health care providers can take a number of actions to promote successful medication error reporting in their respective settings. First, they

Resources	Advantages	Disadvantages
Trained reviewers (nurses, pharmacists)	Most likely to identify events resulting in patient harm; detects more events than self-reports (Jha et al., 1998)	More time-consuming if computer-generated signals are unavailable
Software, trained reviewers	Helps focus reviewer time by using triggers; has the highest positive predictive value for ADEs (see Field et al., 2004); identifies more events than self-reports (Jha et al., 1998)	Best at finding events associated with numbers (Gandhi et al., 2000); availability of electronic data required
Software, trained reviewers	Detects high percentage of ADEs in an efficient manner (see Field et al., 2004)	Electronic record or discharge summaries needed
Providers, report monitoring system and staff	With sufficient data, can identify error and ADE trends; description of event can help trained staff find cause	Detects very small percentage of events
Trained staff to conduct interviews	In addition to advantages of voluntary self-reports, can be performed by attending rounds and nurse shift changes	Detects small percentage of events

TABLE 5-2 Medication Error Detection Methods: Inpatient Setting

Detection Method	Description	Source of Data
Chart review	Data sources are screened for evidence that an error occurred	Medical record
Observation	Observer records medications administered and compares with orders, or observer shadows physician (Rothschild et al., 2005)	Personnel actions
Self-report, voluntary	Providers submit data about events	Patients, medical record
Self-report, prompted	Providers are interviewed to see whether any incidents have occurred	Providers

can create a learning system whereby errors and recommended preventive measures are reported and used as a tool for learning. Second, they can make a commitment to learning about error problems, monitoring national trends and reports, and implementing plans designed to prevent similar errors from occurring at their site. When errors and ADEs are identified, reporting should be encouraged. For example, the Institute for Safe Medication Practices' (ISMP) *Medication Safety Alert* newsletter, United States Pharmacopeia (USP) MedMARx reports, and case studies from AHRQ's Web M&M (http://www.webmm.ahrq.gov) should be required reading for health care practitioners, including community pharmacists, who can learn about errors that have occurred and take action to avoid them. Recommended preventive actions, based on expert review, are included in the ISMP newsletter.

As noted, voluntary reporting is valuable for identifying large problems and providing a stimulus for change, but has recognized limitations for evaluating the true frequency of medication errors and ADEs. In a comparison of voluntary reports against observation in 36 health care facilities, observation detected 456 times more errors (Flynn et al., 2002).

Resources	Advantages	Disadvantages
Trained reviewers	Detects more events than self-reports (Flynn et al., 2002)	More time-consuming if computer-generated signals are unavailable
Trained observers (nurses, pharmacists)	Detects greatest number of medication administration errors (Flynn et al., 2002); identifies clues to causes of errors that may not be found with other methods	Focuses on administration errors
All providers, report monitoring system and staff	With sufficient data, can identify error and ADE trends; description of event can help trained staff find cause	Detects small percentage of events
Trained staff to conduct interviews	In addition to advantages of voluntary self-report, they can be performed during attending rounds and nurse shift changes	Detects small percentage of events

To increase the strength of the evidence that errors truly are being reduced (or are increasing), additional, more robust error detection methods are needed.

Chart Review

Chart review to identify medication errors involves looking for events in patient documentation that indicate a medication error may have occurred, for example, a change in mental status, a new rash or diarrhea, or orders for antidotes. Chart review is an effective way of finding medication errors and ADEs, but is costly to perform and requires special training for the chart reviewers. Recently, chart review has begun to make use of an ADE trigger tool designed by the Institute for Healthcare Improvement (Rozich et al., 2003), which is based on the automated surveillance methodology created at LDS Hospital, Salt Lake City (Classen et al., 1991). Such ADE trigger tools do not require computerized technology and have been used successfully to demonstrate the benefits of low-cost error prevention

TABLE 5-3 ADE and Medication Error Detection Methods: Outpatient Setting

Detection Method	Description	Source of Data
Chart review (Gandhi et al., 2003; Morimoto et al., 2004)	Review of patient's clinic medical record for evidence of an ADE	Medical record
Computer-generated signals (Field et al., 2004)	Computer screens orders, laboratory values, and other data for indicators that an ADE may have occurred; reviewer follows up on results	Triggers from computerized laboratory data
Evaluation of prescriptions (Flynn et al., 2003)	Contents and labels of filled prescriptions are compared against the original order for discrepancies (detects dispensing errors)	Filled prescriptions
Reports, voluntary	Patients or providers may identify an error and report it to the provider or other organization	Patients (symptoms or filled prescriptions)
Survey of patients (Wertheimer, 1973; Forster et al., 2003; Morimoto, 2004)	Patients are interviewed after care or receipt of a prescription to find evidence of ADEs or dispensing errors	Patients

strategies focused on high-risk medications in community hospitals (Cohen et al., 2005).

Computerized Detection Methods

Electronic detection of ADEs should be included in clinical software programs in all areas of health care by 2010. This capability can support early detection of patient harm, with subsequent intervention to correct the problem and treat the patient. Incorporation of this critical feature is important today, at a time when CPOE and EHRs are being developed and implemented. The IOM's *Patient Safety* report describes the functional requirements for electronic ADE detection systems, including rules for detecting possible ADEs using automated surveillance (Evans et al., 1991; Classen et al., 1991; Bates et al., 2001; IOM, 2004).

Resources	Advantages	Disadvantages
Trained reviewer	Most likely to identify events resulting in patient harm	Fewer ADEs detected compared with patient surveys
Software; trained reviewers	Most likely to identify events resulting in patient harm	Limited availability of software in this setting in the short term
Pharmacist	Good measure of dispensing errors; provides clues to causes of errors	Dependent on availability of staff and time
Health care provider	Can provide clues to the causes of errors	Small numbers involved; should not be used for rate calculations
Health care provider	Can be used to follow up on symptoms, obtain additional information	May be time-consuming if no electronic screening is available

Computerized detection of ADEs is based on the use of screening criteria for triggering events. Techniques used by such systems include examining medication orders for antidotes (indicating a wrong dose or wrong drug) and screening clinical laboratory data for results that exceed critical values. These techniques may be employed at various levels of sophistication (Bates et al., 2003). Once a potential ADE has been identified, clinical review is necessary to confirm whether it was in fact such an event.

Observation of Medication Administration

Since 1960, studies have used nurses to observe medication administration in hospitals because the results provide an accurate measure of how often medication administration errors actually occur (Flynn et al., 2002). Observation involves a trained nurse or other health care professional shadowing the nurse who administers medications, recording the medications prepared and administered, and comparing this information with what the prescriber ordered. Any discrepancy between what the patient received and what the prescriber ordered is an administration error. These data have been used to evaluate the accuracy of the output of the entire medication distribution system—whether the patient received the right drug, dose, form, and route—from the patient's point of view (Barker et al., 2002). An important advantage of observation over voluntary reporting is that it does not rely on the heath care provider's being aware of the error (providers typically do not realize they have made an error, and if they do, they may be reluctant to report it). Observation is best performed by nurses or pharmacists, although less costly resources, such as pharmacy residents, pharmacy or nursing students, or experienced pharmacy technicians, can also be used. The average cost of observation per dose was measured in one study as $6.65 when performed by a registered nurse and $4.56 by a licensed practical nurse (Flynn et al., 2002). Observation has been recommended for studying ADEs as well (Rothschild et al., 2005).

To derive the benefits of the lessons that can be learned from observation while keeping the process affordable, observation is best conducted for limited or periodic studies of settings of interest. The number of observations depends on the goal of the study, ranging from 100 per nursing unit over a day or two to see whether there is an error problem to over 1,000 for evaluations of technology effects. A hospital might conduct an observation on several nursing units selected as "typical" every few months to learn from the errors detected and determine whether there is a serious error problem. This process would be part of the hospitals routine quality monitoring program.

Audits of Prescriptions Filled in Community Pharmacies

Detection of medication errors and ADEs in ambulatory care settings is a fairly recent development. For example, incident reports and review of patient records have been used to study ADEs among elderly ambulatory patients (Gurwitz et al., 2003). Medication dispensing errors on prescriptions filled in community pharmacies have been studied using a double-check by an independent observer pharmacist (Flynn et al., 2003); however, the standard in pharmacies is to rely on self-reports of errors detected by patients who notify the pharmacist. National databases of voluntary reports contain few error reports from the ambulatory setting, in part because of unawareness of such errors and in part because pharmacies do not want this information reported to external organizations. With the enactment of the Patient Safety and Quality Improvement Act of 2005 (P.L. 109-41), protecting such data reported to patient safety organizations, community pharmacies should start sharing this information.

Audits in community pharmacies involve random inspections of prescriptions waiting to be picked up. A double-check of the contents of the prescription vial compared with the drug and strength listed on the label can help detect wrong-drug and wrong-strength errors that may have avoided detection during the normal processes. The patient name on the vial can be compared with the identifying information on the bag to help detect wrong-patient errors. An additional audit technique is to review information entered into the computer for new prescriptions for accuracy. Use of such a quality improvement process at a VA outpatient pharmacy resulted in a decrease in serious errors (ones that could have led to patient harm) from 0.6 percent to 0.1 percent of prescriptions over a 1-year period (Boneberg et al., 1991).

Analysis of Safety Data

Time spent detecting, reporting, and analyzing medication errors and ADEs is wasted if the resulting information is not used to prevent future errors and injuries. USP publishes focused analyses based on voluntary reports made to the MedMARx database, which are helpful in identifying problem areas and can serve as one model for how to use this type of data (Young, 2002; Hicks et al., 2004; Santell et al., 2004). As noted earlier, the ISMP newsletter contains not only descriptions of problems reported, but also suggestions for preventing future errors (ISMP, 2005a). And AHRQ's Web M&M site also provides clinically useful analyses of medication errors. Medication error databases at all levels should have a greater ability to track effective methods for preventing the errors described, with a requirement to report on follow-up actions taken and their effectiveness.

An important benefit of using the techniques of computerized detection and observation described above is that they can be used to evaluate interventions (Evans et al., 1994a, 1998). Observation, for example, enables valid measurement of the effects of error prevention efforts on medication administration errors. Studies that use voluntary reports to assess interventions cannot determine whether an intervention led to a decrease in errors or whether staff were unaware of errors that occurred.

The knowledge base on effective error prevention techniques should be advanced at all levels (local, state, and national). The ultimate goal is to have in place a system that facilitates the identification of best practices for preventing errors and dissemination of this information to providers across settings of care.

ELECTRONIC PRESCRIBING

By 2010, all prescribers should write and all pharmacies should be able to receive prescriptions electronically. By 2008, all prescribers should have plans in place to implement electronic prescribing. Providers should subject prescriptions to evidence-based, current clinical decision support.

Increasing evidence demonstrates that paper-based prescribing is associated with high error rates (Bates et al., 1995a; Kaushal et al., 2003) and that electronic prescribing is safer (Bates et al., 1998). Electronic prescribing has a number of advantages (Bates et al., 1999; Teich et al., 2005): it eliminates handwriting, helps ensure that the key fields (for example, drug name, dose, route, and frequency) contain meaningful data, and makes it possible to suggest a default dose. More important, however, computerized prescribing enables a range of clinical decision support (Teich et al., 2005), including checks for allergies, drug–drug interactions, overly high doses, clinical conditions, drug–laboratory issues, and pregnancy-related issues, as well as suggestions about dose given the patient's level of renal function and age.

While all decision-support checks contribute to an effective medication-use system, results of recent studies suggest that dose adjustment may be especially important. It is clear that 10-fold dosage calculation errors in particular are a major clinical issue, especially in pediatrics (Rowe et al., 1998). One inpatient study found that suggesting a dose appropriate for a patient's level of renal function substantially improved the likelihood that the patient would receive the appropriate dose of medication (Chertow et al., 2001); another demonstrated that alerts decreased the likelihood that patients would receive too high a dose of medication given their level of renal function (Galanter et al., 2005). Another study (Peterson et al., 2005) demonstrated that suggesting an appropriate starting dose of medication for geriatric inpatients improved the likelihood that the recommended daily dose would be prescribed, reduced the likelihood of 10-fold overdose, and was associated with a lower rate of falling.

It is not easy to implement decision supports, however, and problems can arise with all of them. For example, many issues remain to be addressed with regard to allergy checking, although some best practices have been suggested (Hsieh et al., 2004). Drug–drug interactions are especially complex since so many have been identified, but the number that are clinically important is more modest (Hansten et al., 2001; Peterson and Bates, 2001; Glintborg et al., 2005). Fewer data are available regarding the frequency of problems in such areas as diagnoses contraindicating drugs, generic checks for overly high doses, and drug–laboratory decision support.

It is also essential that any decision support be practical. Overalerting is a frequent and important problem (Teich et al., 2005), especially for drug–drug interactions. To avoid this problem, it would be helpful if decision support rules were available in a publicly available location. AHRQ should consider approaches for developing a database to which organizations could contribute decision-support rules, expressed in a standard format, that could then be accessed by interested parties. This database would require periodic external vetting to ensure that it included only appropriate rules and to update the decision-support knowledge base. The need for such quality checks is illustrated by ISMP's recent audit of pharmacy decision support, which found a very high rate of deficiencies and no improvement over a 6-year period (ISMP, 2005b).

An important adjunct to electronic prescribing is that all pharmacies should be able to receive prescriptions in coded form—a much lower-risk method than current paper or oral approaches (Bates, 2001), which are error-prone and require transcription and verification. A commonly used approach in the outpatient setting, for example, is to call prescriptions in to the pharmacy. These prescriptions are frequently left on voice mail. This approach, while efficient in some respects, has several limitations: there is no possibility of readback; if there is a problem, the pharmacist must contact the prescriber later; and the prescription cannot be checked at the time it is delivered to the pharmacy. Similarly, in the reverse direction, most communication by the pharmacist to the prescriber's office must be left on voice mail, and sometimes the prescriber's staff do not respond appropriately to queries requiring a clinical response. At the same time, a number of issues must be addressed for electronic transmission of prescriptions to be practical. Many of these issues are regulatory. For example, a number of states have laws that preclude the practice, particularly for narcotics, although there is no evidence that handwritten prescriptions are safer. In other situations, pharmacies can decide whether they will accept electronic transmission, a situation that creates substantial problems for providers attempting to implement safer prescribing practices.

It is also important to recognize that any technology can induce new errors as well as prevent them, and that computerization of prescribing thus does not represent a panacea (Koppel et al., 2005). When any intervention is introduced, it must be monitored, problems it creates must be identified, and appropriate changes must be made in the application and underlying databases to eliminate these problems. Typically, insufficient resources and energy are dedicated to this process, yet results of human factors research clearly demonstrate that it is more efficacious than training staff to work around difficulties (Gosbee, 2004).

Finally, to achieve the desired safety benefits, electronic prescribing must include basic clinical decision support (Bates et al., 1999; Gandhi et al., 2005), which in turn requires a defined set of clinical data—the patient's age, gender, allergies, other medications, problems, and selected laboratory results. Thus to achieve major safety benefits, electronic prescribing should be linked with electronic health records. It should be carried out using a device such as a desktop, laptop, or tablet computer. To date, it has been impossible to deliver adequate clinical decision support on palm-top platforms, primarily because of the infeasibility of incorporating sufficient clinical information in these devices in a timely fashion, the shortage of space on palm-top screens, lack of interoperability, and issues related to transmission speed. The tablet PC provides more screen space than the palm-top device at the cost of some portability.

MULTIDISCIPLINARY TEAMS

Providers should have the appropriate competencies for each step of the medication-use process.

The use of multidisciplinary teams to care for patients receiving complex medication regimens offers the potential to improve substantially the quality of drug therapy and reduce the occurrence of medication errors and ADEs (Leape et al., 1999). Such teams may include nurses, clinical pharmacists, and other health professionals, complementing and extending the efforts of the physician. In most instances, it is useful to enlist the patient and family members as part of the overall team. In certain instances, having specific individuals on the team can be beneficial. For example, having a pharmacist conduct rounds with the team has been found to reduce ADE rates in the intensive care unit setting (Leape et al., 1999). While it probably does not make sense to have pharmacists present during rounds with all teams because of the cost of their services, their input on teams providing care that involves high medication use (for example, chemotherapy units) is likely to provide important benefit.

Multidisciplinary approaches have been employed to optimize pharmacotherapeutic management of patients across a variety of clinical settings, from the intensive care unit to the ambulatory setting. These approaches have often focused on specific medical conditions, such as diabetes mellitus and congestive heart failure (Rich et al., 1995; Whellan et al., 2005), or specific drug therapies, such as anticoagulant therapy.

Cohesive health care teams possess five key characteristics (Grumbach and Bodenheimer, 2004):

- Clear goals with measurable outcomes
- Clinical (e.g., for prescription refills) and administrative (e.g., for making patient appointments) systems

- Division of labor—identifying which people on the team perform which tasks
- Training for the functions each team member routinely performs
- Effective communication (e.g., minute-to-minute communication through brief verbal interactions among team members)

How these characteristics play out in the care of patients on drug therapy can be illustrated by the example of anticoagulation therapy with warfarin. Such therapy is risky, for example, because of the possibility of bleeding due to drug interactions and suboptimal dosing. Specialized anticoagulation clinics employ a team approach to optimize the treatment (Ansell et al., 1997). Such an approach can help achieve improvements in anticoagulation control (Samsa et al., 2000) and reductions in bleeding and thromboembolic event rates (Chiquette et al., 1998; Hamby et al., 2000). One measurable outcome for patients on warfarin therapy is whether the level of anticoagulation has been maintained within the target therapeutic range at least 80 percent of the time, so as to reduce the risk of bleeding and provide optimal therapeutic benefit. Accordingly, key features of effective warfarin therapy teams are as follows:

- A clinical system with a set of procedures for informing patients of laboratory results and of any needed changes in the warfarin dose.
- An administrative system with procedures for scheduling the next laboratory test and notifying the nurse and scheduler when a patient does not present for the test.
- Adequate training of each team member in the specific functions each must perform. For example, the nurse or pharmacist managing the care of patients on warfarin must be trained in the use of protocols and computer programs for dosing and monitoring of the therapy, as well as in surveillance for important drug interactions.
- Communication structures for promptly conveying information to the physician when there is a need for decisions regarding response to a warfarin-related bleeding event or complex dosing and monitoring decisions not encompassed by the usual protocols.

It is important to note that despite the potential benefits of multidisciplinary approaches and their increasing use in the care of patients with a variety of medical conditions, such approaches have not always proven to be more effective than conventional care (Matchar et al., 2002; Strom and Hennessy, 2002). Furthermore, multidisciplinary teams are used most commonly in care for a single medical condition or management of a single type of therapy. Care provided by several different multidisciplinary teams may not be the optimum way to care for patients with multiple chronic medical conditions. Indeed, such a fragmented approach could place patients at increased risk for medication errors, similar to the risk that results from having multiple different health care providers each independently prescribing medications in their own discipline. An example of an alternative is the Program of All-Inclusive Care for the Elderly (PACE), which has shown great promise for providing comprehensive care for the very frail elderly using a multidisciplinary approach (Bodenheimer, 1999).

The committee believes that a team approach to medication use is essential. Different providers will be involved at each step of the process. But all providers who are prescribing, whether a physician, nurse practitioner, or physician's assistant, or administering, whether a registered nurse or licensed practical nurse, need to have the appropriate competencies, which should be determined by their professional organizations and the care organization for which they work.

EFFECTIVE USE OF WELL-DESIGNED TECHNOLOGIES

Providers should make effective use of well-designed technologies, which will vary by setting.

Judicious use of technology will be important in improving medication safety (Bates and Gawande, 2003). While the evidence supporting this statement is strongest for the inpatient setting (AHRQ, 2005), the use of technology will undoubtedly result in major improvements in all settings, although the specific technologies and relative benefits will likely differ by setting. Much remains to be learned in all settings. Moreover, as noted earlier, any technology can introduce errors as well as prevent them (Ash et al., 2004), and it is essential to monitor any new technology and make appropriate midcourse corrections. And even highly promising technologies may not yield the desired safety benefits if issues of safety culture and efficiency are not adequately addressed (Rothschild, 2004).

Inpatient Setting

In the inpatient setting, strong evidence demonstrates that CPOE reduces rates of serious medication errors in adults (Bates et al., 1998; AHRQ, 2005), although the impact on preventable ADEs is uncertain since a large randomized controlled trial has not been conducted. A key issue regarding CPOE is the depth and breadth of the decision support provided. Moroever, the main impact of CPOE is on ordering and transcription errors; the technique has relatively little impact on administration errors. For reducing the frequency of the latter errors, machine identification techniques such as bar coding—especially when linked to an electronic medication administration record—hold substantial promise, although the evidence for their efficacy is less strong than is the case for CPOE (AHRQ, 2005). Bar coding will likely be especially important for medications taken orally, although it will probably also be important for intravenous medications. The latter are particularly risky because they are especially potent, have rapid action, and are given to critically ill patients, and because it is easy to give an intravenous dose that exceeds the norm by 10 (or more) times. Another technology that appears likely to have an impact on improving the safety of intravenous medications is "smart" pumps. These pumps can be programmed according to the medication being given, warn the nurse if the dose is too high, and record what happens if the dose is overridden. The first large trial of this technology demonstrated that it could be used to identify many instances in which doses were too high, but it did not reduce the rate of serious medication errors because nurses often ignored even important warnings (Rothschild, 2004).

Although dispensing appears to be relatively safe compared with other steps in the medication-use process, it, too, can be made safer by bar coding (Poon et al., 2005). The use of robots for filling prescriptions in pharmacies may also have the potential to improve dispensing (Bates, 2000). Automated dispensing devices on clinical units may improve safety as well, although the one study evaluating their impact failed to demonstrate any benefit (Barker, 1995; Barker et al., 1998).

Monitoring should also benefit from computerization in two ways. One is that the standard approach to identifying ADEs—spontaneous reporting on paper—should be replaced by on-line reporting, which has many advantages (Bates, 2002). Specifically, on-line reporting makes it possible to use branching logic; makes it easier to update the reporting scheme; and facilitates collection of the data in standard formats, which in turn facilitates analysis. Much more important, though, is implementation of computerized ADE monitoring (Classen et al., 1991) that uses signals to identify situations in which an ADE has occurred or is likely to occur. In many instances, it may be possible for someone—usually a pharmacist—to intervene either before the event occurs or before it becomes as severe as it might otherwise have been.

There have been a few studies of override problems related to technologies designed to reduce medication errors. As noted above, a smart pump can fail to reduce serious medication error rates because nurses ignore important warnings (Rothschild, 2004). At the prescribing stage, Hsieh and colleagues found that overrides of allergy warnings were common, and 1 in 20 of these overrides, while appearing to be clinically appropriate, resulted in an ADE (Hsieh et al., 2004). At the pharmacist order entry stage, Grisso and colleagues (2004) found that 6.5 percent of overdose and underdose warnings for pediatric patients were inappropriate, and a daily review of pharmacist overrides is now performed to correct problems early in the process. At the medication administration stage, Oren and colleagues (2002) studied overrides of antimicrobial withdrawals from an automated dispensing machine and found that medication errors occurred in 21 percent of cases. Kester (2005) found that 12 percent of overrides were associated with variances from written orders, and 2 percent were related to medication errors or near misses. A unit-based pharmacist can help decrease medication errors resulting from overrides (Haas et al., 2004), and a well-implemented system should include education about the possible implications of overriding system warnings.

Ultimately, it will be important to implement all of the above technologies at the same time and link them electronically. Orders can then be transmitted electronically to the pharmacy, where they can be evaluated and filled. It should be possible to do this for many medications, with manual filling being checked using bar coding for a small minority of medications. The electronic medication record can then be populated. Nurse administration of medications taken orally can be checked through bar coding, while intravenous medications can be screened using smart pumps. All of these techniques should be able to communicate wirelessly. Many of these approaches, especially CPOE and automated dispensing in the pharmacy, will be easier to support in larger, rather than smaller, hospitals. With this combined approach, it might be possible to reduce the medication error rate in hospitals on the order of 100-fold.

Nursing Home Setting

In nursing homes, electronic prescribing will likely be important, although there are few data to date regarding its efficacy in this setting, and the key decision support required will likely differ somewhat from that in the inpatient setting (Gurwitz et al., 2005; Rochon et al., 2005). Therefore, CPOE is likely to yield substantial benefits, especially if it can be done remotely, enabling the physician to review the patient's medication list and perform checks, such as those for drug–drug interactions, in real time (Rochon et al., 2005). This is a particular problem in nursing homes as many residents are taking multiple medications, and most physicians are not located at the site. Nonetheless, implementation of CPOE in this setting will be challenging since most nursing homes have very limited resources, and many have relationships with large numbers of physicians who spend relatively little time at each site.

Bar coding and computerized medication administration records can also be expected to have an impact in this setting. Barker and colleagues

(1982) demonstrated relatively high rates of medication administration errors in nursing homes and the potential of bar coding to decrease these rates, although controlled trials of this technology have not been conducted in this setting.

Outpatient Setting

In the outpatient setting, electronic prescribing will be important (Gandhi et al., 2003), although evidence to date for its effectiveness in this setting is limited, and electronic prescribing without associated decision support is unlikely to yield the potential safety benefits (Gandhi et al., 2005). Indeed, it may be more important to improve communication between patients and providers; the available evidence suggests that many ADEs might have been prevented or ameliorated had communication occurred earlier in the medication-use process (Gandhi et al., 2003). In this regard, personal health records that are linked to provider EHRs represent one attractive approach that deserves further evaluation (Katz et al., 2004). Other technologies, such as on-line communications, also warrant further investigation. In addition, automation may be useful in pharmacies to improve the likelihood that prescriptions will be filled accurately, and to free pharmacists to do more counseling with patients, which too often does not occur today.

Return on Investment

The adoption of CPOE with computerized decision support has been slow (Kaushal et al., 2005). High upfront capital costs and the difficulty of demonstrating the financial benefits have been major barriers to the adoption of CPOE. A recent study demonstrated that the investment in CPOE with decision support at the Brigham and Women's Hospital, Boston, Massachusetts, has resulted in substantial operating budget savings (Kaushal et al., 2006). Over the period 1993–2002, the hospital invested $11.8 million to develop, implement, and operate a CPOE system and achieved net operating budget savings of $9.5 million. The majority of the savings were derived from a relatively small number of interventions. The annual savings generated in 2002 dollars were from renal dosing guidance ($2.24 million), ADE ($1.05 million), improved nursing time utilization ($0.96 million), and specific/expensive drug guidance ($0.88 million).

A key lesson from the implementation of CPOE with computerized decision support at Brigham and Women's Hospital is that hospitals should focus initially on a small number of high-impact interventions (for example, renal dosing guidance, ADE prevention, and specific/expensive drug guidance). There are other high-impact interventions not implemented at Brigham and Women's Hospital, such as the antibiotic assistant implemented at LDS Hospital, Salt Lake City (Evans et al., 1994b). More research is needed to identify further high-impact interventions, particularly regarding the use of intravenous medications because of their high toxicity.

Another key lesson from the implementation of CPOE at Brigham and Women's Hospital is that hospitals should pay careful attention to workflow design to save nursing and physician time. At Brigham and Women's Hospital, the greatest efficiency was achieved through automation of the medication administration record. Other savings were derived from reduced rework of problematic orders to avoid medication errors or ADEs since the CPOE system was performing many of these checks at the time of order creation.

Further cost/benefit studies are urgently needed. The system implemented at Brigham and Women's Hospital was developed in house, so studies of vendor-based systems are particularly desirable. Also needed are studies addressing care settings other than hospitals and a broader range of decision-support tools.

Implementation of Systems

The overall design and implementation of new technologies are fundamental to a successful outcome. Groups of researchers have documented implementation problems for electronic prescribing systems and unintended consequences arising from the implementation of such systems (Ash et al., 2004; Han et al., 2005; Berger and Kichak, 2004; Koppel et al., 2005; Fernando et al., 2004). Achieving the safety benefits of any technological intervention, but perhaps especially CPOE, requires that it be implemented well and routinely maintained. A number of best practices for implementing CPOE and the associated clinical decision support have been described:

- There are many CPOE systems available, and careful analysis is needed to identify the best system to meet the needs of the clinical situation. Entry and retrieval of information is an aspect of CPOE that must be examined with particular care (Ash et al., 2004).
- The success of the implementation of information systems in health care is determined by organizational factors (Aarts et al., 2004). Care delivery processes and the technologies to support these processes need to be designed in conjunction. A corollary is that significant effort must be devoted to staff training in the use of CPOE systems.
- All electronic prescribing applications should be subjected to usability testing and evaluation with test scripts before implementation. Leapfrog is developing a tool for evaluating hospital CPOE systems with decision support (Kilbridge et al., 2006). Currently, EHRs are being certified by the

Certification Commission on Health Information Technology, which will be certifying electronic prescribing applications if they are part of EHRs. It is also useful to pilot the CPOE in a limited setting prior to full implementation to identify and rectify any problems.

• During the implementation period, it is best to include as many order sets as possible at the outset and to provide intensive support to all users so that any problems can be rapidly addressed.

• After implementation, use of the CPOE system must undergo a continuous quality improvement process (Bates, 2005) with frequent evaluation to determine whether the system is functioning as intended, and new errors that are introduced must be tracked and addressed. The clinical processes involved are complex. Errors and problems will continue to occur. Sufficient resources must be available to analyze problems and implement process improvements. Several models of successful quality improvement in clinical units have been documented (IOM, 2004; Batalden et al., 2003; Pronovost et al., 2002). The above practices apply for any clinical decision support system as well.

Care Transitions

Data increasingly suggest that care transitions are associated with high levels of risk (Forster et al., 2003), especially for ADEs (Forster et al., 2005). Many of these ADEs are due in part to the changes in medication that are made at the time of admission or discharge. Thorough reconciliation of medications is crucial in these situations (Rozich et al., 2004), but difficult to achieve. Technology can assist in this process. In addition, outreach to patients who have recently been discharged will likely be necessary, and it appears likely that technology such as telemedicine and personal health records can be used to leverage this outreach.

Conclusions

In the future, it is inevitable that technologies will serve as increasingly important tools for improving medication safety in all settings, though the specific technologies involved will differ by setting. For inpatients, the core challenge appears to be accurately delivering the appropriate and intended medications. Outside the hospital, improving the safety and efficacy of prescribing is essential, together with improving monitoring and communication. In all settings, safety culture is pivotal, and there are many things that individual providers can do to that end, though achieving high levels of safety will demand that providers have tools appropriate for their setting. These tools must be implemented well, and all carry the potential for unintended consequences.

REFERENCES

Aarts J, Doorewaard H, Berg M. 2004. Understanding implementation: The case of a computerized physician order entry system in a large Dutch university medical center. *Journal of the American Medical Informatics Association* 11(3):207–216.

Abarca J, Malone DC, Armstrong EP, Grizzle AJ, Hansten PD, Van Bergen RC, Lipton RB. 2004. Concordance of severity ratings provided in four drug interaction compendia. *Journal of the American Pharmacists Association* 44(2):136–141.

Abookire SA, Teich JM, Sandige H, Paterno MD, Martin MT, Kuperman GJ, Bates DW. 2000. Improving allergy alerting in a computerized physician order entry system. *Proceedings of the American Medical Informatics Association Symposium* 2–6.

AHRQ (Agency for Healthcare Research and Quality). 2005. *Advances in Patient Safety: From Research to Implementation* (Volumes 1–4). Rockville, MD: AHRQ.

Allan EL, Barker KN. 1990. Fundamentals of medication error research. *American Journal of Hospital Pharmacy* 47(3):551–571.

Alper BS, Stevermer JJ, White DS, Ewigman BG. 2001. Answering family physicians' clinical questions using electronic medical databases. *The Journal of Family Practice* 50(11):960–965.

Andrews LB, Stocking C, Krizek T, Gottlieb L, Krizek C, Vargish T, Siegler M. 1997. An alternative strategy for studying adverse events in medical care. *Lancet* 349(9048):309–313.

Anglemyer BL, Hernandez C, Brice JH, Zou B. 2004. The accuracy of visual estimation of body weight in the ED. *The American Journal of Emergency Medicine* 22(7):526–529.

Ansell JE, Buttaro ML, Thomas OV, Knowlton CH. 1997. Consensus guidelines for coordinated outpatient oral anticoagulation therapy management. *The Annals of Pharmacotherapy* 31(5):604–615.

Ash JS, Berg M, Coiera E. 2004. Some unintended consequences of information technology in health care: The nature of patient care information system-related errors. *Journal of the American Medical Informatics Association* 11(2):104–112.

Baker HM. 1997. Rules outside the rules for administration of medication: A study in New South Wales, Australia. *Image—The Journal of Nursing Scholarship* 29(2):155–158.

Ballinger BR, Simpson E, Stewart MJ. 1974. An evaluation of a drug administration system in a psychiatric hospital. *The British Journal of Psychiatry: The Journal of Mental Science* 125:202–207.

Barker KN. 1995. Ensuring safety in the use of automated medication dispensing systems. *American Journal of Health-System Pharmacy* 52(21):2445–2447.

Barker KN, Mikeal RL, Pearson RE, Illig NA, Morse ML. 1982. Medication errors in nursing homes and small hospitals. *American Journal of Hospital Pharmacy* 39:987–991.

Barker KN, Felkey BG, Flynn EA, Carper JL. 1998. White paper on automation in pharmacy. *The Consultant Pharmacist* 13:256–293.

Barker KN, Flynn EA, Pepper GA. 2002. Observation method of detecting medication errors. *American Journal of Health-System Pharmacy* 59(23):2314–2316.

Barrett JR, Strayer SM, Schubart JR. 2004. Assessing medical residents' usage and perceived needs for personal digital assistants. *International Journal of Medical Informatics* 73(1):25–34.

Barrie AR, Ward AM. 1997. Questioning behaviour in general practice: A pragmatic study. *British Medical Journal* 315(7121):1512–1515.

Batalden P, Nelson EC, Edwards WH, Godfrey MM, Mohr JJ. 2003. Microsystems in health care: Part 9. Developing small clinical units to attain peak performance. *Joint Commission Journal on Quality and Safety* 29(11):575–585.

Bates DW. 2000. Using information technology to reduce rates of medication errors in hospitals. *British Medical Journal* 320(7237):788–791.

Bates DW. 2001. A 40-year-old woman who noticed a medication error. *Journal of the American Medical Association* 285(24):3134–3140.

Bates DW. 2002. Invited commentary. *Baylor University Medical Center Proceedings* 15: 208–209.

Bates DW. 2005. Computerized physician order entry and medication errors: Finding a balance. *Journal of Biomedical Informatics* 38(4):259–261.

Bates DW, Gawande AA. 2003. Improving safety with information technology. *New England Journal of Medicine* 348(25):2526–2534.

Bates DW, Boyle DL, Vander Vliet MB, Schneider J, Leape L. 1995a. Relationship between medication errors and adverse drug events. *Journal of General Internal Medicine* 10(4): 199–205.

Bates DW, Cullen DJ, Laird N, Petersen LA, Small SD, Servi D, Laffel G, Sweitzer BJ, Shea BF, Hallisey R, Vander Vliet M, Nemeskal R, Leape LL. 1995b. Incidence of adverse drug events and potential adverse drug events. Implications for prevention. ADE Prevention Study Group. *Journal of the American Medical Association* 274:29–34.

Bates DW, Leape LL, Cullen DJ, Laird N, Petersen LA, Teich JM, Burdick E, Hickey M, Kleefield S, Shea B, Vander Vliet M. 1998. Effect of computerized physician order entry and a team intervention on prevention of serious medication errors. *Journal of the American Medical Association* 280(15):1311–1316.

Bates DW, Teich JM, Lee J, Seger D, Kuperman GJ, Ma'luf N, Boyle D, Leape L. 1999. The impact of computerized physician order entry on medication error prevention. *Journal of the American Medical Informatics Association* 6:313–321.

Bates DW, Cohen M, Leape LL, Overhage JM, Shabot MM, Sheridan T. 2001. Reducing the frequency of errors in medicine using information technology. *Journal of the American Medical Informatics Association* 8(4):299–308.

Bates DW, Evans RS, Murff H, Stetson PD, Pizziferri L, Hripcsak G. 2003. Detecting adverse events using information technology. *Journal of the American Medical Informatics Association* 10(2):115–128.

Beattie JW. 2003. Web-based PDA downloads for clinical practice guidelines and decision support tools. *Medical Reference Services Quarterly* 22(4):57–64.

Benson L, Westphal RG. 2005. Emergency department preparedness trainings in New York State: A needs assessment. *Journal of Public Health Management and Practice* 11(Suppl. 6):S135–S137.

Benson DS, Van Osdol W, Townes P. 1988. Quality ambulatory care: The role of the diagnostic and medication summary lists. *Quality Review Bulletin* 14(6):192–197.

Berger RG, Kichak JP. 2004. Computerized physician order entry: Helpful or harmful? *Journal of the American Medical Informatics Association* 11(2):100–103.

Bodenheimer T. 1999. Long-term care for frail elderly people: The On Lok Model. *New England Journal of Medicine* 341(17):1324–1328.

Boneberg RF, Kellick KA, Pudhorodsky TG, Vitell SJ, Jones GE. 1991. Results of a retrospective outpatient medication error prevention program at a Department of Veterans Affairs Medical Center. *ASHP Midyear Clinical Meeting* 26:325E.

Bower A. 2005. *Katrina's Lingering Medical Nightmare, Time, September 22, 2005.* [Online]. Available: http://www.time.com/time/nation/printout/0,8816,1107826,00.html [accessed December 12, 2005].

Brushwood DB. 2003. Maximizing the value of electronic prescription monitoring programs. *The Journal of Law, Medicine & Ethics* 31(1):41–54.

Burack RC, Gimotty PA. 1997. Promoting screening mammography in inner-city settings. The sustained effectiveness of computerized reminders in a randomized controlled trial. *Medical Care* 35(9):921–931.

Carpenter JD, Gorman PN. 2002. Using medication list—problem list mismatches as markers of potential error. *Proceedings of the American Medical Informatics Association Symposium* 106–110.

CC (The Cochrane Collaboration). 2005. *What Is the Cochrane Collaboration?* [Online]. Available: http://www.cochrane.org/docs/descrip.htm [accessed October 6, 2005].

CDC (Centers for Disease Control and Prevention). 2005. Surveillance for illness and injury after Katrina; New Orleans, Louisiana, September 8–25, 2005. *Morbidity and Mortality Weekly Report* 54(40):1018–1021.

Chertow GM, Lee J, Kuperman GJ, Burdick E, Horsky J, Seger DL, Lee R, Mekala A, Song J, Komaroff AL, Bates DW. 2001. Guided medication dosing for inpatients with renal insufficiency. *Journal of the American Medical Association* 286(22):2839–2844.

Chiquette E, Amato MG, Bussey HI. 1998. Comparison of an anticoagulation clinic with usual medical care: Anticoagulation control, patient outcomes and health care costs. *Archives of Internal Medicine* 158(15):1641–1647.

Classen DC, Pestotnik SL, Evans RS, Burke JP. 1991. Computerized surveillance of adverse drug events in hospital patients. *Journal of the American Medical Association* 266:2847–2851.

The Cochrane Library. 2004. *Cochrane Collaboration.* [Online]. Available: http://www.cochrane.org [accessed October 10, 2005].

Cohen MM, Kimmel NL, Benage MK, Cox MJ, Sanders N, Spence D, Chen J. 2005. Medication safety program reduced adverse drug events in a community hospital. *Quality and Safety in Health Care* 14(3):169–174.

CoSI (Commission on Systemic Interoperability). 2005. *Ending the Document Game: Connecting and Transforming Your Healthcare through Information Technology.* Washington, DC: U.S. Government Printing Office.

Covell DG, Uman GC, Manning PR. 1985. Information needs in office practice: Are they being met? *Annals of Internal Medicine* 103(4):596–599.

Croskerry P, Shapiro M, Campbell S, LeBlanc C, Sinclair D. 2004. Profiles in patient safety: Medication errors in the emergency department. *Academic Emergency Medicine* 11(3):289–299.

CTFPHC (Canadian Task Force on Preventive Health Care). 2005. *Canadian Task Force on Preventive Health Care: Evidence-Based Clinical Prevention.* [Online]. Available: http://www.ctfphc.org [accessed October 6, 2005].

Cunningham MC, Basile SB, Timmons VL, Schauben PB. 1996. *Categorizing Errors on the Medication Administration Record.* Paper presented at ASHP Midyear Clinical Meeting, New Orleans, LA.

DHHS (U.S. Department of Health and Human Services). 2005. *U.S. Preventive Services Task Force (USPSTF).* [Online]. Available: http://www.ahrq.gov/clinic/uspstfix.htm [accessed October 6, 2005].

Ebell M. 1999. Information at the point of care: Answering clinical questions. *The Journal of the American Board of Family Practice* 12(3):225–235.

Ebell MH, Slawson D, Shaughnessy A, Barry H. 2002. Update on InfoRetriever software. *Journal of the Medical Library Association* 90(3):343.

eHI (eHealth Initiative). 2004. *Electronic Prescribing: Toward Maximum Value and Rapid Adoption.* Washington, DC: eHI.

Ely JW. 2001. Why can't we answer our questions? *The Journal of Family Practice* 50(11):974–975.

Ely JW, Osheroff JA, Ebell MH, Bergus GR, Levy BT, Chambliss ML, Evans ER. 1999. Analysis of questions asked by family doctors regarding patient care. *British Medical Journal* 319(7206):358–361.

Ely JW, Osheroff JA, Chambliss ML, Ebell MH, Rosenbaum ME. 2005. Answering physicians' clinical questions: Obstacles and potential solutions. *Journal of the American Medical Informatics Association* 12(2):217–224.

Epocrates. 2005. *All-One-Guide to Drugs, Diseases and Diagnostics.* [Online]. Available: http://www2.epocrates.com [accessed October 6, 2005].

Estabrooks CA, Chong H, Brigidear K, Profetto-McGrath J. 2005. Profiling Canadian nurses' preferred knowledge sources for clinical practice. *The Canadian Journal of Nursing Research* 37(2):119–140.

Evans RS, Pestotnik SL, Classen DC, Bass SB, Menlove RL, Gardner RM, Burke JP. 1991. Development of a computerized adverse drug event monitor. *Proceedings of the Annual Symposium on Computer Application in Medical Care* 23–27.

Evans RS, Classen DC, Pestotnik SL, Lundsgaarde HP, Burke JP. 1994a. Improving empiric antibiotic selection using computer decision support. *Archives of Internal Medicine* 154(8):878–884.

Evans RS, Pestotnik SL, Classen DC, Horn SD, Bass SB, Burke JP. 1994b. Preventing adverse drug events in hospitalized patients. *The Annals of Pharmacotherapy* 28(4):523–527.

Evans RS, Pestotnik SL, Classen DC, Clemmer TP, Weaver LK, Orme JF, Lloyd JF, Burke JP. 1998. A computer-assisted management program for antibiotics and other antiinfective agents. *New England Journal of Medicine* 338(4):232–238.

Farris KB, McCarthy AM, Kelly MW, Clay D, Gross JN. 2003. Issues of medication administration and control in Iowa schools. *The Journal of School Health* 73(9):331–337.

Fernando B, Savelyich BSP, Avery AJ, Sheikh A, Bainbridge M, Horsfield P, Teasdale S. 2004. Prescribing safety features of general practice computer systems: Evaluation using simulated test cases. *British Medical Journal* 328(7449):1171–1172.

Field TS, Gurwitz JH, Harrold LR, Rothschild JM, Debellis K, Seger AC, Fish LS, Garber L, Kelleher M, Bates DW. 2004. Strategies for detecting adverse drug events among older persons in the ambulatory setting. *Journal of the American Medical Informatics Association* 11(6):492–498.

Finnell JT, Overhage JM, Dexter PR, Perkins SM, Lane KA, McDonald CJ. 2003. Community clinical data exchange for emergency medicine patients. *Proceedings of the American Medical Informatics Association Annual Symposium* 235–238.

Flynn EA, Barker KN, Pepper GA, Bates DW, Mikeal RL. 2002. Comparison of methods for detecting medication errors in 36 hospitals and skilled-nursing facilities. *American Journal of Health-System Pharmacy* 59(5):436–446.

Flynn EA, Barker KN, Carnahan BJ. 2003. National observational study of prescription dispensing accuracy and safety in 50 pharmacies. *Journal of the American Pharmaceutical Association* 43(2):191–200.

Forster AJ, Murff HJ, Peterson JF, Gandhi TK, Bates DW. 2003. The incidence and severity of adverse events affecting patients after discharge from the hospital. *Annals of Internal Medicine* 138(3):161–167.

Forster AJ, Murff HJ, Peterson JF, Gandhi TK, Bates DW. 2005. Adverse drug events following hospital discharge. *Journal of General Internal Medicine* 20:317–323.

FPIN (Family Physicians Inquiries Network). 2005. *About FPIN*. [Online]. Available: http://www.fpin.org/about [accessed October 6, 2005].

Galanter WL, Didomenico RJ, Polikaitis A. 2005. A trial of automated decision support alerts for contraindicated medications using computerized physician order entry. *Journal of the American Medical Informatics Association* 12(3):269–274.

Galloway M, Woods R, Whitehead S, Gedling P. 2002. Providing feedback to users on unacceptable practice in the delivery of a hospital transfusion service—a pilot study. *Transfusion Medicine* 12(2):129–132.

Galt KA, Rule AM, Houghton B, Young DO, Remington G. 2005. Personal digital assistant-based drug information sources: Potential to improve medication safety. *Journal of the Medical Library Association* 93(2):229–236.

Gandhi TK, Seger DL, Bates DW. 2000. Identifying drug safety issues: From research to practice. *International Journal for Quality in Health Care* 12(1):69–76.

Gandhi TK, Weingart SN, Borus J, Seger AC, Peterson J, Burdick E, Seger DL, Shu K, Federico F, Leape LL, Bates DW. 2003. Adverse drug events in ambulatory care. *New England Journal of Medicine* 348(16):1556–1564.

Gandhi TK, Weingart SN, Seger AC, Borus J, Burdick E, Poon EG, Leape LL, Bates DW. 2005. Outpatient prescribing errors and the impact of computerized prescribing. *Journal of General Internal Medicine* 20(9):837–841.

GAO (Government Accountability Office). 2005. *Hurricane Katrina: Providing Oversight of the Nation's Preparedness, Response, and Recovery Activities. Statement of Norman J. Rabkin, Managing Director, Homeland Security and Justice Issues.* Washington, DC: GAO.

Gift MG, Mavko LE, Vanderpool WH. 1996. *Evaluating Returned Doses as an Approach to Improving Medication Use.* Paper presented at ASHP Midyear Clinical Meeting, New Orleans, LA.

Giuse NB, Huber JT, Giuse DA, Brown CW, Bankowitz RA, Hunt S. 1994. Information needs of health care professionals in an AIDS outpatient clinic as determined by chart review. *Journal of the American Medical Informatics Association* 1(5):395–403.

Glintborg B, Andersen SE, Dalhoff K. 2005. Drug-drug interactions among recently hospitalised patients: Frequent but mostly clinically insignificant. *European Journal of Clinical Pharmacology* 61(9):675–681.

Gorman PN. 1995. Information needs of physicians. *Journal of the American Society for Information Science* 46(10):729–736.

Gorman PN, Helfand M. 1995. Information seeking in primary care: How physicians choose which clinical questions to pursue and which to leave unanswered. *Medical Decision Making* 15(2):113–119.

Gosbee JW. 2004. Conclusion: You need human factors engineering expertise to see design hazards that are hiding in "plain sight!" *Joint Commission Journal on Quality and Safety* 30(12):696–700.

Grandage KK, Slawson DC, Shaughnessy AF. 2002. When less is more: A practical approach to searching for evidence-based answers. *Journal of the Medical Library Association* 90(3):298–304.

Grasso BC, Rothschild JM, Genest R, Bates DW. 2003. What do we know about medication errors in psychiatry? *Joint Commission Journal on Quality and Safety* 29(8):391–400.

Grisso AG, Pingel JS, Wright L, Hargrove FR. 2004. Monitoring for medication dosing errors through the daily review of a pharmacist override list. *ASHP Midyear Clinical Meeting* 39:276E.

Grumbach K, and Bodenheimer T. 2004. Can health care teams improve primary care practice? *Journal of the American Medical Association* 291(10):1246–1251.

Gurwitz JH, Field TS, Avorn J, McCormick D, Jain S, Eckler M, Benser M, Edmondson AC, Bates DW. 2000. Incidence and preventability of adverse drug events in nursing homes. *The American Journal of Medicine* 109(2):87–94.

Gurwitz JH, Field TS, Harrold LR, Rothschild J, Debellis K, Seger AC, Cadoret C, Fish LS, Garber L, Kelleher M, Bates DW. 2003. Incidence and preventability of adverse drug events among older persons in the ambulatory setting. *Journal of the American Medical Association* 289(9):1107–1116.

Gurwitz JH, Field TS, Judge J, Rochon P, Harrold LR, Cadoret C, Lee M, White K, LaPrino J, Mainard JF, DeFlorio M, Gavendo L, Auger J, Bates DW. 2005. The incidence of adverse drug events in two large academic long-term care facilities. *The American Journal of Medicine* 118(3):251–258.

Haas D, Griffiths L, Severing J. 2004. Impact of a unit-based clinical generalist pharmacist on patient care. *ASHP Midyear Clinical Meeting* 39:69D.

Hamby L, Weeks WB, Malikowski C. 2000. Complications of warfarin therapy: Causes, costs, and the role of the anticoagulation clinic. *Effective Clinical Practice* 3(4):179–184.

Han YY, Carcillo JA, Venkataraman ST, Clark RSB, Watson RS, Nguyen TC, Bayir H, Orr RA. 2005. Unexpected increased mortality after implementation of a commercially sold computerized physician order entry system. *Pediatrics* 116(5):1506–1512.

Hansten P, Horn J, Hazlet T. 2001. ORCA: OpeRational ClassificAtion of drug interactions. *Journal of the American Pharmaceutical Association (Washington, D.C.)* 41:161–165.

Hayes C, O'Herlihy B, Hynes M, Johnson Z. 1999. The impact of reminder letters on attendance for breast cancer screening. *Irish Journal of Medical Science* 168(1):29–32.

Hicks RW, Cousins DD, Williams RL. 2004. Selected medication-error data from USP's MEDMARX program for 2002. *American Journal of Health-System Pharmacy* 61(10): 993–1000.

Hofmans-Okkes IM, Lamberts H. 1996. The International Classification of Primary Care (ICPC): New applications in research and computer-based patient records in family practice. *Family Practice* 13(3):294–302.

Hsieh TC, Kuperman GJ, Jaggi T, Hojnowski-Diaz P, Fiskio J, Williams DH, Bates DW, Gandhi TK. 2004. Characteristics and consequences of drug allergy alert overrides in a computerized physician order entry system. *Journal of the American Medical Informatics Association* 11(6):482–491.

IOM (Institute of Medicine). 2000. *To Err Is Human: Building a Safer Health System.* Washington, DC: National Academy Press.

IOM. 2004. *Patient Safety: Achieving a New Standard for Care.* Washington, DC: The National Academies Press.

Isetts BJ, Brown LM, Schondelmeyer SW, Lenarz LA. 2003. Quality assessment of a collaborative approach for decreasing drug-related morbidity and achieving therapeutic goals. *Archives of Internal Medicine* 163(15):1813–1820.

ISMP (Institute for Safe Medication Practice). 2005a. *Institute of Safe Medication Practices.* [Online]. Available: http://www.ismp.org [accessed August 22, 2005].

ISMP. 2005b. *Safety Still Compromised by Computer Weaknesses. Comparing 1999 and 2005 Pharmacy Computer Field Test Results.* [Online]. Available: http://www.ismp.org/MSAarticles/20050825.htm [accessed September 2, 2005].

James B. 2005. E-Health: Steps on the road to interoperability. *Health Affairs (Millwood)* Suppl. Web Exclusives W5-26–W5-30.

JCAHO (Joint Commission on Accreditation of Healthcare Organizations). 2005. *2006 Critical Access Hospital and Hospital National Patient Safety Goals.* [Online]. Available: http://www.jcipatientsafety.org/show.asp?durki=10293&site=164&return=10289 [accessed August 22, 2005].

JFP (Journal of Family Practice). 2005. *POEMs: Patient Oriented Evidence That Matters.* [Online]. Available: http://www.jfponline.com [accessed October 6, 2005].

Jha AK, Kuperman GJ, Teich JM, Leape L, Shea B, Rittenberg E, Burdick E, Seger DL, Vender Vliet M, Bates DW. 1998. Identifying adverse drug events: Development of a computer-based monitor and comparison with chart review and stimulated voluntary report. *Journal of the American Medical Informatics Association* 5(3):305–314.

Kaboli PJ, McClimon BJ, Hoth AB, Barnett MJ. 2004. Assessing the accuracy of computerized medication histories. *The American Journal of Managed Care* 10(11 Pt. 2):872–877.

Kamel Boulos MN, Roudsari AV, Carson ER. 2002. A dynamic problem to knowledge linking Semantic Web service based on clinical codes. *Medical Informatics and the Internet in Medicine* 27(3):127–137.

Katz SJ, Nissan N, Moyer CA. 2004. Crossing the digital divide: Evaluating online communication between patients and their providers. *The American Journal of Managed Care* 10(9):593–598.

Kaushal R, Shojania KG, Bates DW. 2003. Effects of computerized physician order entry and clinical decision support systems on medication safety: A systematic review. *Archives of Internal Medicine* 163(12):1409–1416.

Kaushal R, Bates DW, Poon EG, Jha AK, Blumenthal D. 2005. Functional gaps in attaining a national health information network. What will it take to get there in five years? *Health Affairs* 24(5):1281–1289.

Kaushal R, Jha AK, Franz C, Shetty KD, Jaggi T, Glaser J, Middleton B, Kuperman GJ, Khorasani R, Tanasijevic M, Bates DW. 2006. Return on investment for a computerized physician order entry system. *Journal of the American Medical Informatics Association* 13(3):261–266.

Kester KA. 2005. Errors associated with medications removed from automated dispensing machines using override function. *ASHP Summer Meeting* 62:31E.

Kilbridge PM, Welebob EM, Classen DC. 2006. Development of the Leapfrog methodology for evaluating hospital implemented inpatient computerized physician order entry systems. *Quality and Safety in Health Care* 15(2):81–84.

Kobusingye OC, Hyder AA, Bishai D, Hicks ER, Mock C, Joshipura M. 2005. Emergency medical systems in low- and middle-income countries: Recommendations for action. *Bulletin of the World Health Organization* 83(8):626–631.

Koppel R, Metlay JP, Cohen A, Abaluck B, Localio AR, Kimmel SE, Strom BL. 2005. Role of computerized physician order entry systems in facilitating medication errors. *Journal of the American Medical Association* 293(10):1197–1203.

Kuyper AR. 1993. Patient counseling detects prescription errors. *Hospital Pharmacy* 28(12): 1180–1181, 1184–1189.

Lappa E. 2005. Undertaking an information-needs analysis of the emergency-care physician to inform the role of the clinical librarian: A Greek perspective. *Health Information and Libraries Journal* 22(2):124–132.

Leape LL, Cullen DJ, Clapp MD, Burdick E, Demonaco HJ, Erickson JI, Bates DW. 1999. Pharmacists participation on physician rounds and adverse drug events in the intensive care unit. *Journal of the American Medical Association* 282(3):267–270.

Lu YC, Lee JK, Xiao Y, Sears A, Jacko JA, Charters K. 2003. Why don't physicians use their personal digital assistants? *Proceedings of the American Medical Informatics Association Annual Symposium* 404–405.

Matchar DB, Samsa GP, Cohen SJ, Oddone EZ, Jurgelski AE. 2002. Improving the quality of anticoagulation of patients with atrial fibrillation in managed care organizations: Results of the managing anticoagulation services trial. *The American Journal of Medicine* 113(1):42–51.

Maviglia SM, Yoon CS, Bates DW, Kuperman G. 2005. KnowledgeLink: Impact of context sensitive information retrieval on clinicians' information needs. *Journal of the American Medical Informatics Association*.

McDonald CJ, Hui SL, Smith DM, Tierney WM, Cohen SJ, Weinberger M, McCabe GP. 1984. Reminders to physicians from an introspective computer medical record. A two-year randomized trial. *Annals of Internal Medicine* 100(1):130–138.

McDonald CJ, Overhage JM, Barnes M, Schadow G, Blevins L, Dexter PR, Mamlin B, INPC Management Committee. 2005. The Indiana network for patient care: A working local health information infrastructure. An example of a working infrastructure collaboration that links data from five health systems and hundreds of millions of entries. *Health Affairs* 24(5):1214–1220.

Meyer TA. 2000. Improving the quality of the order-writing process for inpatient orders and outpatient prescriptions. *American Journal of Health-System Pharmacy* 57(Suppl. 4): S18–S22.

Mohr JJ, Batalden PB. 2002. Improving safety on the front lines: The role of clinical microsystems. *Quality and Safety in Health Care* 11(1):45–50.

Morimoto T, Gandhi TK, Seger AC, Hsieh TC, Bates DW. 2004. Adverse drug events and medication errors: Detection and classification methods. *Quality and Safety in Health Care* 13(4):306–314.

Murff HJ, Forster AJ, Peterson JF, Fiskio JM, Heiman HL, Bates DW. 2003. Electronically screening discharge summaries for adverse medical events. *Journal of the American Medical Informatics Association* 10(4):339–350.

NCPDP (National Council for Prescription Drug Programs, Inc.). 2005. *National Council for Prescription Drug Programs, Inc.* [Online]. Available: http://www.ncpdp.org [accessed November 22, 2005].

Neilson EG, Johnson KB, Rosenbloom ST. 2004. The impact of peer management on test-ordering behavior. *Annals of Internal Medicine* 141(3):196–204.

NQF (National Quality Forum). 2003. *Safe Practices for Better Healthcare: A Consensus Report*. Washington, DC: NQF.

Okkes IM, Groen A, Oskam SK, Lamberts H. 2001. Advantages of long observation in episode-oriented electronic patient records in family practice. *Methods of Information in Medicine* 40(3):229–235.

Oren E, Griffiths LP, Guglielmo BJ. 2002. Characteristics of antimicrobial overrides associated with automated dispensing machines. *American Journal of Health-System Pharmacy* 59(15):1445–1448.

Overhage JM, Tierney WM, McDonald CJ. 1995. Design and implementation of the Indianapolis Network for Patient Care and Research. *Bulletin of the Medical Library Association* 83(1):48–56.

Oxman AD, Sackett DL, Guyatt GH. 1993. Users' guides to the medical literature. I. How to get started. The Evidence-Based Medicine Working Group. *Journal of the American Medical Association* 270(17):2093–2095.

Pauker SD, Gorry G, Kassirer J, Schwartz W. 1976. Towards the simulation of clinical cognition: Taking a present illness by computer. *The American Journal of Medicine* 60(7):981–996.

Payne TH, Nichol WP, Hoey P, Savarino J. 2002. Characteristics and override rates of order checks in a practitioner order entry system. *Proceedings of the American Medical Informatics Association Symposium* 602–606.

Petersen LA, Orav EJ, Teich JM, O'Neil AC, Brennan TA. 1998. Using a computerized sign-out program to improve continuity of inpatient care and prevent adverse events. *The Joint Commission Journal on Quality Improvement* 24(2):77–87.

Peterson JF, Bates DW. 2001. Preventable medication errors: Identifying and eliminating serious drug interactions. *Journal of the American Pharmaceutical Association (Washington, D.C.)* 41(2):159–160.

Peterson JF, Kuperman GJ, Shek C, Patel M, Avorn J, Bates DW. 2005. Guided prescription of psychotropic medications for geriatric inpatients. *Archives of Internal Medicine* 165(7): 802–807.

Peth HA. 2003. Medication errors in the emergency department: A systems approach to minimizing risk. *Emergency Medicine Clinics of North America* 21(1):141–158.

Phillips DP, Christenfeld N, Glynn LM. 1998. Increase in U.S. medication-error deaths between 1983 and 1993. *Lancet* 351(9103):643–644.

Phillips MA. 2002. Voluntary reporting of medication errors. *American Journal of Health-System Pharmacy* 59(23):2326–2328.

Poon EG, Cina JL, Churchill W, Featherstone E, Rothschild JM, Keohane CA, Bates DW, Gandhi TK. 2005. Effect of barcode technology on the incidence of medication dispensing errors and potential adverse drug events in a hospital pharmacy. *Proceedings of the American Medical Informatics Association Symposium* 1085.

Porter SC, Kohane IS, Goldmann DA. 2005. Parents as partners in obtaining the medication history. *Journal of the American Medical Informatics Association* 12(3):299–305.

Pronovost P, Wu AW, Dorman T, Morlock L. 2002. Building safety into ICU care. *Journal of Critical Care* 17(2):78–85.

Pronovost P, Weast B, Schwarz M, Wyskiel RM, Prow D, Milanovich SN, Berenholtz S, Dorman T, Lipsett P. 2003a. Medication reconciliation: A practical tool to reduce the risk of medication errors. *Journal of Critical Care* 18(4):201–205.

Pronovost P, Berenholtz S, Dorman T, Lipsett PA, Simmonds T, Haraden C. 2003b. Improving communication in the ICU using daily goals. *Journal of Critical Care* 18(2): 71–75.

Rich MW, Beckham V, Wittenberg C, Leven CL, Freedland KE, Carney RM. 1995. A multidisciplinary intervention to prevent the readmission of elderly patients with congestive heart failure. *New England Journal of Medicine* 333(18):1190–1195.

Rochon PA, Field TS, Bates DW, Lee M, Gavendo L, Erramuspe-Mainard J, Judge J, Gurwitz JH. 2005. Computerized physician order entry with clinical decision support in the long-term care setting: Insights from the Baycrest Centre for Geriatric Care. *Journal of the American Geriatrics Society* 53(10):1780–1789.

Rothschild J. 2004. Computerized physician order entry in the critical care and general inpatient setting: A narrative review. *Journal of Critical Care* 19(4):271–278.

Rothschild JM, Lee TH, Bae T, Bates DW. 2002. Clinician use of a palmtop drug reference guide. *Journal of the American Medical Informatics Association* 9(3):223–229.

Rothschild JM, Landrigan CP, Cronin JW, Kaushal R, Lockley SW, Burdick E, Stone PH, Lilly CM, Katz JT, Czeisler CA, Bates DW. 2005. The Critical Care Safety Study: The incidence and nature of adverse events and serious medical errors in intensive care. *Critical Care Medicine* 33(8):1694–1700.

Rowe C, Koren T, Koren G. 1998. Errors by pediatric residents in calculating drug doses. *Archives of Disease in Childhood* 79(1):56–58.

Rozich JD, Haraden CR, Resar RK. 2003. Adverse drug event trigger tool: A practical methodology for measuring medication related harm. *Quality and Safety in Health Care* 12(3):194–200.

Rozich JD, Howard RJ, Justeson JM, Macken PD, Lindsay ME, Resar RK. 2004. Standardization as a mechanism to improve safety in health care. *Joint Commission Journal on Quality and Safety* 30(1):5–14.

Samsa GP, Matcher DB, Goldstein LB, Bonito AJ, Lux LJ, Witter DM, Bian J. 2000. Quality of anticoagulation management among patients with atrial fibrillation: results of a review of medical records from 2 communities. *Archives of Internal Medicine* 160:967–973.

Santell JP, Protzel MM, Cousins D. 2004. Medication errors in oncology practice. *U.S. Pharmacist* 29(4).

Shablinsky I, Starren J, Friedman C. 1999. What do ER physicians really want? A method for elucidating ER information needs. *Proceedings of the American Medical Informatics Association Symposium* 390–394.

Shah NR, Seger AC, Seger DL, Fiskio JM, Kuperman GJ, Blumenfeld B, Recklet EG, Bates DW, Gandhi TK. 2005. Improving acceptance of computerized prescribing alerts in ambulatory care. *Journal of the American Medical Informatics Association* 13(1):5–11.

Shea S, DuMouchel W, Bahamonde L. 1996. A meta-analysis of 16 randomized controlled trials to evaluate computer-based clinical reminder systems for preventive care in the ambulatory setting. *Journal of the American Medical Informatics Association* 3(6):399–409.

Shuttleworth TA, Ruelle S. 1996. *Detecting Medication Errors with Automated Distribution.* Paper presented at ASHP Midyear Clinical Meeting, New Orleans, LA.

Simon GE, Ludman EJ, Tutty S, Operskalski B, Von Korff M. 2004. Telephone psychotherapy and telephone care management for primary care patients starting antidepressant treatment: A randomized controlled trial. *Journal of the American Medical Association* 292(8):935–942.

Simon GE, Ludman EJ, Unutzer J, Bauer MS, Operskalski B, Rutter C. 2005. Randomized trial of a population-based care program for people with bipolar disorder. *Psychological Medicine* 35(1):13–24.

Smith PC, Araya-Guerra R, Bublitz C, Parnes B, Dickinson LM, Van Vorst R, Westfall JM, Pace WD. 2005. Missing clinical information during primary care visits. *Journal of the American Medical Association* 293(5):565–571.

Smith R. 1996. What clinical information do doctors need? *British Medical Journal* 313(7064):1062–1068.

Solet DJ, Norvell JM, Rutan GH, Frankel RM. 2005. Lost in translation: Challenges and opportunities in physician-to-physician communication during patient handoffs. *Academic Medicine* 80(12):1094–1099.

Strom BL, Hennessy S. 2002. Pharmacist care and clinical outcomes for patients with reactive airways disease. *Journal of the American Medical Association* 288(13):1642–1643.

Stupalski KA, Russell GE. 1999. Reported medication errors in community residences for individuals with mental retardation: A quality review. *Mental Retardation* 37(2):139–146.

Sung NS, Crowley WF, Genel M, Salber P, Sandy L, Sherwood LM, Johnson SB, Catanese V, Tilson H, Getz K, Larson EL, Scheinberg D, Reece EA, Slavkin H, Dobs A, Grebb J, Martinez RA, Korn A, Romoin D. 2003. Central challenges facing the national clinical research enterprise. *Journal of the American Medical Association* 289(10):1278–1287.

Sutcliffe KM, Lewton E, Rosenthal MM. 2004. Communication failures: An insidious contributor to medical mishaps. *Academic Medicine* 79(2):186–194.

Tafreshi MJ, Melby MJ, Kaback KR, Nord TC. 1999. Medication-related visits to the emergency department: A prospective study. *The Annals of Pharmacotherapy* 33(12):1252–1257.

Taylor PP. 2005. Use of handheld devices in critical care. *Critical Care Nursing Clinics of North America* 17(1):45–50, x.

Teich JM, Osheroff JA, Pifer EA, Sittig DF, Jenders RA, The CDS Expert Review Panel. 2005. Clinical decision support in electronic prescribing: Recommendations and an action plan: Report of the joint clinical decision support workgroup. *Journal of the American Medical Informatics Association* 12(4):365–376.

Thompson C, McCaughan D, Cullum N, Sheldon TA, Mulhall A, Thompson DR. 2001. Research information in nurses' clinical decision-making: What is useful? *Journal of Advanced Nursing* 36(3):376–388.

Torre D. 2004. Remote access simplified. A large healthcare provider shares some practical lessons learned. *Healthcare Informatics* 21(4):45–46.

Tufo HM, Bouchard RE, Rubin AS, Twitchell JC, VanBuren HC, Weed LB, Rothwell M. 1977. Problem-oriented approach to practice. I. Economic impact. *Journal of the American Medical Association* 238(5):414–417.

Volpp KG, Grande D. 2003. Residents' suggestions for reducing errors in teaching hospitals. *New England Journal of Medicine* 348(9):851–855.

Waldron I. 1977. Increased prescribing of Valium, Librium, and other drugs—an example of the influence of economic and social factors on the practice of medicine. *International Journal of Health Services* 7(1):37–62.

Wallace S. 2005. Mean what you say. Before achieving IT interoperability, leaders must agree on a definition. *Modern Healthcare* 35(12):22.

Weed L. 2004. Shedding our illusions: A better way of medicine. *Fertility and Sterility* 81(Suppl. 2):45–52.

Weingart SN, Toth M, Sands DZ, Aronson MD, Davis RB, Phillips RS. 2003. Physicians' decisions to override computerized drug alerts in primary care. *Archives of Internal Medicine* 163(21):2625–2631.

Weingart SN, Toth M, Eneman J, Aronson MD, Sands DZ, Ship AN, Davis RB, Phillips RS. 2004. Lessons from a patient partnership intervention to prevent adverse drug events. *International Journal for Quality in Health Care* 16(6):499–507.

Wertheimer AI, Ritchko C, Dougherty DW. 1973. Prescription accuracy: Room for improvement. *Medical Care* 11(1):68–71.

Whellan DJ, Hasselblad V, Peterson E, O'Connor CM, Schulman KA. 2005. Metaanalysis and review of heart failure disease management randomized controlled clinical trials. *American Heart Journal* 149(4):722–729.

Woodwell DA, Cherry, DK. 2004. *National Ambulatory Medical Care Survey: 2002 Summary. Advance Data from Vital and Health Statistics; No. 346.* Hyattsville, MD: National Center for Health Statistics.

Woolf SH, Kuzel AJ, Dovey SM, Phillips RL. 2004. A string of mistakes: The importance of cascade analysis in describing, counting, and preventing medical errors. *Annals of Family Medicine* 2(4):317–326.

Young D. 2002. More hospitals report medication errors, but USP finds few changes. *American Journal of Health-System Pharmacy* 59(13):1233.

6

Action Agenda for the Pharmaceutical, Medical Device, and Health Information Technology Industries

CHAPTER SUMMARY

Pharmaceutical, medical device, and health information technology companies represent the chief drug product-related industry sectors of the medication-use system. If designed well, their products can improve the health and well-being of consumers, advance medical science, and enhance clinical practice. As with other components of the medication-use system, however, certain features of design processes and communication mechanisms warrant significant improvement to better serve the health needs of consumers and the practice needs of providers and, most important, prevent medication errors. This chapter provides an action agenda for the pharmaceutical, medical device, and health information technology industries that, in collaboration with appropriate government agencies, can begin to address key problems that affect the safety and quality of the medication-use system.

This chapter presents an action agenda first for the pharmaceutical industry, and then for the medical device and health information technology industries.

PHARMACEUTICAL INDUSTRY

As discussed in Chapter 2, improving the safety of medication use requires improving the quality of information generated by industry and other researchers regarding drug products and their use in clinical practice. Also required are improvements in the way drug information is presented to providers and consumers through labeling and packaging since such materials have a direct effect on medication errors and adverse drug events (ADEs). This section reviews key problems involved in the generation and presentation of information that should be addressed by the pharmaceutical industry and the Food and Drug Administration (FDA).

Generation of Information

Current methods for generating information about medications are insufficient to meet the changing medical needs of the population, particularly given expected increases in the numbers of elderly people with multiple chronic conditions (IOM, 2000, 2001). While a comprehensive review of the drug research and development process and recommendations for its redesign are beyond the scope of this report, certain key aspects of information generation germane to medication safety merit discussion here.

Clinical Data

Determining that a medication error has occurred presumes that the correct dose of a drug for a given patient at a particular time is known, and that the indication for that drug is correct relative to alternative approaches to treatment. Unfortunately, this fundamental presumption is too often unwarranted.

The benefits of drugs can be categorized as improvement in longevity, improvement or stabilization of symptoms (improvement in quality of life), prevention of adverse events, or reduction in the costs of other medical interventions. To determine whether the benefits of a drug outweigh its risks, both the benefits and the risks must be measured in the population to whom the drug will be given for a relevant period of time (Yusuf et al., 1984; Prentice, 1989; Fleming and DeMets, 1996). Ideally, after these measurements have been made, individuals should be informed about both the benefits that can be expected and the potential risks. Since the benefits and risks are measured with different metrics, it is important to recognize that in the end, a subjective judgment regarding the balance of benefit and risk is necessary, since a ratio cannot be calculated (CERTS, 2003; Tsintis and La Mache, 2004; Edwards et al., 2005).

Over the past several decades, our understanding of therapeutic evaluation has advanced significantly. Nonetheless, the balance of benefit and risk of a drug compared with alternative treatments usually is not known. A variety of examples can be used to illustrate this point. Hormone replacement therapy, for instance, was once the most prevalent drug prescription globally, with its most common indication for use being prevention of cardiovascular disease in postmenopausal women. Many years after the therapy was marketed, however, both the HERS (Heart and Estrogen/progestin Replacement study) Trial and the Women's Health Initiative demonstrated its association with an *excess* of vascular events (Hulley et al., 1998; WHI Steering Committee, 2004). As a second example, the COX-2 (cyclo-oxygenase-2) inhibitors were expected to be a safer alternative to nonsteroidal anti-inflammatory drugs (NSAIDs). Vioxx and Bextra (among others), however, were removed from the market after the FDA Advisory Committee meeting in February 2005. Some experts believed the true balance of benefit and risk was not known for *any* of the COX-2 inhibitors (Psaty and Furberg, 2005). Perhaps even more startling, it was pointed out at the hearing that the same could be said for the traditional NSAIDs, which had been considered safe enough to sell over the counter. As a final example, a variety of antihypertension drugs have been developed and marketed as superior to the older, generic drugs used for this indication. However, when the National Institutes of Health (NIH) funded a pragamatic clinical trial involving more than 40,000 patients, it was found that the newer drugs provided no greater protection against stroke, heart failure, or death than the generic drug chlorthalidone (ALLHAT, 2002). Given that these examples involve some of the most commonly used and intensively studied drugs, there is uncertainty that drugs receiving less attention are better characterized. Since the only way to be confident about the balance of benefit and risk is empirical measurement, this information is lacking for most prescriptions that are written, especially those for chronically administered drugs.

The above issues are magnified in certain populations that bear much of the risk of drug prescription and administration:

• The majority of prescriptions written for children are off label,[1] with no empirical demonstration of safety and efficacy (Roberts et al., 2003). The Best Pharmaceuticals Act for Children has stimulated a major increase in clinical trials in children, but the legacy of sparse evidence remains substantial, and few of these trials have provided definitive information about indications and doses for the drugs involved. Pediatric oncology has been at the forefront in terms of enrolling a significant number of children in trials and could possibly be used as a model for other drug categories.

• Almost nothing is known about the balance of benefit and risk in the fastest-growing segment of the population—those over age 80. These patients have only recently been enrolled in clinical trials (Alexander and

---

[1]The FDA permits the prescribing of approved medications for other than their intended indications. This practice is known as off-label use.

Peterson, 2003). Given the major changes in organ physiology that occur in the elderly, people over age 80 have unique characteristics related to drug metabolism and pharmacodynamics.

• Patients with renal dysfunction represent a large and growing population requiring more comprehensive studies. Over 10 percent of the population now has a creatinine clearance below 60 milligrams per deciliter (mg/dl), indicating moderate or worse renal function (Reddan et al., 2003). The fact that many drugs are excreted by the kidneys raises obvious issues about dosing as a function of renal clearance. In addition, however, almost everyone with impaired renal function is either elderly or chronically ill, so that a simple mathematical calculation of clearance will not yield an accurate estimate of the balance of the benefit and risk of a drug at a particular dose.

• Patients with multiple comorbidities are typically excluded from premarketing clinical trials, yet many of the major problems involving drug toxicity have occurred in those taking multiple medications because of multiple diseases (Gurwitz, 2004). Drug interactions and additive toxic effects are common, and while they can be anticipated based on studies in other populations, the cumulative effects of multiple drugs cannot be predicted accurately without empirical study.

• Drugs for patients with psychiatric illnesses are particularly controversial. Most studies in these populations have been small and incapable of providing pragmatic, comparative information (March et al., 2005). Recent studies funded by the National Institute of Mental Health (NIMH) have fueled concern about the basic knowledge base for treatment of depression, manic-depressive illness, and schizophrenia.

The theory of clinical pharmacology has not been well supported by the academic community or the NIH. In particular, the characteristics of patients that determine the manner in which the pharmacokinetics and pharmacodynamics of drugs will be manifest are poorly understood and often overlooked (Fitzgerald, 2005). As a result of marketing considerations, the industry has tended to attempt to develop drugs that are given once a day and intravenous formulations that have fixed doses for ease of administration. Thus recommended doses are not specifically tailored to the needs of the individual patient.

The field of clinical pharmacology needs to be invigorated. Few training programs in this area exist today in the United States, prompting the Institute of Medicine (IOM) to initiate its own national course in drug development. With the anticipated availability of pharmacogenomic data, a cadre of experts will be needed to evaluate the modifiers of drug concentration and activity.

A large increase in the number of patients for whom clinical outcomes are measured is needed to elucidate the proper dosing of drugs in individuals (Califf and DeMets, 2002a,b). The case of anticoagulant drugs illustrates this need. These drugs are characterized by a complex balance of benefit (prevention of blood clots) and risk (bleeding) (Schünemann et al., 2004). Aspirin has been available for over 100 years and heparin for over 50 years. Yet the best dose of each for preventing arterial thrombosis remains controversial. Multiple new drugs, including direct antithrombins, low-molecular-weight heparins, P2Y12 inhibitors, and glycoprotein IIb/IIIa inhibitors, have been developed in the past two decades and have been demonstrated to provide a net balance of benefit on average in patients entered into clinical trials. Yet little is known about the appropriate dose of these agents in children, the very elderly, and patients with renal impairment. The adjusted dosing regimens for heparin and coumadin, each of which has been marketed for more than four decades, were delineated relatively recently after thousands of patients had been entered into clinical trials that included outcome measurement to determine the degree of anticoagulation with each agent that led to prevention of thrombosis without unacceptable bleeding.

Once a drug is on the market, the expansion to new indications continues throughout its life cycle. Most postmarket studies funded by industry are intended specifically to expand the market for a drug, and such studies are usually not undertaken unless the calculated probabilities indicate that the study will yield a positive financial return (Tunis et al., 2003). Direct comparisons of a drug with an alternative drug or other treatment rarely meet this financial test because there is too great a risk of finding that there is no difference or that the competing treatment is better.

An increasing number of reports over the past several decades have called for a marked increase in pragmatic clinical trials that answer questions relevant to clinical practice (Crowley et al., 2004). A new approach is needed that includes industry participation, but also independent oversight to stimulate more such trials. Lacking the results of such trials, neither prescriber nor patient can know what treatment plan is best.

A critical issue is where to draw the line between the premarketing development phase and the point at which the drug is allowed on the market. Scientifically, the gaining of knowledge about a drug should be a continuous process in which new information is used to refine understanding of the drug's uses, benefits, and risks at particular doses in particular patients. In actuality, however, the development of scientific knowledge about drugs is quite discontinuous, and the process is dependent on clearing a series of hurdles with defined criteria. In particular, tremendous effort and expense go into the New Drug Application (NDA) required to obtain initial approval for marketing (see Chapter 2). Ideally, at the time of initial marketing, the balance of a drug's benefit and risk would be known so that the label for its use could be clear. In reality, however, the costs of drug development and the length of time required to develop this information, particularly for drugs used to treat chronic diseases, make this impractical (Wood, 1999). Accordingly, an increasing number of experts advocate greater use of provisional drug approval to allow access to new therapies, with the requirement for long-term studies in heterogeneous populations after the drug is on the market.

Key Finding

Providers require better-quality information about medications and their effects if they are to meet the needs of their patients. For example, to facilitate safety and quality in the medication-use system, there is a need for more comprehensive benefit/risk information, clinical outcome data, and effectiveness data. Open access to such data is important not only for developing clinical understanding, but also for populating clinical knowledge and decision-support systems.

Disclosure of Clinical Data

The current state of disclosure of the findings of clinical studies is inadequate to support safety and quality in medication use, although the situation is improving. Of the multitude of drug products on the market, mandatory registration of clinical trial data applies only to those used for serious and life-threatening conditions. Moreover, requirements do not include disclosure of the results of Phase III trials—a key tool for educating patients and health care providers about drug benefits and risks—while results for only selected Phase IV studies are voluntarily included. Registration of clinical trial data is done at http://www.ClinicalTrials.gov, a federal government website operated through the NIH.

Until recently, information about other drugs was scattered over several database systems operated by different entities (IOM, 2006). However, the International Consortium of Medical Journal Editors now requires registration of clinical trial data at ClinicalTrials.gov as a condition for journal publication. Until this new requirement and its associated public scrutiny, the overall quality of the information reported was low in terms of usefulness, comprehensiveness, and standardization. A recent report from ClinicalTrials.gov documents improvement in the quality of reporting, but considerable progress is still needed (Zarin et al., 2005).

Providers and others have historically relied on medical journals publications to obtain results of different types of clinical studies and compensate for the limitations of repositories. While medical journals will remain important to the dissemination of objective clinical trial and practice information, a more flexible system is needed to ensure that the demands of the public for complete disclosure of drug benefits and risks are met.

The recently released IOM workshop report *Clinical Trial Registration: Developing a National Registry to Improve Public Access and Reliability* states that the best course of action to build the nation's repository of information about therapeutics and improve the quality of that information may be a broad expansion of the ClinicalTrials.gov database (IOM, 2006). A single national registry populated with information generated through clinical studies of *all* drug products would be a critically important resource for all stakeholders in the medication-use system. Each stakeholder group (e.g., patients, providers, researchers, medical journal editors, pharmaceutical companies, health insurers, information technology vendors, and regulators) has different needs and uses for the information contained in such a registry (see Box 6-1) (IOM, 2006). For optimal functioning, the registry should serve several purposes:

- List and track the status of ongoing clinical trials.
- Provide information on patient recruitment.
- Report results of clinical trials, including late Phase II, Phase III, and postmarketing studies; "head-to-head" comparisons of drugs; comparisons of drugs and alternative treatments; and effectiveness studies.

Full disclosure of the results of all clinical trials and postmarket studies in a national registry is particularly important to fill the current knowledge gaps that affect clinical practice, patient self-management, and medication safety. The distortion of information that results from the design of postmarketing studies has been described above. Well beyond this distortion, however, positive study results are much more likely to be published than negative results. This publication bias yields an incomplete picture of the drug characteristics that must be known for more accurate medication use and error prevention, and can therefore have a detrimental effect on patients. This has clearly been a major issue with COX-2 inhibitors and NSAIDs (see the discussion above). Thus all clinical trial results must be disseminated in a comprehensive, objective, and unbiased manner (IOM, 2006). Clear communication of risk information (not just benefits) is essential to preventing errors and potential adverse reactions.

The same holds true for other study results that should be incorporated into a national registry (i.e., postmarket, comparison, and effectiveness studies). Postmarket studies are especially important in relaying new safety information revealed as a drug is used in clinical practice. Comparative and effectiveness studies contribute further to understanding a drug's characteristics and therapeutic value. Given the proposed national registry, patients, providers, and others would not have to search multiple database systems for these study results but could easily maneuver within one comprehensive

---

BOX 6-1
Diverse Expectations and Perceived Needs
for a National Registry of Clinical Trial Data

The public and various entities within the medical community have different expectations and perceived needs regarding a public registry of clinical trial data:

- **Individuals suffering from various diseases**—and their family members—want to know that appropriate therapies are being offered and that patient safety is being ensured. Patients today want to be able to search on their own for research results that pertain to their disease and potentially to enroll in a clinical trial if appropriate.
- **Health care professionals** need both unbiased summary information derived from all trials conducted on a drug or therapy and the capacity to review the clinical data from any single study. They do not want to confine their review to the approved drug labeling or articles published in medical journals.
- **Researchers** may generate new ideas for investigation or look for data trends by accessing all the trials conducted on a drug or therapy.
- **Medical journals** have an enormous impact on clinical practice and medical policy. When journal editors receive clinical trial manuscripts for publication, they are concerned that they understand the research fully. They want to know whether clinical trials exist that may conflict with the submitted manuscript. And they want to know whether the authors failed to follow the original research plan, because such discrepancies may reflect serious defects in the research. Indeed, the integrity of the journal is at stake, as is the entire scientific enterprise, when research is published through the peer-review process.
- **Regulators** would use the information in a registry to develop policies regarding clinical research.
- **Health insurers** want to remain abreast of evidence-based results as the basis for insurance coverage policy.
- **Sponsors of research** aimed at developing a new therapy or drug incur great expense. Some of the information involved is highly proprietary and confidential to the sponsor. Companies are concerned that if all such proprietary information were required to be made broadly available to the public at the outset of clinical trials, they could not recoup their investment because competitors in the United States or abroad could copy their innovations. At the same time, industry recognizes its responsibility to do everything possible to ensure patient safety and secure the public trust.

---

system to learn more about a particular medication. The registry would also facilitate more efficient use of clinical data for such purposes as cross-referencing patients' response to a drug during clinical trials and their response in clinical practice, patients' response to one drug and their response to another, and patients' response to a drug and their response to other treatment options. Also, a drug's overall effectiveness in terms of patient outcomes is becoming a valuable measure of therapeutic success.

Further discussion and recommendations concerning such a national registry will be provided in the forthcoming report of the IOM Committee on the Assessment of the U.S. Drug Safety System.

Communication of Information

Drug information is communicated to providers and consumers through labeling and packaging, marketing practices, and advertisements. Poorly designed materials and inadequate representation of drug benefits and risks has led to errors across the medication-use continuum, such as inappropriate prescribing, confusion among products affecting dispensing and administration, and compromised ability to monitor a drug's effects adequately. This section addresses these issues.

> Recommendation 4: Enhancing the safety and quality of the medication-use process and reducing errors requires improved methods for labeling drug products and communicating medication information to providers and consumers. For such improvements to occur, materials should be designed according to designated standards to meet the needs of the end user. Industry, the Agency for Healthcare Research and Quality (AHRQ), the FDA, and others as appropriate (e.g., U.S. Pharmacopeia, Institute for Safe Medication Practices) should work together to undertake the following actions to address labeling, packaging, and the distribution of free samples:

> • The FDA should develop two guidance documents for industry: one for drug naming and another for labeling and packaging. The FDA and industry should collaborate to develop (1) a common drug nomenclature that standardizes abbreviations, acronyms, and terms to the extent possible, and (2) methods of applying failure modes and effects analysis to labeling and packaging.
> • Additional study of optimum designs for all drug labeling and information sheets to reflect human and cognitive factors should be undertaken. Methods for testing and measuring the effects of these materials on providers and consumers should also be established, including methods for field testing of the materials. The FDA, the National Library of Medicine (NLM), and industry should work with consumer and patient safety organizations to improve the nomenclature used in consumer materials.
> • The FDA, the pharmaceutical industry, and other stakeholders should collaborate to develop a strategy for expanding unit-of-use packaging for consumers to new therapeutic areas. Studies should be undertaken to evaluate different unit-of-use packaging

and design approaches that will best support various consumer groups in their medication self-management.

• AHRQ should fund studies to evaluate the impact of free samples on overall patient safety, provider prescribing practices, and consumer behavior (e.g., adherence to the medication regimen), as well as alternative methods of distribution that can improve safety, quality, and effectiveness.

Naming, Labeling, and Packaging

Drug names that look or sound alike increase the risk of medication errors (Cohen, 2000). Confusion over the similarity of drug names for prescription, generic, and over-the-counter (OTC) products accounts for up to 25 percent of all errors reported to the U.S. Pharmacopeia (USP) (NCC MERP, 2001). Abbreviations, acronyms, certain dose designations, and other symbols used for labeling also have caused a number of errors (FDA, 2005b). Even the layout and presentation of drug information on the drug container or package label can be visually confusing, particularly when designed for the marketplace instead of clinical practice. From January 2000 to March 2004, close to 32,000 reports were submitted to USP's MedMarx Reporting System that linked errors to look-alike or sound-alike drug names (Santell and Camp, 2004). The Joint Commission on Accreditation of Healthcare Organizations' (JCAHO) National Patient Safety Goals reference several look-alike/sound-alike generic drug names that have contributed to 9 of 10 serious medication errors in the hospital setting (JCAHO, 2006). And labeling and packaging issues were cited as the cause of 33 percent of errors, including 30 percent of fatalities, reported to the USP–Institute for Safe Medication Practices (ISMP) Medication Error Reporting Program (MERP) database (USP, 1998). Box 6-2 outlines the major problems in drug naming, labeling, and packaging that contribute to medication errors. Addressing these problems requires understanding the processes and requirements involved in naming, labeling, and packaging drug products.

Drug naming is a complex process. Each drug has multiple names assigned by different organizations for different purposes (Berman, 2004). The *chemical name* is assigned by the International Union of Pure and Applied Chemistry and identifies molecular structure. It serves the needs of scientific researchers. The *nonproprietary* or *generic name* is assigned by the United States Adopted Name Council (USAN) using a series of guidelines to ensure uniformity and safety.[2] These guidelines require that the

---

[2]The World Health Organization (WHO) coordinates international efforts to create a single worldwide standard and has established an International Nonproprietary Name (INN) for every product (Berman, 2004).

BOX 6-2
Examples of Major Naming, Labeling,
and Packaging Problems

- **Brand names that look alike or sound alike**—Celebrex® (celecoxib), Cerebryx® (fosphenytoin), and Celexa® (citalopram) (Zoeller, 1999). Celebrex® is a nonsteroidal anti-inflammatory drug; Cerebryx® is an intravenous antiepileptic; and Celexa® is an antidepressant.
- **Generic names that look alike or sound alike**—Amrinone (used to treat heart failure) and Amiodarone (an antiarrythmic). Amrinone was renamed Inamrinone to avoid confusion with Amiodarone (FDA, 2005b).
- **Different formulations with the same brand name**—Dulcolax (bisacodyl—a stimulant laxative) and Dulcolax (docusate—a stool softener).
- **Different formulations of a generic drug**—Four different versions of amphotericin B products are on the market—conventional amphotericin B (Amphocin®, Fungizone®, and a generic), amphotericin B cholesteryl sulfate complex (Amphotec®), amphotericin B lipid complex (Abelcet®), and amphotericin B liposomal (AmBisome®) (USP, 2005).
- **Multiple abbreviations to represent the same concept**—The extended-release version of a drug can use any number of different suffixes (e.g., LA, XL, XR, CC, CD, ER, SA, CR, XT, SR) to indicate long-acting or slow, delayed, or extended release (Berman, 2004).
- **Word derivatives or abbreviations that can be confused**—Similar prefixes (e.g., chlor-, clo-) (Aronson, 2004) can be misinterpreted, as can abbreviations used for labeling (e.g., AD [aura dexter or right ear] can be confused with "as directed," OD [oculus dexter or right eye], QD [once daily], and PO [by mouth]) (ISMP, 2002).
- **Unclear dose concentration/strength designations**—The contents of a 20 ml, 40 mg/ml gentamicin vial can be mistaken for a 40 mg/ml vial single dose (Cohen, 2000).
- **Lack of terminology standardization**—Use of the term "concentrate" for oral morphine sulfate products is inconsistent among manufacturers. Roxanol Concentrated Oral Solution and Roxanol-T Concentrated Oral Solution (with tinting and flavoring) both contain morphine sulfate 20 mg/ml, but one is expressed as 20 mg/5 ml. A nurse could easily misread the label and think they are the same.
- **Use of symbols that can be confused**—Symbols such as the ampersand (&) and the slash mark (/) can be misidentified as numbers (Cohen, 2000; JCAHO, 2003).
- **Cluttered labeling, small font, and serif typeface resulting in poor readability of printed information**—Containers with labels that have line after line of small print, identical-looking text, and extraneous, unnecessary commercial information are difficult to read and to differentiate from others that look similar (Cohen, 2000). Serif typeface is more difficult to read correctly than sans serif. At home, older adults also have difficulty reading cluttered labels (Wogalter and Vigilante, 2003).
- **Lack of adequate background contrast**—Drug information printed directly on a clear product container (e.g., vial, intravenous bag) is extremely difficult

to read and violates an established standard.[*] Depending on the color of the print, the background, and lighting conditions, labeling may be illegible (Cohen, 2000).
  • **Inadequate prominence of reminders and warnings**—In some cases, warnings are nonexistent or not prominently displayed.
  • **Overemphasis on company logos and trade dress**—Occasionally, company information is more prominent than information identifying the product, concentration/strength, and total volume (Berman, 2004).

[*]Standard D4267-89, established by the American Society for Testing and Materials, requires manufacturers to use contrasting type for the proprietary and established names of a drug, and for the amount of the drug per unit and either the immediate drug container or an opaque background (ASTM, 1988).

---

appropriate name stem from a standardized list and be incorporated into the generic name to give clinicians some indication of the chemical and/or therapeutic characteristics of the drug (USAN, 2005). The *official title* of a medication is determined by the USP Expert Committee on Nomenclature using the nonproprietary name plus dosage, formulation, and route of administration.[3] The *proprietary* or *brand name* is created by pharmaceutical companies to facilitate brand recognition and promote brand loyalty (Berman, 2004). The brand name for a drug may be different among countries, and drugs marketed by more than one pharmaceutical company may have more than one brand name (Hoffman and Proulx, 2003). Nevertheless, all drugs are promoted and marketed in the United States to providers and consumers under their brand name, although many providers and payers prefer to use the nonproprietary name.

Mixups resulting in medication errors can occur with either generic or brand names. In cases where the generic names are similar, the brand name can be used to differentiate products. Brand names are almost always easier to pronounce, spell, and remember than generic names (Cohen, 2002). The reverse is also true: similar brand names can be differentiated by using or including the generic name. In very rare cases the generic and brand names are similar for a particular drug. Thus, using both the generic and brand name is one of the easiest means of decreasing the likelihood of medication errors due to name confusion (Cohen, 2000; Hoffman and Proulx, 2003; Berman, 2004). It is particularly important to use both names when a drug has been involved in a name mix-up that led to an adverse event.

---

[3]USP also works with WHO and USAN to assess the utility and safety of generic drug names.

Because generic names are assigned from a limited list of word stems, there are a limited number of ways to represent a drug, increasing the likelihood that a name similar to that of another drug will be selected. Analysis is usually based on peer review. In contrast, brand names are cleared and trademarked[4] through the U.S. Patent and Trademark Office. In addition, brand names are analyzed by pharmaceutical companies themselves and the FDA (after submission of a regulatory approval application) using failure modes and effects analysis (FMEA). FMEA is a systematic approach used to identify and prevent product and process problems before they occur (IOM, 2004). With FMEA, a topic (e.g., drug name) is analyzed using a flow diagram of each step involved in the processes and subprocesses affecting the end user (e.g., using the drug in the clinical setting). A failure analysis is conducted to identify all possible points (i.e., modes) and causes of an error, and the severity and probability of each error. The final evaluation determines which modes to eliminate, control, or accept, and actions that can be taken to eliminate or reduce the error. If the company decides that the benefit/risk of the drug name is acceptable, it obtains a trademark for that name and includes the name in its application for regulatory approval.

From that point, the FDA's Division of Medication Errors and Technical Support (DMETS) reviews brand names for prescription and certain OTC drugs to determine the potential for naming-related medication errors (FDA, 2005b).[5] The FDA's FMEA review includes several evaluations. First, FDA staff undertake a handwriting and verbal analysis (through internal testing) to determine the degree of confusion in visual appearance or pronunciation between the brand name and the names of other products on the market. Second, the FDA uses a computer software tool, the Phonetic Orthographic Computer Analysis (POCA) program, to identify names with similar spelling, letter strings, or syllables. Third, additional risk information (e.g., overlapping strengths, dosage forms, dosing recommendations, indications for use) and container labeling/packaging are evaluated (but not using FMEA) to identify areas of potential confusion and improvement (FDA, 2005a). When errors occur after approval, DMETS has limited ability to require manufacturers to make name or labeling changes.

Generally, FMEA is not used by either pharmaceutical companies or the FDA to evaluate external labeling and packaging. As a result, many of the problems listed in Box 6-2 (e.g., cluttered labeling, small font, serif

---

[4]The U.S. Patent and Trademark Office examines the similarity between new and existing trademarks in terms of appearance to avoid infringing on an established trademark (Berman, 2004).

[5]Brand names for OTCs are analyzed only for a drug that is a prescription-to-OTC switch for which an NDA exists, or for an NDA or Abbreviated New Drug Application (ANDA). The brand names of monograph drugs do not undergo FMEA analysis.

typeface, lack of background contrast, inadequate prominence of reminders and warnings, overemphasis on company logos and trade dress) continue to have a direct effect on the readability and comprehensibility of product labels, and hence on rates of medication errors (Cohen, 2000; Berman, 2004). An important example is the redesign of the labels for potassium chloride concentrate. The older bottle label was poorly designed and looked very similar to the label for dextrose. Many mix-ups between potassium chloride concentrate and dextrose occurred that resulted in fatalities (Cohen, 2000). The labeling was redesigned to eliminate clutter and emphasize the drug name, concentration, and warnings. Another example is lidocaine hydrochloride, used for cardiac arrhythmias, which is administered via a loading dose followed by a continuous intravenous infusion (Berman, 2004). The prefilled 100 mg syringes (most common loading dose) were frequently confused with the prefilled 1 or 2 g syringes (for injection into a bag of 5 percent dextrose) because of similarities in appearance and design.

When problems with labeling and packaging do occur, they are usually addressed on a case-by-case basis, if at all. An exception to this policy is related to the labeling for small vials and injection syringes and for high-alert medications, which are particularly susceptible to errors due to such problems (Cohen, 2000). In 1994, a USP–FDA advisory panel made a number of recommendations for improving labeling and safety for injectable medications (http://www.nccmerp.org/council/council1997-09-16.html). Because USP functions as a standards organization for medication safety, most companies are complying with these recommendations and a few others cited in the Code of Federal Regulations (e.g., replacing "Federal Law Prohibits Dispensing without a Prescription" by "Rx Only"). In 1997, following the USP–FDA lead, the National Coordinating Council for Medication Error Reporting Programs developed a set of general recommendations for improving the labeling and packaging of all drug products. However, these are just recommendations and not formal requirements or standards, and compliance is inconsistent.

Once a product is on the market, adjustments to naming, labeling, and packaging are made only when providers and patient safety experts exert significant effort to get problems acknowledged and accepted by industry and FDA representatives. In many instances, however, known problems continue to be inadequately addressed over extended periods of time. For example, from 2000 until the present, ISMP, USP, and the Centers for Disease Control and Prevention (CDC) have notified the manufacturer and the FDA about repeated medication errors due to labeling confusion between tetanus toxoid and tuberculin vaccines (ISMP, 2005). Vaccine mix-ups can place hundreds, if not thousands, of patients at risk for serious ADEs. For about a year, the response by industry and the FDA to the error notification was that "providers should read the label." The FDA did produce a safety video on the vaccine mix-up, but errors continued to be reported. When the manufacturer sent the FDA a revised label for approval, it remained at the agency for 6 months without action being taken. Moreover, when the change in labeling was finally approved, the FDA would not discuss it and did not notify patient safety organizations or the public about it. This example illustrates the problems that can occur when human factors issues are not incorporated into labeling and packaging designs, and communications about problems are not transparent.

The FDA has held public meetings to address some of the problems identified above (e.g., naming, need for color coding). Progress is being made incrementally on certain naming issues. For example, the FDA has instituted a requirement that medications have bar codes to facilitate accurate drug dispensing and administration. And at the FDA's request, the generic drug industry agreed to use a mix of upper- and lowercase letters to highlight the differences between similar generic names, such as vinBLAStine and vinCRIStine (FDA, 2005b). Still, an overall guidance document that formally and comprehensively advises companies on naming, labeling, and packaging for safety has not yet been produced. As a consequence, there is great inconsistency among products and companies as regards follow-through on the detailed aspects of labeling and packaging that can reduce medication errors. In contrast, the National Health Service in the United Kingdom recently released *Guidance Note 25: Best Practices for Labeling and Packaging of Medicines*, which expanded requirements to increase the clarity and safety of drug labeling on external packaging and blister pacs (MHPRA, 2003). This document addresses several of the issues (e.g., font size, color, design) discussed at FDA public meetings.

The proliferation of manufacturers, medications, formulations, and doses will likely continue, increasing providers' difficulties in differentiating drug products (Berman, 2004). Thus, a formal action plan to address naming, labeling, and packaging problems is critical to improving the safety of medication use.

The committee believes strongly that industry and the FDA should take several specific actions to address the remaining key problems with drug naming, labeling, and packaging (see Box 6-3). This proposed action plan is founded on two overarching principles:

- Product naming, labeling, and packaging should be designed for the end user—the provider in the clinical environment and/or the consumer.
- Safety should always take precedence over commercial interests.

Unit-of-Use Packaging

Chapter 4 examines one possible way of improving consumers' medication self-management—redesigning pharmacy containers and warning

BOX 6-3
Actions to Improve Drug Naming, Labeling, and Packaging

• Drug-naming terms should be standardized to the extent possible to im-prove safety and minimize misinterpretation. Thus, a controlled vocabulary for certain drug-naming terms should be developed and implemented. Organizations that have been working in this area (i.e., U.S. Pharmacopeia [USP], Institute for Safe Medication Practices [ISMP], Joint Commission on Accreditation of Health-care Organzations [JCAHO]) should work with industry and the Food and Drug Administration (FDA) to formalize a single vocabulary. All companies should be required to use the controlled naming terminology. The terms decided upon should be integrated with the efforts of the National Committee on Vital and Health Statis-tics to formulate standardized drug terminologies for the national health informa-tion network (NCVHS, 2003).

• Failure modes and effects analysis (FMEA) should be required as part of the design and assessment of labeling and packaging for all prescription drug products. For example, warnings and reminders should be clearly displayed and highlighted, and logo size and placement should not interfere with readability. In-dustry, the FDA, third-party organizations (e.g., USP, ISMP), and others should collaborate to develop FMEA methods for drug labeling and packaging. This effort should involve practitioners as well as expert panels external to the FDA and the drug sponsor to ensure that real-world conditions are considered in the analysis. In turn, industry should fulfill these requirements and submit the results of FMEA as a required part of the New Drug Application (NDA)/Abbreviated New Drug Ap-plication (ANDA). When the safety of proposed labels and packaging remains a concern to the FDA, additional requirements should be imposed.

• A new coordinated effort should be undertaken by the FDA, USP, ISMP, and Pharmaceutical Research and Manufacturers of America (PhRMA) to exam-ine the problems associated with drug naming, labeling, and packaging, and to develop a plan of action for addressing those problems by the end of 2007. This effort should include regular meetings among the parties involved to address newly reported medication errors related to these problems. A means should be devel-oped for effectively communicating about medication errors to practitioners, regu-latory authorities, standards organizations, and manufacturers when such errors are reported by consumers or providers, as well as for obtaining a response from the manufacturer to the FDA and the other parties that identifies necessary steps to resolve the problem(s) identified. The plan also should establish time limits on negations, voting, and implementation of new measures.

• By the end of 2006 or early 2007, the FDA should publish two comprehen-sive guidance documents: one on naming, and the other on labeling and packag-ing. The agency should work with USP, ISMP, and PhRMA to develop specific measures for each of these documents. The documents should address such is-sues as acceptable and nonacceptable naming practices; the procedure for chang-ing names, labeling, and packaging after marketing as a result of high rates of medication errors; how warnings should appear on labels; the use of suffixes to modify various dosage forms that share the same drug name; and the placement of information, such as company names and logos, that may distract readers.

• The FDA should improve communication between Office of Drug Safety staff and others at all levels within the agency. In addition, the FDA's expert group

continued

for product-related safety issues should have a greater say in final decision making on such issues. The agency also needs to engage in more interactive communication with patient safety organizations (e.g., USP, ISMP) about known/reported serious drug safety problems.

• Industry should provide patient safety organizations (e.g., ISMP, USP) with complete contact information (i.e., names and telephone numbers) for specific company representatives or a company division to improve communication about reported product-related safety issues (e.g., labeling and packaging). Currently on official correspondence, company representatives may use a first name only and/ or omit a contact number.

• Additional research applying the principles of human factors engineering and cognitive psychology should be undertaken to study error prevention strategies such as the use of color, contrast, tall man letters,* and hazard statements and warnings on labels.

• For all consumer-related materials, research should engage experts in communications and health literacy to facilitate the development of designs and ways of presenting information that support readability, comprehensibility, and usefulness.

*The printing/writing of sections of words in capital ("tall man") letters to emphasize differences between similar words (e.g., EPINEPHrine and ePHEDdrine).

labels. Another method is the provision of medications to consumers in unit-of-use packaging. Unit-of-use packaging refers to drug products supplied in containers that provide enough medication for patients' use during a specified time interval (Szeinbach et al., 2003). The unit can be dispensed directly to a patient without pharmacists' repackaging or modification other than the application of a prescription label[6] (USP, 1993).

The most common forms of unit-of-use packaging for solid medications (tablets or capsules) are (1) the blister pack—a sheet of 10 to 30 individually wrapped doses of a particular medication (more than one sheet may be dispensed to the consumer); (2) the calendar blister pack of individually wrapped doses, organized for administration according to a calendar, such as that used for oral contraceptives; and (3) the multidose packet or sachet, which contains doses of more than one medication (Ientile et al., 2004). Semisolids (creams) and liquids are typically packaged in unit-of-use plastic tubes or ampoules.

---

[6]Unlike a unit-dose package or container that holds just enough medication for one dose, a unit-of-use package contains enough medication for the duration of a specified therapeutic regimen (Szeinbach et al., 2003).

Unit-of-use packaging is employed broadly for both prescription and nonprescription drugs in Europe, Australia, Asia, and Latin America as an important part of product approval requirements (Ientile et al., 2004). There are several reasons for instituting unit-of-use packaging standards. First, such packaging promotes child safety by providing greater protection against death or serious injury from accidental poisoning (HCPC, 2003). Second, because medicines are often distributed in the manufacturer's original packaging, errors that occur as a result of repackaging at the pharmacy can be minimized or prevented (HCPC, 2003). Third, several studies have shown that unit-of-use packaging is easier for consumers to use, facilitates more accurate self-administration, and improves adherence to treatment regimens (including complex regimens) and health outcomes (Becker et al., 1986; Wright et al., 1999; Huang et al., 2000; Simmons et al., 2000). Lastly, unit-of-use packaging is "tamper evident" (i.e., it is easy to detect product tampering), which can reassure consumers of product safety amidst growing concern about contamination or counterfeits (Allen, 2002).

In the United States, only certain medicines, such as oral contraceptives, azithromycin, prednisone, and many OTCs, are packaged in this manner (Schneider et al., 2006). Some vitamin and supplement combinations are available in multidose packets. Though the positive effect of unit-of-use packaging on many aspects of medication use are well documented in Europe and other regions, fewer than 20 percent of all prescription and OTC drugs in the United States are produced in blister packs (Erickson, 1998). Until recently, a few practical issues hindered more widespread adoption in the United States: (1) the cost to shift manufacturing from bulk distribution to unit-of-use packaging; (2) limited space and storage in community pharmacies; (3) rigidity of dispensing, making it more difficult to customize doses for patients; and (4) the lack of regulatory requirements (Allen, 2002). Changes taking place in the marketplace are now addressing many of these issues: (1) passage of the FDA's final rule requiring unit-dose packaging and bar codes for all medicines distributed to hospitals (FR, 2004); (2) growth in the number of repackaging companies, resulting in competitive pricing for such services; (3) a shift among community pharmacies to just-in-time inventories; (4) advances in packaging machinery, making unit-of-use packaging more efficient and less costly; and (5) revisions to and adoption of international packaging standards by manufacturers (Allen, 2002; HCPC, 2003; FG, 2003). Some are even predicting that the higher costs of unit-of-use packaging could be offset by increased adherence and decreased waste (Valero, 2005). Current trends suggest that unit-of-use packaging will generate the highest worldwide growth prospects among all pharmaceutical packaging products (FG, 2003) and gain momentum in the United States, possibly achieving the same level of use as in European and other countries where it is standard (Szeinbach et al., 2003).

The potential to improve patient safety and prevent errors has generated interest among U.S. regulators, providers, consumers, industry representatives, and other stakeholders in expanding unit-of-use packaging to medications for chronic conditions (Schneider et al., 2006). The strategy of using calendar blister packs could help large numbers of patients (including seniors, children, and those challenged by cognitive, physical, or functional impairment) take their medication more reliably and safely and enhance their treatment outcomes. In a 2003 survey of state boards of pharmacy, two-thirds of respondents expressed their belief that unit-of-use packaging would improve efficiency, reduce errors in dispensing, improve patient compliance, and increase opportunities for patient counseling (Szeinbach et al., 2003). Schneider and colleagues (2006) believe that packaging prescription medicines in easy-to-remember forms should be an important component of health care redesign for quality and safety.

The committee believes that stakeholders should collaborate to develop a strategy for expansion of unit-of-use packaging to new therapeutic areas. Additional head-to-head studies should be undertaken to evaluate various approaches to unit-of-use packaging and determine optimum designs to support different consumer groups in their medication self-management.

Distribution of Free Samples

The prescription drug industry defines a drug sample as ". . . a package containing a limited quantity of pharmaceutical product sufficient to evaluate clinical response, distributed to authorized health care practitioners free of charge, for patient treatment" (Groves et al., 2003). Such distribution of samples to physicians during detailing visits is the number one promotional tool used by industry. According to IMS Health, the estimated retail value of free product samples distributed in 2003 was over $16 billion (IMS Health, 2004). The actual cost to the manufacturer is much less, however— about 20 to 30 percent of the retail price (Petersen, 2000).

Few studies have been conducted to evaluate the true impact of the distribution of drug samples (Groves et al., 2003). Those studies that have been carried out have found conflicting attitudes about the use of free samples (Chew et al., 2000). Some early studies emphasized the benefits of the practice, including allowing physicians to start patients on medications quickly, to evaluate early effectiveness or adverse effects, to adjust prescribed doses before a full prescription is filled, to offset the cost of drugs to indigent and underinsured patients, and to demonstrate appropriate use to patients (Rasmussen, 1988; Weary, 1988). One more recent study highlighted the benefits of a sample pack in helping consumers detect a drug dispensing error because of visual familiarity with the product (Dodds-Ashley et al., 2002). Visual familiarity can change, however, when a generic product is dispensed, particularly since generics are manufactured by multiple different vendors, and have different colors (and sometimes shapes) to differentiate among competitors.

Historically, concerns about the safety of sample use were focused on the products themselves—on diversion of samples to the wholesale market for repackaging and retail sale, as well as outright counterfeiting (Rasmussen, 1988). Attempts by Congress to pass legislation banning or regulating the distribution of free samples were unsuccessful, and these concerns persist. In general over the past decade, there has been growing unease among the provider community and others about the use of samples and their direct effects on physician behavior and medication safety (see Box 6-4) (Chew et al., 2000).

Because sampling is reserved for newer, higher-priced, brand-name drugs, prescribing is skewed toward these drugs (versus generics, older drugs, or OTC medications). Overall health expenditures increase as a result of the cost of additional office visits to obtain more samples or the higher cost of the prescription (Taira et al., 2003).

In efforts to lower prescription drug costs to payers, several insurers, such as BlueCross BlueShield, have recently started to provide free samples of generics to health care providers to encourage use of these products (Davia, 2003; Sipkoff, 2003). The free generic samples are supplied on a trial basis for consumers who are currently using a brand name version or

---

BOX 6-4
Safety Issues Related to the Distribution of Free Samples

A number of critical medication safety and quality-of-care issues related to the distribution of product samples can contribute to errors:

- Physician disregard of evidence-based guidelines
- Prescribing based on samples rather than clinical appropriateness or the physician's preferred drug choice
- Prescribing of products not in hospital or managed care formularies
- Drug switching based on availability of samples rather than clinical need
- Inability of patients to receive the benefit of pharmacy services (e.g., drug interaction checking) and counseling
- Information gaps in health plan and pharmacy database systems
- Poor documentation in medical records
- Nonreporting of adverse effects
- Unregulated handling and dispensing of samples by physicians

SOURCE: Chew et al., 2000; Groves et al., 2003; Taira et al., 2003.

are about to start a new treatment. Other practices traditionally in the realm of brand name manufacturers, including aggressive advertising and voucher campaigns, are being used by payers to promote generics. Insurers mail thousands of vouchers to members, along with educational materials to help consumers understand the FDA review process for approving generics, as well as brand–generic comparative pricing information. Consumers bring the vouchers to their provider and receive the generic sample if clinically appropriate.

Comprehensive change in the delivery of free samples for prescription drugs is important to ensuring safety and quality in the medication-use system. Increasing numbers of health care providers are either banning drug samples altogether or experimenting with alternative means of dispensing them (Blumenthal, 2004; Simon et al., 2005; Brennan et al., 2006). Alternatives being evaluated include the use of coupons or vouchers to receive a sample dispensed by the pharmacy, policies restricting samples, and a smart-card system (Paterson and Anderson, 2002; Groves et al., 2003). Brennan and colleagues (2006) recently advocated a total ban on the direct provision of samples to physicians, and the institution of a voucher system for low-income patients or other arrangements that would distance a company and its products from physicians (Brennan et al., 2006). Some health care organizations have already instituted voucher systems. For example, the University of Wisconsin Hospital now uses a voucher program to replace free samples from drug companies (Charatan, 2001). Vouchers issued to patients at the hospital cover part of the cost of their prescription drugs. Participating manufacturers reimburse the hospital pharmacy for brand-name drugs, but the hospital pays for generic medications. The Everett Clinic in Washington State also has implemented a voucher program, which it believes has allowed greater assistance to the uninsured and financially impoverished (Charatan, 2001). Technology companies such as TrialCard Inc. (smart cards) and eMedRx (electronic prescribing) are developing systems to deliver pharmaceutical company coupons and vouchers electronically to physicians and/or pharmacies (Levy, 2002; Security Biometrics, Inc., 2004). Extensive studies are needed to evaluate the impact of free samples on physician and consumer behavior and patient safety and determine alternative methods of distribution.

MEDICAL DEVICE AND HEALTH INFORMATION TECHNOLOGY INDUSTRIES

Information technology systems and applications are valuable tools that can improve the safety and quality of care across the medication-use continuum. Some drug-related technologies are already in use, including knowledge-based systems used for laboratory and pharmacy data, patient safety reporting systems, infusion pumps, and applications for computerized provider order entry (CPOE) and electronic prescribing (IOM, 2004). Bar code medication administration systems have been implemented in some institutions. A key feature of pharmacy database systems, infusion pumps, and bar code and decision-support applications is the alert function that warns clinicians of potential medication safety problems. In general, a fully developed set of drug alerts includes drug–dose defaults, drug–dose checking, allergy checking, drug interaction checking, drug–laboratory checking, drug–condition checking, and drug–diet (food) checking. Other rule-based alerts (e.g., a required laboratory test for the use of particular drug) and automated surveillance for ADEs and near misses also are important to improving safety and reducing errors. Yet most providers currently use these technologies as independent, stand-alone systems rather than as integrated components of comprehensive clinical information systems—the overarching goal in building the national health information infrastructure (IOM, 2004). Nurses rely on the medication administration record generated by infusion and bar code systems to administer medications; physicians rely on CPOE and, if linked, pharmacy database systems for prescribing; and pharmacists rely on their databases for preparation and dispensing of prescriptions. As a result, each component of the medication use-system remains compartmentalized, increasing safety risks.

The lack of common drug information standards and integration of pharmacy database, decision-support, infusion, and bar code systems can have particularly devastating effects on patient safety (Patterson et al., 2002; Han et al., 2005; Koppel et al., 2005). For example, Koppel and colleagues (2005) found that medication errors increased as a result of data fragmentation, failures of system integration, and poorly designed human–machine interfaces. Because all of the above systems produce medication administration records, they must be able to communicate with each other to produce a comprehensive view of the patient's medication regimen. If they operate as stand-alone systems, no one has the full medication administration record, and clinicians have incomplete information.

Recommendation 5: Industry and government should collaborate to establish standards affecting drug-related health information technologies. Specifically:

- **The NLM should take the lead in developing a common drug nomenclature for use in all clinical information technology systems, based on standards for the national health information infrastructure.**

• AHRQ should take the lead in organizing mechanisms for safety alerts according to severity, frequency, and clinical importance to improve clinical value and acceptance.

• AHRQ should take the lead in developing intelligent prompting mechanisms specific to a patient's unique characteristics and needs; provider prescribing, ordering, and error patterns; and evidence-based best-practice guidelines.

• AHRQ should take the lead in developing user interface designs based on the principles of cognitive and human factors and the context of the clinical environment.

• AHRQ should support additional research to determine specifications for alert mechanisms and intelligent prompting, as well as optimum designs for user interfaces.

Data Standards

Unresolved problems with data standards inhibit the development and use of drug-related technologies, especially the alert functions described above. Data standards serve as the basis for representing and exchanging information electronically. Uniform data standards act as a common language, allowing communication and interoperability between different technologies. For example, a CPOE application on a handheld personal digital assistant (PDA) must be able to communicate with a pharmacy database system to process an electronic prescription. Although different types of data standards serve different functions, uniformity in the representation of similar data is required to optimize the usefulness and efficiency of technologies among systems and institutions.

Four problems are associated with data standards for drug information. First, there is no complete, standardized set of terms, concepts, and codes to represent drug information. Providers compensate for this lack of standards by piecing together different, incomplete datasets from multiple vendors, standards organizations, and internal sources. Second, there is no standardized method for presenting safety alerts, which should be ranked according to severity and/or clinical importance. Instead, providers are inundated with too many nonrelevant alerts, resulting in alert fatigue and high rates of alert overrides (Glassman et al., 2002; Hsieh et al., 2004). Third, systems lack intelligent or intuitive mechanisms for recognizing patient-specific data and relating those data to allowable overrides, such as those associated with a particular patient and drug allergy alert or duplicate therapy request (Abookire et al., 2000). Fourth, the bar codes stamped on drug packaging labels are designed differently by each vendor. Resolving these problems requires standardization on several levels: drug nomenclature, organization of alerts, intelligent prompting, and bar coding.

Drug Nomenclature

As the group overseeing the development of national data standards to support the technologies composing electronic health record systems, the National Committee on Vital and Health Statistics (NCVHS) should ensure that the appropriate organizations formulate a comprehensive set of standards for drug information (IOM, 2004). These standards should accomplish the following:

- Representation of all attributes of a drug needed for electronic communication about prescriptions, medication administration, and monitoring
- Representation of drug data specified according to the clinical needs of a specific patient population (e.g., pediatric, geriatric, pregnant women, those with renal or hepatic impairment)

RxNORM, developed by the NLM, standardizes certain components of the clinical drug nomenclature—active ingredient, strength, physical form, and dosage form. Work also is being carried out by the Veterans Health Administration (VHA) and the NLM to complete the national drug file reference terminology (NDF-RT), which will standardize many additional components (see Figure 6-1 and Box 6-5). NCVHS has designated RxNORM and NDF-RT as the core clinical drug nomenclature for electronic health records and the national health information network. However, these terminologies have not been widely adopted by most technology vendors or provider groups. Moreover, critical information needed for alert functions and for specific patient populations (e.g., dose limits, units of measure) have not been developed for NDF-RT. In the interim, proprietary standards for drug alerts developed by different pharmacy database vendors (e.g., First Data Bank, Multium) are being used in decision-support applications since they are the terminologies that cover the widest range of attributes listed in Table 6-1. To facilitate the transition to a standardized drug nomenclature, the NLM is planning to map the NDF-RT terminology to pharmacy database terminologies.

A similar effort is needed to address the lack of standardization among the drug terminologies used in medical devices (i.e., infusion pumps, patient-controlled analgesia [PCA]) and bar code medication administration systems. Infusion pumps with smart-pump technology contain datasets for drug libraries and error reduction software that facilitates programming of standardized concentrations, approved dosing units, general drug information, and dose limits (Vanderveen, 2005). The needs of specific populations (e.g., neonates, pediatric populations) can be addressed within one infusion system by programming the drug libraries to reflect the characteristics of the patient. However, the drug libraries used in smart-pump software are

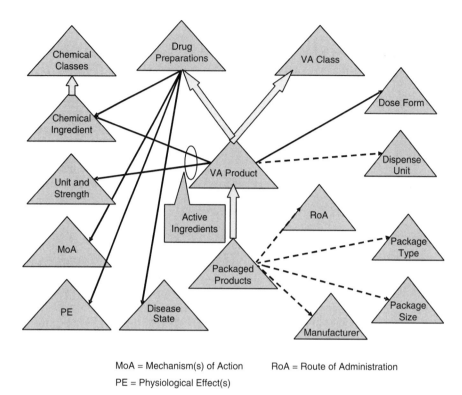

MoA = Mechanism(s) of Action   RoA = Route of Administration
PE = Physiological Effect(s)

FIGURE 6-1 Veterans Health Administration's national drug formulary reference terminology.
NOTE: See Box 6-5 for a discussion of this figure.
SOURCE: Brown, 2006

uploaded by each hospital using drug terminology from the pharmacy database system of choice. The device's software program helps organize the data, but each hospital determines how the drug terminology will be used by its staff. Bar code medication administration systems are no different; they rely on the National Drug Code (NDC) for the bar code used on external package labels and on software programs that allow hospitals to upload drug terminology to generate drug alerts.

The lack of common data standards among provider organizations not only prevents systems from communicating with one another, but also compromises the comparability of data from one organization to another, as well as epidemiological analysis of medication errors and ADEs in all health care settings. To remedy this problem, the NCVHS, the NLM, and the VHA need to develop a strategy for completing the development of all attributes of a comprehensive drug nomenclature. Once this standardized

> ## BOX 6-5
> ## Overview of the Veterans Health Administration's National Drug Formulary Reference Terminology (NDF RT)
>
> Figure 6-1 depicts NDF-RT, a drug terminology knowledge base derived from the U.S. Department of Veterans Affairs' (VA) National Drug File. NDF-RT was developed over the past 5 years with input from a variety of government and other stakeholders. The figure outlines NDF-RT's structure, and may be interpreted as follows. Each triangle represents a hierarchy of related concept definitions, with labels explained below. Thick arrows represent additional hierarchical connections. Solid black and dotted arrows represent semantic relationships. The triangles represent data contained in NDF-RT.
>
> The heart of NDF-RT is labeled VA Product, such as ASPIRIN 325MG ORAL TABLET. The VA Product is generally equivalent to the RxNORM Semantic Clinical Drug. Each VA Product is a "child" of two separate parents, a VA Class (e.g., ANALGESICS) and a Drug Preparation (e.g., ASPIRIN PREPARATIONS). Drug Preparations are described by relationships to their Mechanism(s) of Action (MoA triangle) (function at the cellular or subcellular level), Physiologic Effect(s) (PE triangle) (function at the organ, tissue, or body system level), and Disease State actions (diseases treated, caused, or prevented by the drug).
>
> Each VA Product also is characterized by its therapeutically active Chemical Ingredient(s), which in turn are characterized according to a structural class. In addition, each VA Product has a Dose Form (e.g., ORAL TABLET); a VA Dispense Units entry (e.g., TABLET); and a variety of other attributes, including links to RxNORM and commercial drug knowledge bases (not shown).
>
> For each active ingredient in a VA Product, there is an entry in the Unit Str. (Unit and Strength) hierarchy (325MG in the aspirin example).
>
> Each VA Product also encompasses some number of Packaged Products, which are identified by National Drug Code (NDC) numbers from the Food and Drug Administration (FDA).
>
> Each Packaged Product includes dispensing information, such as Route of Administration (RoA) (e.g., ORAL, INTRAMUSCULAR), Package Type (Pkg. Type) (e.g., BOX or BOTTLE), Package Size (Pkg. Size) (e.g., 500, 8 FL OZ), and Manufacturer (e.g., LILLY, SEARLE).
>
> NDF-RT's multiaxial hierarchical structure is designed to provide a balance of rigor in terminology and compatibility with deployed systems, while simultaneously streamlining the maintenance required to keep pace with the thousands of changes to drug products that occur each month. Existing and planned extensions to NDF-RT (not shown) support a variety of clinical decision-support cases, such as dose adjustment based on individual pharmacogenomic characteristics. Currently, the VA is extending a commercial terminology management system to support the semiautomated integration of data from pharmacy personnel, the FDA's Structured Product Label (SPL) project, and commercial drug knowledge sources.

TABLE 6-1 Attributes Requiring Standardization for Drug Nomenclature

Basic Attributes	Therapeutic Attributes	Alert Attribute	Payment Attributes	Commercial Attributes
• Active ingredient	• Mechanism of action	• Therapeutic duplication	• Cost of drug	• Brand name
• Strength	• Physiologic effect	• Drug–drug interaction	• Plan authorization	• Packaged product
• Dose forms	• Pharmacokinetics	• Drug allergy	• Cost of care	• Product kit
• Route of administration	• Therapeutic intent	• Drug–food interaction		
• Frequency	• Chemical structure	• Single and cumulative dose limits/contraindications based on patient age and weight		
• Units of measure		• Drug–laboratory checking (dose limits or contraindications)		
• Drug family		• Drug–condition checking (dose limits or contraindications)		
• Patient medication list		• Drug–radiology checking (dose limits or contraindications)		
		• Contraindicated route of administration		
		• Corollary		

drug nomenclature is completed, the NCVHS should ensure that all vendors incorporate it into their technology software.

Organization of Alerts

Standardizing the organization of alerts in pharmacy database systems, infusion pumps, and decision-support applications is required to reduce alert fatigue. The knowledge bases from which drug-related technologies derive their alerts are often highly inclusive, placing more emphasis on breadth of coverage than on clinical relevancy or severity of adverse events (Reichley et al., 2005). Unless alerts are ranked according to a severity–frequency scale and clinical importance, too many alerts tend to be delivered. The need to override excessive, inappropriate, nonspecified alerts can cause clinicians to miss critical safety alerts or to refuse the application altogether because of disruptions in workflow (van Bemmel and Musen, 1997). By the same token, many overrides are clinically appropriate and do not lead to ADEs (Hsieh et al., 2004).

Several studies have demonstrated improvements in clinician acceptance and reductions in inappropriate alerts through the ranking of alerts for all technologies (Kilbridge et al., 2001; DHA, 2002; Weingart et al., 2003; Shah et al., 2006). For example, a study of CPOE systems conducted by Shah and colleagues (2006) used a three-tiered alert structure:

- Level 1—alerts of the highest severity (i.e., life-threatening or with the potential to cause permanent damage). Clinicians could not proceed with a prescription without either eliminating the contraindication or responding to specific information requested about the patient.
- Level 2—alerts of strong severity (i.e., serious, capable of aggravating the patient's condition). Clinicians could proceed if they provided a reason for an override.
- Level 3—alerts of significant severity (i.e., important for the clinician to know). Clinicians could view clinical information in the alert, but the alert was noninterruptive.

Rather than using an all-inclusive knowledge base to determine the alerts, the researchers used a subset of only the most clinically relevant contraindications that pertained to the ambulatory care setting. Alerts of moderate to low severity were not included. The result was a significantly higher rate of acceptance among clinicians (67 percent) than that found in other studies (11 percent), although acceptance rates differed substantially by alert type (Weingart et al., 2003; Shah et al., 2006).

Alert fatigue and frequent overrides experienced with infusion pumps and bar code medication administration systems are no different than those experienced with CPOE and pharmacy database systems. Alerts with infusion systems can be of particular concern since the highest percentage of medication errors is associated with intravenous medicines (Cohen, 2000; Billman, 2004). Smart-pump alerts may occur during programming or administration regardless of whether infusion rate limits are available for the drug (Malashock et al., 2004). The most common override occurs when the infusion rate is either above or below the maximum/minimum rate limit (Malashock et al., 2004). Other alerts can include informing the programmer of a duration change, a secondary stop, cancellation of drug selection, weight change–related dose recalculation, and same-drug infusion on multiple channels. Alerts can also occur for low battery power, venous occlusion, and similar conditions. The development of methods to rank the alert functions of infusion pumps could improve their functioning and safety.

While studies have clearly indicated that a tiered severity structure is important, additional work on how to differentiate, select, and integrate a separate tier for certain moderate-level alerts is required. A moderate-level warning may not be clinically important to one patient but may be for another, or may be important to a patient's quality of life and adherence to medication therapy (Ahern and Kerr, 2003). A method for ranking the most frequent types of ADEs for each severity level also should be incorporated into the alert structure (Kilbridge et al., 2001; Miller et al., 2005). There have been many evidence-based studies identifying the frequency and severity of ADEs that can be used to determine these parameters (Classen et al., 1997; Forester et al., 2003, 2004; Gurwitz et al., 2005). Miller and colleagues (2005) suggest that the frequency rating might be based on percentage of total administrations, or 100 and 1,000 administrations. Table 6-2 provides a sample of the most common occurrences of alerts and the reasons for overriding them.

Standardization, however, does not imply rigidity. The alert configuration must remain flexible enough to reflect the inherent variability in clinical practice, such as the off-label use of a drug. In addition to severity and frequency, clinical importance is a third essential element of an alert structure. Alert ranking should be flexible enough to target the needs of specific patient populations (e.g., pediatric, geriatric) and medical disciplines (e.g., oncology, psychiatry) (Fortescue et al., 2003; Grasso et al., 2003). Most drug-related technologies allow for alert configurations according to patient age and weight, but are not designed to incorporate other individualized patient information. Hospital pharmacy database systems are the exception where laboratory test values can be linked to the patient's medication management profile (IOM, 2004). As in the ambulatory care setting, alert rankings should reflect considerations specific to a patient's condition or provider's medical discipline (e.g., the alert ranking related to drug toxicity may be different for oncology than for nephrology). Such considerations do not

TABLE 6-2 Sample of Alert Types, Most Common Occurrences, and Most Common Reasons for Alert Override

Alert Type	Most Common Occurrences of Highest Alerts	Most Common Reasons for Alert Override
Therapeutic duplication	• Analgesic (29%) • Psychiatric (26%) • Gastrointestinal (19%) • Cardiac (17%) • Endocrine (9%)	• Transitioning from one drug to another (42%) • Long-term therapy with combination (21%) • Short-term combination (7%) • Advice from consultant (5%)
Drug–drug interaction	• Sildenafil and isorbide mononitrate • Gatifloxacin and levofloxacin • Linezolid and methylphenidate	• Clinician would monitor patient (49%) • Patient previously tolerated drug (21%) • Clinician would adjust dose as recommended (14%) • No reasonable alternatives (4%)
Drug–laboratory	Not documented	• Clinician would monitor/manage as recommended (67%) • Most recent laboratory test results available (18%) • Patient on dialysis (11%)
Drug–disease	• Hepatic disease contraindications • Seizure disorder contraindications • Coronary artery disease contraindications	• Patient previously tolerated drug (56%) • New evidence for use (22%) • Advice from consultant • No reasonable alternative (11%)
Drug–pregnancy	• Isotretinoin • Leflunomide • Misprostol	• Patient is not pregnant (93%) • Advice from consultant (1%) • No reasonable alternative (1%) • Patient previously tolerated drug (1%) • Short-term use (1%)

SOURCE: Shah et al., 2006

imply that known dangerous drug interactions or contraindications will change; instead, they reflect a recognition that in some cases, certain clinical preferences should take precedence. Thus, ranking of alerts according to all three dimensions—severity, frequency, and clinical importance—is necessary.

Intelligent Prompting

Technology that could use intelligent or intuitive mechanisms to prompt alerts would require the application of additional parameters beyond severity and frequency ranking and generalized patient data delineated only by age and weight. Such intelligent mechanisms would generate alerts specific to a patient's unique characteristics and needs; physician prescribing, ordering, and error patterns; and evidence-based best-practice guidelines. For example, a patient might be allergic to one medication in a drug class but not others (Abookire et al., 2000). The software configuration should recognize the patient's unique drug allergy without requiring that an alert be generated for every drug ordered in that class. As another example, a physician might have a preference for therapeutic duplication in transitioning a patient being prepared for discharge. The software configuration should accommodate the duration of the therapeutic duplication and the specific dosing transition of the two drugs without issuing repeated alerts requesting the same information. For this type of intelligent prompting to be possible, drug-related technologies must be linked not only to each other, but also to more comprehensive clinical information systems.

Incorporating rule-based physician monitoring features within prescribing systems is considered important for safety and learning. Anton and colleagues (2004) designed a more structured ranking of message severity according to seven categories, and system capabilities for monitoring based on storage functions and unique numbers for each prescription, provider, and patient. The system creates warnings using the incorporated rules and maintains a record of every occasion on which an alert is displayed. Each message can be linked to the user, the individual prescription key, and the outcome of the warning. Queries of the data were used to assess providers' proficiency in preventing errors with the system and overall skill in using it (Anton et al., 2004).

In addition, evidence-based decision-support algorithms are necessary to ensure the adequacy of software configurations that incorporate specific protocols for real-time decision making and clinical action (Cole and Stewart, 1994; Sawa and Ohno-Machado, 2001; Fields and Peterman, 2005; Miller et al., 2005). Ideally, the algorithms should be developed according to three principles: (1) they should be system tested before full implementation; (2) they may have to be facility tailored based on process and workflow; and (3) they should be monitored and updated over time (Sawa and Ohno-Machado, 2001; Bates et al., 2003; Reichley et al., 2005). The algorithms, similar to any computer program, can never be finished or finalized as medicine is always changing; therefore, expiration labeling or update notices may be helpful to maintain currency.

One method for testing systems is to develop and test software configurations as well as train clinicians using simulation programs. The Anesthesia Patient Safety Foundation is the first medical community to adopt this technique successfully and apply it to anesthesia information management systems (AIMS) (Sawa and Ohno-Machado, 2001; Weinger and Slagle,

2002; Wachter et al., 2003; Pierce, 2006). Anesthesiologists administer anesthetics and observe the condition of their patients aided by multiple electronic monitors (e.g., electrocardiograph, pulse-oximeter, blood pressure monitors), which determine real-time decision making and actions. The AIMS records electronically all data generated by these technologies. The simulation programs allow clinicians to test themselves under various surgical situations. More recently, the Leapfrog Group commissioned the development of a simulation application both to test the decision-support algorithms of CPOE systems implemented in health care organizations and to train clinicians (Kilbridge et al., 2006). The methodology simulates different clinical scenarios using a wide variety of test patients and orders to evaluate how a hospital's CPOE system responds to unsafe medication ordering and clinical situations.

Bar Coding

Another area requiring standardization is the bar codes used for drug labels and bar code medication administration systems. The ability of bar coding to affect medication error rates depends largely on the ability of hospitals to scan and interpret the data in the bar codes. A commonly used standard that scanners can easily read will have a greater impact on patient safety than a unique symbology that few scanners are programmed to read (FR, 2004).

A number of different stakeholders—drug manufacturers, distributors, repackagers/relabelers, manufacturers of bar code medication administration systems, and hospitals—use bar codes on drug products. As with the lack of a common drug nomenclature, there is no single, common bar code standard or symbology. Among hospitals, repackagers, and vendors of bar code medication administration systems, up to six different bar code standards are being used, each with its own special characteristics, features, and methods for encoding product information (see Figure 6-2). This situation creates several problems. First, the lack of a common standard drives costs up throughout the drug delivery system, particularly for hospitals that incur the expense of repackaging/relabeling drugs to the unit dose level and/or purchasing additional software or technology to read the different bar codes. Second, error rates associated with hospital relabeling are estimated at 17 percent nationwide, increasing the risk of ADEs (FR, 2004). Third, the multitude of standards inhibits integration of clinical systems. Designation of a single, common bar code standard could resolve these problems.

Efforts to standardize bar codes are linked to a rule establishing federal requirements for labeling of products down to the unit dose level. In the rule, the FDA requires all stakeholders using bar codes to choose one of two standards: (1) European Article Number/Uniform Code Council (EAN/

Code 128

RSS 14

RSS Composite

2 D

Data Matrix

FIGURE 6-2 Bar code symbologies.
SOURCE: Combes, 2004.

UCC) or (2) Health Industry Business Communications Council (HIBCC). The NDC drug code must be incorporated into the bar code as it will serve as the unique product identifier. The different codes serve different purposes. The EAN/UCC standard was originally developed by the medical device industry, which uses Universal Product Numbers to meet the needs of retailers (HIBCC, 2001). Because no other standard was available at the time, drug manufacturers adopted the standard and integrated the NDC codes. However, many stakeholders consider the EAN/UCC standard to be inadequate for the specific applications and needs of the health care environment, especially those associated with patient safety (HIBCC, 2001). The HIBCC standard was designed to allow for more extensive and precise encoding and quicker tracking and tracing of specific drug products.

While narrowing choices down to two standards represents improvement, stakeholders believe that other aspects of the FDA rule need revision. In particular, the rule states that bar code symbology will be limited to a linear model that constrains the ability to encode a significant amount of information. This capability will be needed as health information technologies and clinical information systems advance. Therefore, these stakeholders are seeking to have the rule revised to allow for the use of three-dimensional models as well.

In addition, there are sizable cost implications when a hospital implements a bar code medication administration system. Thus, software programs will be required to be compatible with both the EAN/UCC and HIBCC standards, to accommodate various dimensional encoding models, and to be easily upgraded to meet demands for the encoding of additional information. Further, radio frequency identification (RFID) technology may replace bar codes on external packaging altogether, particularly in light of the growing problems with counterfeit drug imports entering the U.S. market. However, RFID will not replace the need for standardized bar code systems for patient care.

User Interface

The ability of clinicians to use a medical device or decision-support system successfully depends on how well the technologies have been designed at the level of the human–machine interaction (i.e., user interface). From the user's perspective, the interface *is* the system (Shortliffe et al., 2001). When interacting with technology, clinicians aim to carry out tasks in which information is assessed, manipulated, or created (van Bemmel and Musen, 1997). The quality and style of the interface directly affect this processing of information. Well-organized information that is presented in a logical and meaningful way results in a higher degree of usability, whereas the display of information in a cluttered, illogical, or confusing manner leads to decreases in user performance and satisfaction (van Bemmel and Musen, 1997). Most important, a poorly designed user interface can even contribute to medication errors for all drug-related technologies (Patterson et al., 2002; Ash et al., 2004; Koppel et al., 2005).

As noted earlier, several studies have confirmed that many medication errors resulting in patient harm involve intravenous infusion devices, with the most common cause of the errors being incorrect programming (Kaushal et al., 2001; Taxis and Barber, 2003; Tourville, 2003). Several problems with the interface design for these devices in terms of programming keys, display screens, and menu structure have contributed to these high rates of ADEs. In an effort to simplify programming and reduce pump size, a limited number of programming keys are provided on the pumps. Each key serves multiple functions, and clinical protocol is selected through scroll menus. However, menu structures are so complex that even skilled users could easily get confused (Nemeth, 2003). Device programming is often further complicated by small display screens that are difficult to read and follow. As a result, the state of the infusion pump is not always obvious during each step of the process. Even small data entry errors can result in numerous unforeseen medical complications that cause patient harm. Clinicians frequently must power down the pumps and start over to clear programming mistakes. Device manufacturers have been working to improve the user interface by incorporating the principles of human factors engineering into the pumps' design structure. Standards for human factors design have been established by the Association for the Advancement of Medical Instrumentation (AAMI) and approved by the American National

Standards Institute (ANSI), and are a part of the FDA's Good Manufacturing Practices (GMP) regulatory requirements (IOM, 2004). The standards do not go far enough to address user interface issues, however, and additional work is needed.

Medication errors also result from comparable problems in the user interface design for decision-support systems. A recent study of CPOE systems found that human–machine interface flaws facilitated 22 types of medication errors (Koppel et al., 2005).

A number of factors affect the ability of clinicians to interact effectively and efficiently with decision-support systems (whether CPOE, electronic health records, or pharmacy database). First, most of the commercial systems on the market were designed according to rigid machine rules that do not correspond appropriately to the clinician's workflow and behavior (Koppel et al., 2005). The natural chain of clinical events is disrupted while clinicians are forced to accommodate the rigid data requirements of the technology (Han et al., 2005). Often, a second physician devoted solely to entering orders is needed when time-sensitive therapeutic interventions must be administered, such as in emergency or intensive care. Second, many interface designs are highly impractical or outdated. Information is presented in numerous lines of identical-looking text, without a windows-based structure or intuitive graphical navigation aids (Ash et al., 2004). Even when the information is there, it is difficult to find. Clinicians must click on multiple different screens to either retrieve all of a patient's information or enter new clinical information. Information becomes fragmented, and clinicians lose their ability to develop a more comprehensive overview and conceptual understanding of the case (Ash et al., 2004). For example, in many inpatient CPOE systems, patient names are grouped alphabetically rather than by clinical staff or rooms. Thus similar names, combined with small fonts, hectic workstations, and interruptions, can easily be confused (Koppel et al., 2005). Equally troubling, a patient's medication information is seldom synthesized on one screen; a clinician may need to access up to 20 screens to view all the medications included in the patient's regimen. Although decision-support systems use standard computer monitors to display information, a significant amount of work is needed to develop optimal user interface designs that can make data capture and manipulation easier for clinicians and more accurate for patient safety.

Data presentation and the user interface affect the usability of bar code medication administration systems as well. Although there are no studies indicating that the design of such systems directly caused medication errors (Johnson et al., 2002), several studies have confirmed that negative unintended consequences resulting from the introduction of these systems may create new paths to ADEs (Patterson et al., 2002; Patterson, 2003). The information display of the systems is much like that of other decision-support systems that rely on computer-based monitors and graphical interfaces. Specific issues with interface design vary depending on the vendor, but generally relate to the incompleteness of the medication information displayed and its effect on clinical coordination (Cipriano, 2003; Patterson, 2003). For example, the more inflexible systems require a long, confusing sequence of programming activities for a simple change to medication administration times. Moreover, important medication information is either not available or not displayed in a timely manner. Key problems identified include (1) pending and discontinued medication orders not displayed; (2) inability to document medications not displayed as administered when they had been administered; (3) automated removal of medications from bar code medication administration systems, resulting in confusion; (4) inability to view changes to medication orders without opening a patient record; (5) difficulty of undoing actions: (6) difficulty of revising database information once entered; and (7) poorly organized data screens, resulting in missed medications (Patterson et al., 2002; Rogers et al., 2005). The fragmentation of patient data also contributes to clinicians' inability to obtain at a glance a comprehensive overview of patients' medication information, as well as to degraded coordination between physicians and nurses—one of the more noted negative side effects of bar code medication administration systems (Patterson et al., 2002).

Efforts in the United Kingdom have started to address user interface issues through an agreement with Microsoft Corporation. Microsoft will develop a health-specific user interface for clinical systems used by the National Health Service to improve patient care and safety. Under the terms of the agreement, Microsoft will supply code based on the full shipping versions of its desktop software that can be used by independent vendors and supply customized versions of Office and Windows (NHS, 2004). However, use of common coding to link and present data is only one aspect of improving the user interface.

Addressing user interface issues will require greater attention to the cognitive and social factors influencing clinicians in their daily workflow and interaction with technologies (van Bemmel and Musen, 1997). Yet little emphasis has been placed on physicians' ability to learn and use these systems or on the technologies' effects on physicians' reasoning. From the perspective of cognitive psychology, designers must develop a better understanding of how clinicians best comprehend information, as well as of the limits of human perception and memory. The context of the clinical environment, in which clinicians must perform multiple tasks simultaneously and manage numerous interruptions by beepers, telephones, and colleagues, must be taken into account (Ash et al., 2004). Designers should understand that cognitive overload can result from overemphasizing complete information entry or retrieval.

A prime example of how comprehensive design strategies such as these have been successful in transforming health technology interfaces to improve patient safety is in the high-risk area of anesthesia (IOM, 2000; Hallinan, 2005; Pierce, 2006). Anesthesiology has reduced anesthesia mortality rates from two deaths per 10,000 administrations to one death per 300,000 administrations (JCAHO, 1998). This success was accomplished through a combination of the following:

- Technical changes (new monitoring equipment, standardization of existing equipment)
- Information-based strategies, including the development and adoption of guidelines and standards
- Application of human factors to improve performance, such as the use of simulators for training
- Formation of the Anesthesia Patient Safety Foundation to bring together stakeholders from different disciplines (physicians, nurses, manufacturers)
- Having a leader who could serve as a champion for the cause (Leape et al., 1998; IOM, 2000)

No single one of these changes has been sufficient to have a clear-cut impact on mortality, yet, the application of human factors principles in conjunction with the other factors has been highly effective (Leape at al., 2002; Sawa and Ohno-Machado, 2002; Wachter at al., 2003). Measuring progress over time and regularly integrated lessons learned into clinical systems created a dynamic process for ongoing quality and safety improvement.

It can be challenging to capture the richness and complexity of clinical data in a manner that is concise and precise, but still comprehensive enough for medical care (Cimino et al., 2001). Screen layout and the visual salience of the information presented critically affect the way the information is interpreted by clinicians using decision-support systems (Kushniruk et al., 1996; Kaufman et al., 2003). Menus, graphics, and colors can all help differentiate data and make systems more attractive and simpler to learn and use. Interfaces must offer clear presentations, avoid unnecessary detail, and provide consistent interaction to be effective (Shortliffe et al., 2001). Designers also should recognize the inherent differences among clinician user groups, and seek to design multidimensional interfaces that can accommodate the information requirements of individual clinicians and comprehensive conceptual views of patient information.

REFERENCES

Abookire SA, Teich JM, Sandige H, Paterno MD, Martin MT, Kuperman GJ, Bates DW. 2000. Improving allergy alerting in a computerized physician order entry system. *Proceedings of American Medical Informatics Association Symposium* 2–6.

Ahern MD, Kerr SJ. 2003. General practitioners' perceptions of the pharmaceutical decision-support tools in their prescribing software. *Medical Journal of Australia* 179(1):34–37.

Alexander KP, Peterson ED. 2003. Evidence-based care for all patients. *American Journal of Medicine* 114(4):333–335.

Allen D. 2002. *The Next Chapter: Unit-of-Use Packaging. Pharmaceutical and Medical Packaging News.* [Online]. Available: http://www.devicelink.com/pmpn/archive/02/11/004. html [accessed May 27, 2006].

ALLHAT (Antihypertensive and Lipid-Lowering Treatment to Prevent Heart Attack Trial). 2002. Major outcomes in high-risk hypertensive patients randomized to angiotensin-converting enzyme inhibitor or calcium channel blocker vs. diuretic: The Antihypertensive and Lipid-Lowering Treatment to Prevent Heart Attack Trial (ALLHAT). *Journal of the American Medical Association* 288(23):2981–2997.

Anton C, Nightingale PG, Adu D, Lipkin G, Ferner RE. 2004. Improving prescribing using a rule-based prescribing system. *Quality and Safety in Health Care* 13(3):186–190.

Aronson JK. 2004. Medication errors resulting from the confusion of drug names. *Drug Safety* 3(3):167–172.

Ash JS, Berg M, Coiera E. 2004. Some unintended consequences of information technology in health care: The nature of patient care information system-related errors. *Journal of the American Medical Informatics Association* 11(2):104–112.

ASTM (American Society for Testing and Materials). 1988. *Standard D4267-89.* Philadelphia, PA: ASTM.

Bates DW, Kuperman GJ, Wang S, Gandhi T, Kittler A, Volk L, Spurr C, Khorasani R, Tanasijevic M, Middleton B. 2003. Ten commandments for effective clinical decision support: Making the practice of evidence-based medicine a reality. *Journal of the American Medical Informatics Association* 10(6):523–530.

Becker LA, Glanz K, Sobel E, Mossey J, Zinn SL, Knott KA. 1986. A randomized trial of special packaging of antihypertensive medications. *Journal of Family Practice* 22(4):357–361.

Berman A. 2004. Reducing medication errors through naming, labeling, and packaging. *Journal of Medical Systems* 28(1):9–29.

Billman G. 2004. *A Medical Center's Experience Using Smart Infusion Pumps to Manage Medication Administration.* San Diego, CA: ALARIS Center for Medication Safety and Clinical Improvement.

Blumenthal D. 2004. Doctors and drug companies. *New England Journal of Medicine* 351(18): 1885–1890.

Brennan TA, Rothman DJ, Blank L, Blumenthal D, Chimonas SC, Cohen JJ, Goldman J, Kassirer JP, Kimball H, Naughton J, Smelser N. 2006. Health industry practices that create conflicts of interest: A policy proposal for academic medical centers. *Journal of the American Medical Association* 295(4):429–433.

Brown, SH. 2006. Diagram of NDF-RT Data Elements. Personal Communication.

Califf RM, DeMets DL. 2002a. Principles from clinical trials relevant to clinical practice: Part I. *Circulation* 106:1015–1021.

Califf RM, DeMets DL. 2002b. Principles from clinical trials relevant to clinical practice: Part II. *Circulation* 106:1172–1175.

CERTS (Centers for Education and Research on Therapeutics). 2003. Risk assessment of drugs, biologics, and therapeutic devices: Present and future issues. *Pharmacoepidemiology and Drug Safety* 12(8):653–662.

Charatan F. 2001. Hospital bans free drug samples. *Western Journal of Medicine* 174(4): 236–237.

Chew LD, O'Young TS, Hazlet TK, Bradley KA, Maynard C, Lessler D. 2000. A physician survey of the effect of drug sample availability on physicians' behavior. *Journal of General Internal Medicine* 15(7):478–483.

Cimino JJ, Patel VL, Kushniruk AW. 2001. Studying the human-computer-terminology interface. *Journal of the American Medical Informatics Association* 8(2):163–173.

Cipriano PF. 2003. A nursing perspective on bedside scanning systems. *Hospital Pharmacy* 38(11):S14–S15.

Classen DC, Pestotnik SL, Evans RS, Lloyd JF, Burke JP. 1997. Adverse drug events in hospitalized patients. Excess length of stay, extra costs, and attributable mortality. *Journal of the American Medical Association* 277(4):301–306.

Cohen MR. 2000. *Medication Errors: Causes, Prevention, and Risk Management*. Sudbury, MA: Jones and Bartlett Publishers.

Cohen MR. 2002. Trade name, INNs, and medication errors. *Archives of Internal Medicine* 162(22):2636–2637.

Cole WG, Stewart JG. 1994. Human performance evaluation of a metaphor graphic display for respiratory data. *Methods of Information in Medicine* 33(4):390–396.

Combes JR. 2004. Understanding the Challenges of Implementation of Point Care Bar Code Systems. Presentation to the IOM Committee on Identifying and Preventing Medication Errors, March 19, 2004.

Crowley WF, Sherwoo, L, Salber P, Scheinberg D, Slavkin H, Tilson H, Reece EA, Catanese V, Johnson SB, Dobs A, Genel M, Korn A, Reame N, Bonow R, Grebb J, Rimoin D. 2004. Clinical research in the United States at a crossroads: Proposal for a novel public-private partnership to establish a national clinical research enterprise. *Journal of the American Medical Association* 291(9):1120–1126.

Davia J. 2003. *Encourage Use of Generics to Rein in Cost of Medications*. [Online]. Available: http://www.democratandchronicle.com/news/extra/fighting/health/story4.shtml [accessed March 12, 2006].

DHA (Australian Department of Health and Ageing). 2002. *BMMS: Alerts Discussion Paper* (Version 3.0 edition). Canbera, Australia: DHA.

Dodds-Ashley ES, Kirk K, Fowler VG. 2002. Patient detection of a drug dispensing error by use of physician-provided drug samples. *Pharmacotherapy* 22(12):1642–1643.

Edwards R, Faich G, Tilson H, and International Society of Pharmacovigilance. 2005. Points to consider: The roles of surveillance and epidemiology in advancing drug safety. *Pharmacoepidemiology and Drug Safety* 14(9):665–667.

Erickson G. 1998. *Unit-of-Use Packaging: The Wave of the Future? Pharmaceutical and Medical Packaging News*. [Online]. Available: http://www.devicelink.com/pmpn/archive/98/06/003.html [accessed May 27, 2006].

FDA (U.S. Food and Drug Administration). 2005a. *Overview of the Office of Medication Errors and Technical Support*. Submission to the IOM Committee on Identifying and Preventing Medication Errors. Rockville, MD: FDA.

FDA. 2005b, July–August 2005. Drug name confusion: Preventing medication errors. *FDA Consumer Magazine*.

FG (Freedonia Group). 2003. *World Pharmaceutical Packaging: Forecasts to 2007 and 2012*. [Online]. Available: http://www.gii.co.jp/sample/pdf/fd17351.pdf [accessed April 2, 2006].

Fields M, Peterman J. 2005. Intravenous medication safety system averts high-risk medication errors and provides actionable data. *Nursing Administration Quarterly* 29(1):78–87.

Fitzgerald GA. 2005. Opinion: Anticipating change in drug development: The emerging era of translational medicine and therapeutics. *Drug Discovery* 4(10):815–818.

Fleming TR, DeMets DL. 1996. Surrogate end points in clinical trials: Are we being misled? *Annals of Internal Medicine* 125:605–613.

Forester AJ, Murff HJ, Peterson JF, Gandhi TK, Bates DW. 2003. The incidence and severity of adverse events affecting patients after discharge from the hospital. *Annals of Internal Medicine* 138(3):161–167.

Forester AJ, Halil RB, Tierney MG. 2004. Pharmacist surveillance of adverse drug events. *American Journal of Health System Pharmacists* 61(14):1466–1472.

Fortescue EB, Kaushal R, Landrigan CP, McKenna KJ, Clapp MD, Federico F, Goldman DA, Bates DW. 2003. Prioritizing strategies for preventing medication errors and adverse drug events in pediatric inpatients. *Pediatrics* 111(4):722–729.

FR (Federal Register). 2004. *Bar Code Label Requirements for Human Drug Products and Biological Products: Final Rule.* Washington, DC: National Archives and Records Administration.

Glassman PA, Simon B, Belperio P, Lanto A. 2002. Improving recognition of drug interactions: Benefits and barriers to using automated drug alerts. *Medical Care* 40(12):1161–1171.

Grasso BC, Rothschild JM, Genest R, Bates DW. 2003. What do we know about medication errors in psychiatry? *Joint Commission Journal on Quality and Safety* 29(8):391–400.

Groves KEM, Sketris I, Tett SE. 2003. Prescription drug samples: Does this marketing strategy counteract policies for quality use of medicines? *Journal of Clinical Pharmacy and Therapeutics* 28:259–271.

Gurwitz JH. 2004. Polypharmacy: A new paradigm for quality drug therapy in the elderly? *Archives of Internal Medicine* 164(18):1957–1959.

Gurwitz JH, Field TS, Judge J, Rochon P, Harrold LR, Cadoret C, Lee M, White K, LaPrino J, Mainard JF, DeFlorio M, Gavendo L, Auger J, Bates DW. 2005. The incidence of adverse drug events in two large academic long-term care facilities. *The American Journal of Medicine* 118(3):251–258.

Hallinan TJ. 2005. *Once Seen as Risky, One Group of Doctors Changes Its Ways.* [Online]. Available: http://webreprints.djreprints.com/1254400029287.html [accessed May 29, 2006].

Han YY, Carcillo JA, Venkataraman ST, Clark RSB, Watson RS, Nguyen TC, Bayir H, Orr RA. 2005. Unexpected increased mortality after implementation of a commercially sold computerized physician order entry system. *Pediatrics* 116(5):1506–1512.

HCPC (Healthcare Compliance Packaging Council). 2003. *HCPC Response to Public Comments Requested in 68 FR 115, CPSC Petition PP 03-1.* Falls Church, VA: HCPC.

HIBCC (Health Industry Business Communications Council). 2001. *The Use of the Health Industry Bar Code for Product Labeling and Device Tracking.* [Online]. Available: http://www.hibcc.org/PUBS/WhitePapers/HIBCFeatures.pdf [accessed December 19, 2005].

Hoffman JM, Proulx SM. 2003. Medication errors caused by confusion of drug names. *Drug Safety* 26(7):445–452.

Hsieh TC, Kuperman GJ, Jaggi T, Hojnowski-Diaz P, Fiskio J, Williams DH, Bates DW, Gandhi TK. 2004. Characteristics and consequences of drug allergy alert overrides in a computerized physician order entry system. *Journal of the American Medical Informatics Association* 11(6):482–491.

Huang HY, Maguire MG, Miller ER, Appel LJ. 2000. Impact of pill organizers and blister packs on adherence to pill taking in two vitamin supplementation trials. *American Journal of Epidemiology* 152(8):780–787.

Hulley S, Grady D, Bush T, Furberg C, Herrington D, Riggs B, Vittinghoff E. 1998. Randomized trial of estrogen plus progestin for secondary prevention of coronary heart disease in postmenopausal women. Heart and Estrogen/progestin Replacement Study (HERS) Research Group. *Journal of the American Medical Association* 280(7):605–613.

Ientile C, Stokes J, Hendry M, Jensen A, Lewis G. 2004. *Literature Review for the Effectiveness and Cost Effectiveness of Dose Administration Aids Project.* Queensland, Australia: University of Queensland.

IMS Health. 2004. *Total U.S. Promotional Spending by Type, 2003.* Notes: Provided to IOM from PhRMA.

IOM (Institute of Medicine). 2000. *To Err Is Human: Building a Safer Health System.* Washington, DC: National Academy Press.

IOM. 2001. *Crossing the Quality Chasm: A New Health System for the 21st Century.* Washington, DC: National Academy Press.

IOM. 2004. *Patient Safety: Achieving a New Standard for Care.* Washington, DC: The National Academies Press.

IOM. 2006. *Developing a Registry of Pharmacologic and Biologic Clinical Trials.* Washington, DC: The National Academies Press.

ISMP (Institute for Safe Medication Practice). 2002. *ISMP Medication Safety Alert* July 10. Huntington Valley, PA: ISMP.

ISMP. 2005. *Medication Safety Alert.* December 15. Huntington Valley, PA: ISMP.

JCAHO (Joint Commission on Accreditation of Healthcare Organizations). 1998. *Medication Use: A Systems Approach to Reducing Errors.* Oakbrook Terrace, IL: JCAHO.

JCAHO. 2003. *2003 JCAHO National Patient Safety Goals: Practical Strategies and Helpful Solutions for Meeting These Goals (Special Report 2003).* Oakbrook Terrace, IL: JCAHO.

JCAHO. 2006. *National Patient Safety Goals: Look-Alike/Sound-Alike Drug List.* [Online]. Available: http://www.jointcommission.org/PatientSafety/NationalPatientSafetyGoals [accessed June 13, 2006].

Johnson CL, Carlson RA, Tucker CL, Willette C. 2002. Using BCMA software to improve patient safety in Veterans Administration Medical Centers. *Journal of Healthcare Information Management* 16(1):46–51.

Kaufman DR, Patel VL, Hilliman C, Morin PC, Pevzner J, Weinstock RS, Goland R, Shea S, Starren J. 2003. Usability in the real world: Assessing medical information technologies in patients' homes. *Journal of Biomedical Informatics* 36:45–60.

Kaushal R, Bates DW, Landrigan C, McKenna KJ, Clapp MD, Federico F, Goldmann DA. 2001. Medication errors and adverse drug events in pediatric inpatients. *Journal of the American Medical Association* 285(16):2114–2120.

Kilbridge P, Welebob E, Classen D. 2001. *Overview of the Leapfrog Group Evaluation Tool for Computerized Physician Order Entry.* Washington, DC: The Leapfrog Group.

Kilbridge PM, Welebob EM, Classen DC. 2006. Development of the Leapfrog methodology for evaluating hospital implemented inpatient computerized physician order entry systems. *Quality and Safety in Health Care* 15(2):81–84.

Koppel R, Metlay JP, Cohen A, Abaluck B, Localio AR, Kimmel SE, Strom BL. 2005. Role of computerized physician order entry systems in facilitating medication errors. *Journal of the American Medical Association* 293(10):1197–1203.

Kushniruk AW, Kaufman DR, Patel VL, Levesque Y, Lottin P. 1996. Assessment of a computerized patient record system: A cognitive approach to evaluating medical technology. *MD Computing* 13:406–415.

Leape LL, Kabcenell A, Berwick DM, Roessner J. 1998. *Breakthrough Series Guide: Reducing Adverse Drug Events.* Boston, MA: Institute for Healthcare Improvement.

Leape LL, Berwick DM, Bates DW. 2002. What practices will most improve safety? Evidence-based medicine meets patient safety. *Journal of the American Medical Association* 288(4): 501–507.

Levy S. 2002. *TrialCard Puts Drug Samples in R.Ph.'s Hands.* [Online]. Available: http://www.drugtopics.com/drugtopics/article/articleDetail.jsp?id-116704 [accessed January 23, 2006].

Malashock CM, Shull SS, Gould DA. 2004. Effect of smart infusion pumps on medication errors related to infusion device programming. *Hospital Pharmacy* 39(5):460–469.

March JS, Silva SG, Compton S, Shapiro M, Califf R, Krishnan R. 2005. The case for practical clinical trials in psychiatry. *American Journal of Psychiatry* 162(5):836–846.

MHPRA (Medicines and Healthcare Products Regulatory Agency). 2003. *Guidance Note 25: Best Practices for Labeling and Packaging of Medicines.* London, United Kingdom: MHPRA.

Miller RA, Gardner RM, Johnson KB, Hripcsak G. 2005. Clinical decision support and electronic prescribing systems: A time for responsible thought and action. *Journal of the American Medical Informatics Association* 12(4):403–409.

NCC MERP (National Coordinating Council for Medication Error Reporting and Prevention). 2001. *Recommendations to Reduce Medication Errors Associated with Verbal Medication Orders and Prescriptions.* [Online]. Available: http://www.nccmerp.org/council/council2001-02-20.html [accessed December 23, 2005].

NCVHS (National Committee on Vital and Health Statistics), 2003. *Letter to Secretary of DHHS Tommy Thompson: PMRI Terminology Standards.* [Online]. Available: http://www.ncvhs.hhs.gov/reptrecs.htm [accessed May 23, 2006].

Nemeth C. 2003. *Report on Infusion Pump Operation by Healthcare Professionals.* Chicago, IL: Cognitive Technologies Laboratory.

NHS (National Health Service). 2004. *Microsoft and Partners to Invest £40 Million in Development Resources to Improve Clinical Care in the NHS.* [Online]. Available: http://www.connectingforhealth.nhs.uk.news/0311041 [accessed March 15, 2006].

Paterson JM, Anderson GM. 2002. "Trial" prescriptions to reduce drug wastage: Results from Canadian programs and a community demonstration project. *American Journal of Managed Care* 8(2):151–158.

Patterson ES. 2003. Addressing human factors in bar code medication administration systems. *Hospital Pharmacy* 38(11):S16–S17.

Patterson ES, Cook RI, Render ML. 2002. Improving patient safety by identifying side effects from introducing bar coding in medication administration. *Journal of the American Medical Informatics Association* 9(5):540–553.

Petersen M. 2000, November 15. Growing opposition to free drug samples. *New York Times.* Business.

Pierce EC. 2006. *34th Rovenstine Lecture: Enhancing Patient Safety from the 1980's through the Present.* Pittsburgh, PA: Anesthesia Patient Safety Foundation.

Prentice RL. 1989. Surrogate end points in clinical trials: Definition and operational criteria. *Statistics in Medicine* 8:431–440.

Psaty BM, Furberg CD. 2005. COX-2 inhibitors—Lessons in drug safety. *New England Journal of Medicine* 352(11):1133–1135.

Rasmussen JE. 1988. Free drug samples. *Archives of Determatology* 124:135–137.

Reddan D, Szczech LA, O'Shea S, Califf RM. 2003. Anticoagulation in acute cardiac care in patients with chronic kidney disease. *American Heart Journal* 145(4):586–594.

Reichley RM, Seaton TL, Resetar E, Micek ST, Scott KL, Fraser VJ, Dunagan C, Bailey T.C. 2005. Implementing a commercial rule base as a medication order safety net. *Journal of the American Medical Informatics Association* 12(4):383–389.

Roberts R, Rodriguez W, Murphy D, Crescenzi T. 2003. Pediatric drug labeling: Improving the safety and efficacy of pediatric therapies. *Journal of the American Medical Association* 290:905–911.

Rogers ML, Patterson E, Chapman R, Render M. 2005. *Usability Testing and the Relation of Clinical Information Systems to Patient Safety.* [Online]. Available: http://www.ahrq.gov/downloads/pub/advances/vol2/Rogers.pdf [accessed December 20, 2005].

Santell JO, Camp S. 2004. Similarity of drug names, labels, or packaging creates safety issues. *U.S. Pharmacist* 29(7).

Sawa T, Ohno-Machado L. 2001. Generation of dynamically configured check lists for intra-operative problems using a set covering algorithm. *Proceedings of American Medical Informatics Association Symposium* 593–597.

Schneider PJ, Murphy JE, Pedersen CA. 2006, In press. Adherence and treatment outcomes in elderly outpatients with hypertension using specially packaged medications. *Journal of the American Pharmacists Association.*

Schünemann HJ, Cook D, Grimshaw J, Liberati A, Heffner J, Tapson V, Guyatt G. 2004. Antithrombotic and thrombolytic therapy: From evidence to application. *Chest* 126(Suppl.): 688–696.

Security Biometrics, Inc. 2004. *Security Biometrics, Inc. Subsidiary eMedRx, Forms Exclusive Strategic Alliance with Univec.* [Online]. Available: http://findbiometrics.com/viewnews. php?id=831 [accessed January 23, 2006].

Shah NR, Seger AC, Seger DL, Fiskio JM, Kuperman GJ, Blumenfeld B, Recklet EG, Bates DW, Gandhi TK. 2006. Improving acceptance of computerized prescribing alerts in ambulatory care. *Journal of the American Medical Informatics Association* 13(1):5–11.

Shortliffe EH, Perreault LE, Wiederhold G, Fagan LM. 2001. *Medical Informatics: Computer Applications in Health Care and Biomedicine.* 2nd ed. New York: Springer.

Simmons D, Upjohn M, Gamble GD. 2000. Can medication packaging improve glycemic control abd blood pressure in Type 2 diabetes? *Diabetes Care* 23(2):153–156.

Simon SR, Majumdar SR, Prosser LA, Salem-Schatz S, Warner C, Kleinman K, Miroshnik I, Soumerai SB. 2005. Group versus individual academic detaining to improve the use of antihypertensive medications in primary care: A cluster-randomized controlled trial. *American Journal of Medicine* 118:521–528.

Sipkoff M. 2003. *Getting Serious About Generics.* [Online]. Available: http://www.managed caremag.com/archives/0301/0301.generics.html [accessed March 12, 2006].

Szeinbach SL, Baron M, Guschke T, Torkilson EA. 2003. Survey of state requirements for unit-of-use packaging. *American Journal of Health-System Pharmacists* 60(18):1863–1866.

Taira DA, Iwane KA, Chung RS. 2003. Prescription drugs: Elderly enrollee reports of financial access, receipt of free samples, and discussion of generic equivalents related to type of coverage. *American Journal of Managed Care* 9(4):305–312.

Taxis K, Barber N. 2003. Ethnographic study of incidence and severity of intravenous drug errors. *British Medical Journal* 326(7391):684.

Tourville J. 2003. Automation and error reduction: How technology is helping Children's Medical Center of Dallas reach zero-error tolerance. *U.S. Pharmacist* 28:80–86.

Tsintis P, La Mache E. 2004. CIOMS and ICH initiatives in pharmacovigilance and risk management: Overview and implications. *Drug Safety* 27(8):509–517.

Tunis SR, Stryer DB, Clancy CM. 2003. Practical clinical trials: Increasing the value of clinical research for decision making in clinical and health policy. *Journal of the American Medical Association* 290(12):1624–1632.

USAN (United States Adopted Name Council). 2005. *Stem List.* [Online]. Available: http:// www.ama-assn.org/ama1/pub/upload/mm/365/usanstmlist_10_19_05.doc [accessed December 23, 2005].

USP (U.S. Pharmacopeia). 1993. *Unit-of-Use Packaging: Contemporary Issues.* Rockville, MD: USP.

USP. 1998. *USP Quality Review. No. 62.* Rockville, MD: USP.

USP. 2005. *CAPSLink Newsletter*. Rockville, MD: USP.

Valero G. 2005. *Patient Compliance via Unit-Dose Packaging. Pharmaceutical Business Strategies*. [Online]. Available: http://www.pbsmag.com/ArticlePrinterFriendly.cfm?ID=176 [accessed May 27, 2006].

van Bemmel JH, Musen MA. 1997. *Handbook of Medical Informatics*. Heidelberg, Germany: Springer-Verlag.

Vanderveen T. 2005. *Smart Pumps and Patient Controlled Analgesia Machines*. Submission to the IOM Committee on Identifying and Preventing Medication Errors, July 2006.

Wachter SB, Agutter J, Syroid N, Drews F, Weinger MB, Westenskow D. 2003. The employment of an iterative design process to develop a pulmonary graphical display. *Journal of the American Medical Informatics Association* 10(4):363–372.

Weary PE. 1988. Free drug samples: Use and abuse. *Archives of Determatology* 124: 135–137.

Weingart SN, Toth M, Sands DZ, Aronson MD, Davis RB, Phillips RS. 2003. Physicians' decisions to override computerized drug alerts in primary care. *Archives of Internal Medicine* 163(21):2625–2631.

Weinger MB, Slagle J. 2002. Human factors research in anesthesia patient safety. *Journal of the American Medical Informatics Association* 9(6):S58–S63.

WHI Steering Committee (Women's Health Initiative). 2004. Effects of conjugated equine estrogen in postmenopausal women with hysterectomy: The Women's Health Initiative randomized controlled trial. *Journal of the American Medical Association* 29:11701–1712.

Wogalter MS, Vigilante WJ. 2003. Effects of label format on knowledge acquisition and perceived readability by younger and older adults. *Ergonomics* 46(4):327–344.

Wood AJ. 1999. The safety of new medicines: The importance of asking the right questions. *Journal of the American Medical Association* 281(18):1753–1754.

Wright JM, Htun Y, Leong MG, Forman P, Ballard RC. 1999. Evaluation of the use of calendar blister packaging on patient compliance with STD syndromic treatment regimens. *Sexually Transmitted Disease* 26(10):556–563.

Yusuf S, Collins R, Peto R. 1984. Why do we need some large, simple randomized trials? *Statistics in Medicine* 3:409–422.

Zarin DA, Tse T, Ide NC, 2005. Trial registration at ClinicalTrials.gov between May and October 2005. *New England Journal of Medicine* 353(26):2779–2787.

Zoeller J. 1999. Searle weighs Celebrex name change: New cox-2 has been confused with other similarly-named drugs. *American Druggist* 216(5):15.

7

Applied Research Agenda for Safe Medication Use

CHAPTER SUMMARY

In this chapter, the committee proposes an applied research agenda for the safe use of medications across all care settings. This agenda, based on gaps in the medication error knowledge base, encompasses research methodologies, incidence rates, costs of medication errors, reporting systems, and testing of error prevention strategies.

In developing the recommendations presented in this chapter, the committee reviewed the literature on the incidence and costs of medication errors and on error prevention strategies. From this review, the committee identified important methodological issues and gaps in the medication error knowledge base. Overall, the committee believes the emphasis of research on safe medication use should gradually shift away from incidence rates, the current focus, to error prevention strategies. The committee believes the nation should invest about $100 million in research addressing medication safety, starting at $50 million per year.

Recommendation 6: The Agency for Healthcare Research and Quality (AHRQ) should take the lead, working with other government agencies such as the Centers for Medicare and Medicaid Services (CMS), the Food and Drug Administration (FDA), and the National Library of Medicine (NLM), in coordinating a broad

research agenda on the safe and appropriate use of medications across all care settings, and Congress should allocate the funds necessary to carry out this agenda. This agenda should encompass research methodologies, incidence rates by type and severity, costs of medication errors, reporting systems, and in particular, further testing of error prevention strategies.

DEFINITIONS

Researchers use a variety of definitions for medication errors, near misses, and adverse drug events (ADEs). There is a clear need to standardize terminology and measures for these phenomena if the field is going to advance.

Much of the literature reviewed by the committee failed to specify in sufficient detail the definition of a medication error used in the study. When detail was given, the definitions varied widely. Studies of medication errors in pediatric populations illustrate the problem: in one study, the definition of a medication dosing error was any dose greater than 10 percent over the recommended dose, while in another study, the definition was any dose greater than 10 times the recommended dose. In another set of studies examining the entire medication delivery system, some research teams did not include as errors events that were detected before they reached the patient, whereas other researchers counted these events as errors. As another example, some studies counted an order that was lacking a prescriber's signature as a medication error; although this is clearly an error, the potential for harm to patients is substantially different from that resulting from orders with dosage errors. If the definitions of medication errors and their subtypes are not standardized, and outcome data are not collected in a manner that permits assessment of the potential for harm, it is difficult to compare incidence rates across studies and to identify areas of high priority for intervention. The existing variations also result in a broad range of reported frequency and severity of errors.

To address this issue, the committee recommends that an international consensus conference be held to define the terms *medication error, near miss*, and *ADE*, as well as the subtypes of these terms, and to identify the practical applications of these definitions in various care settings. This conference could be similar to a session organized by the American College of Chest Physicians/Society of Critical Care Medicine in August 1991 to agree on a set of definitions that could be applied to patients with sepsis and its sequelae (Bone et al., 1992). The definitions introduced as a result of this conference have been widely used in practice and have served as the foundation for inclusion criteria for many clinical trials of therapeutic interventions (Levy et al., 2003). This uniform set of definitions has also made it much easier to compare results from different sepsis studies and to better understand the various syndromes.

ROLE OF THE PATIENT AND FAMILY

The public at large needs to develop a healthy respect for the risks as well as the benefits of medications. For example, one study revealed that patient-level errors are associated with about 20 percent of ADEs in the ambulatory setting among the elderly (Gurwitz et al., 2003). Engaging the patient as an active participant in decisions about and monitoring of medication use is critically important. Thus the committee recommends pursuit of a research agenda aimed at delineating effective strategies for involving patients and their families in the prevention, early detection, and mitigation of harm due to medication errors (IOM, 2004), with particular focus on the following topics:

- Determining how best to present information to patients to facilitate their understanding of medication use and safety, including the development of a consumer-friendly nomenclature for representing this information.
- Developing improved systems for supporting patients in identifying and eliminating barriers to following the prescribed medication regimen, or in seeking advice before altering the regimen in response to drug side effects or barriers to administration.
- Developing improved systems for supporting surrogates' roles in safe medication use when patients are receiving medications from professionals and are unable (too ill, disabled, or cognitively impaired) to monitor the administration of or their response to the drugs.
- Developing standard approaches to the maintenance of personal medication lists and investigating the effects of these lists on the effectiveness of safety strategies, such as medication reconciliation.
- Developing strategies to inform ambulatory patients of clinically significant abnormal test results, including the use of computerized patient notification of such results.
- Exploring the effectiveness of patient self-monitoring devices, such as home finger-stick devices and nomograms to self-adjust wafarin dosages.

The committee believes medication self-management can be enhanced with tools available through personal health records. In this regard, CMS, the FDA, and the NLM should collaborate to confirm a minimum dataset for personal health records and develop requirements for vendor self-certification of compliance. Vendors should take the initiative to improve the use and functionality of consumer-oriented information technologies by incorporating basic information tools for consumers' medication self-management.

MEDICATION SAFETY RESEARCH: INCIDENCE, COSTS, AND PREVENTION STRATEGIES

Incidence Rates

The committee examined the literature on incidence rates of medication errors. Despite the considerable research on incidence that has already taken place in certain areas, the committee believes much more such research needs to be carried out. In particular, it is important to characterize incidence rates by type and severity. Incidence rates are important for gauging the scope of the problem, for setting priorities for prevention strategies, and for measuring the impact of such strategies. The types of research required are described below for the hospital, nursing home, and ambulatory care settings; for pediatric and psychiatric care; and for the use of over-the-counter (OTC) and complementary and alternative medications.

Hospital Care

Medication error rates in hospitals have been relatively well researched. Thus the committee believes measurement of error rates in this care setting, with the exception of rates for specific populations (pediatric and psychiatric patients; see below), is not a priority for research. As indicated in Chapter 5, methods for detecting errors and ADEs can increasingly be built into electronic health records and other information systems, enabling better estimation of incidence rates for some types of errors and ADEs on an ongoing basis. Furthermore, these systems may be able to identify ADEs early enough in many situations to mitigate harm. However, research aimed at improving and standardizing these methods is a high priority.

Nursing Home Care

The long-term care arena is in need of a broad research agenda, including incidence data and the characterization of high-risk errors. There are more than 1.6 million residents of nursing homes in the United States. Levels of medication use are particularly high in these facilities, and patients are at particular risk for ADEs (Gurwitz et al., 2000, 2005). Recent studies have not focused specifically on medication errors, but have indicated that as many as half of all ADEs in the nursing home setting may be preventable. Nursing home residents taking antipsychotic medications, anticoagulants, and diuretics are at greatest risk for experiencing a preventable ADE. Nursing home residents may also be especially vulnerable to medication errors as they move between different settings of care, such as from the ambulatory setting to the nursing home, and back and forth to the hospital during episodes of acute illness.

Ambulatory Care

In the ambulatory setting, the best-understood aspects of medication error rates are prescribing errors in ambulatory primary care clinics and dispensing errors in community pharmacies. There is some understanding of the incidence of ADEs in ambulatory care and self-care errors. There is limited understanding of incidence rates in care transition situations, medication administration and monitoring in ambulatory care, mail order pharmacy, and school care (Forster et al., 2003). Little information exists as well concerning medication errors associated with prescribing in ambulatory specialty clinics. Specialty clinicians typically prescribe a limited set of medications (for example, chemotherapeutic agents). Nonetheless, specialists often work with incomplete medication data on patients that are referred or transitioning between settings—situations known to increase the risk of errors (Fernald et al., 2004).

New studies should focus especially on error incidence rates associated with care transitions, medication administration in ambulatory care, monitoring of medications in ambulatory care, mail order pharmacy, and school care. In addition, not enough is known about what happens between the time a prescription is filled and the time the patient is supposed to take a particular dose of the medication at a particular time. Such research is difficult for multiple reasons, although technological approaches using smart pill bottles and bioassays can be used. However, the very act of intrusive observation raises questions about the generalizability of results obtained with these approaches.

Pediatric Care

Despite extensive work on medication errors in the hospital setting, the committee found only a handful of studies on medication errors in pediatric patients in the emergency department, ambulatory care, and home environments, all of which are critical targets for future research. The home environment in particular should be a high priority given the growing reliance on home care for increasingly complex medical conditions. All three of the existing studies involving home medication administration (Li et al., 2000; McErlean et al., 2001; Goldman and Scolnik, 2004) focused narrowly on the administration of antipyretics. These studies estimated significant rates of medication errors by parents and guardians. A preliminary report also indicates high rates of prescribing errors in outpatient pediatric clinics (McPhillips et al., 2005b).

Psychiatric Care

The committee found only two studies of medication errors in psychiatry (Senst et al., 2001; Grasso et al., 2003). The committee found no studies of psychiatric care that used an independent audit to identify medication errors and then examine a potential causal link between errors and clinical harm. The committee believes medication errors in inpatient and outpatient psychiatry require more study.

Psychiatrist professional organizations have only recently identified medication errors as a patient safety and quality concern. The American Psychiatric Association (APA) first convened its Task Force on Patient Safety in 2002 (Herzog et al., 2003). ADEs were identified as one of four priority areas. The recommendations of the task force were approved by the board of trustees in November 2002 and by the assembly executive committee in January 2003, leading to the inception of the APA Committee on Patient Safety (Herzog et al., 2003).

The committee believes psychiatrists and other mental health professionals should join with their medical and surgical colleagues to speak a common language regarding the detection, reporting, and management of medication errors and ADEs. Broader incorporation of such terminology might also enable a more objective comparison of quality among psychiatric hospitals.

OTC Medications

Apart from the three highly specialized studies on the administration of antipyretics mentioned in the above discussion of pediatric care, the committee found no studies on incidence rates of medication errors arising from use of OTC drugs. Yet there is a growing literature on OTC drug–disease issues and OTC drug–drug interactions (see Box 3-2 in Chapter 3).

Further, a growing number of OTC drugs are being approved, including some that formerly had prescription status. From 1995 to 2004, there were 84 new approvals or prescription-to-OTC switches, an average of 8.4 per year (CDER, 2005). Looking to the future, it is likely that completely new categories of OTC drugs will become available in the United States. In 2004, the United Kingdom approved the first low-dose statin as an OTC drug, provided that a pharmacist reviews the purchase (Bellingham, 2004)—this even though statins do have drug–drug interactions, and it is difficult for patients to monitor either their effectiveness or their toxicity. This decision came 4 years after failed attempts in the United States to achieve OTC status for low-dose statins (Mitka, 2004). Against this background, the committee believes the time is right for a major study on the use of OTC drugs and the epidemiology of associated medication errors and ADEs, as well as drug–drug and drug–disease interactions.

Complementary and Alternative Medications

An emerging literature suggests that complementary and alternative medications have the potential for adverse interactions with prescription drugs (D'Arcy, 1993; Calis and Young, 2004). The Institute of Medicine's (IOM) recent report *Complementary and Alternative Medicine* (IOM, 2005) recommended that the National Institutes of Health and other public agencies provide the support necessary to develop and implement a sentinel surveillance system (comprising selected sites collecting and reporting data on patterns of use of these and conventional medications), practice-based research networks,[1] and complementary and alternative medication research centers to facilitate the work of the networks (by collecting and analyzing information from national surveys, identifying important questions, designing studies, coordinating data collection and analysis, and providing training in research and other areas). The IOM report also recommended that the National Institutes of Health and other public or private agencies sponsor quantitative and qualitative research to examine adverse events associated with complementary and alternative medications and their interactions with conventional treatments. The committee endorses both of these recommendations.

Costs

There have been few micro-level studies of the costs of medication errors. Most of these studies have estimated either the extra hospital costs of an ADE occurring while the patient is in the hospital or the costs of hospital admissions attributable to earlier ADEs. Two of these studies are now quite dated: one used data from 1990–1993 (Classen et al., 1997) and the other data from 1993 (Bates et al., 1997). Apart from one study relating to ambulatory care (Field et al., 2005), all of the studies related to hospital care. Clearly there are large gaps in our understanding of the costs of

---

[1]These networks are defined by the Agency for Healthcare Research and Quality as a group of ambulatory practices devoted principally to the primary care of patients, affiliated with each other (and often with an academic or professional organization) in order to investigate questions related to community-based practice (IOM, 2005).

medication errors. A better understanding of these costs is important for a number of reasons, including informing decisions about investments in technological interventions designed to reduce the risk of medication errors. Accordingly, the committee recommends that additional studies be carried out on these costs in hospitals, nursing homes, and ambulatory care. These studies should include (1) the costs of medication errors in pediatric and psychiatric care, (2) the costs of errors associated with OTC and complementary and alternative medications, (3) the costs of the failure to receive drugs that should have been prescribed, and (4) the costs of over-utilization of drugs (for example, antibiotics). Moreover, some of these studies should examine not just additional health care costs relating to medication errors, but also the economic and social costs borne by patients and their families.

Prevention Strategies

The committee acknowledges that it is not possible to put forward a fully comprehensive set of corrective medication error strategies. The area best understood is the incidence of medication errors and preventable ADEs in various care settings where significant problems and their causes have been identified. More research is needed to evaluate the impact of system problems in the research and development, regulatory review, and distribution/marketing stages on the incidence of errors in the use of medications and the impact of the underutilization of medications.

As suggested above, the primary focus of research on medication errors should be on informing, developing, and then testing prevention strategies. In the next sections, the committee outlines suggestions for further research on such strategies for hospital care, nursing home care, ambulatory care, pediatric care, psychiatric care, and care transitions.

As reported in Chapter 3, the universe of preventable ADEs is a minority of total ADEs. Although most of the development of error prevention strategies to date has been focused on the ADEs that are known to be preventable today, it will likely be possible in the future to prevent many events currently considered nonpreventable. In particular, better tools for detecting drug sensitivities and the use of pharmacogenomics offer great promise in this regard (Gandhi et al., 2005). In addition, innovations in the way compounds are constructed or delivered may result in a safer drug administration process.

Finally, further cost/benefit studies of all prevention strategies are urgently needed. Most such studies carried out to date have involved hospitals and a limited number of decision-support tools. Particularly needed are studies of vendor-based systems, a broad range of decision-support tools, and care settings other than hospitals. The aim should be to identify a group of high-impact interventions in each care setting that can be implemented first.

Hospital Care

For the most part, interventions that appear to have the strongest evidence are consistently incorporated into recommended best practices for reducing medication error rates, such as the National Quality Forum's (NQF) Safe Practices for Better Healthcare (NQF, 2003). Computerized provider order entry (CPOE) is almost universally recommended, as is incorporating clinical pharmacists into the inpatient medical team during daily rounds and creating specialized protocols for high-alert medications. Other strategies for which the evidence is not as strong but that are commonly recommended include standardizing prescription writing, limiting oral orders, improving medication error identification systems, adopting system-based approaches to reducing medication errors, promoting a culture of safety, implementing bar coding, and using unit dosing.

Bar coding and smart pumps are widely recommended interventions for which more rigorous testing appears warranted. In addition, there is a need to investigate nontechnical strategies that address human factors, such as techniques for combating fatigue (e.g., adequate staffing of professionals involved in medication use); elimination of redundancies (e.g., identifying when double-checks add value in decreasing errors); echoing and readback; the use of reminders, constraints, and color differentiation; and systematic approaches that couple continuous surveillance of error reports/alerts and review of good-practice guidance from internal and external sources with proactive prevention strategies.

Beyond the validation of individual approaches to error reduction, the next steps in research on prevention strategies for hospital care should focus on evaluation of the following:

• How to make a business case for investment in error prevention strategies. CPOE, bar coding, and smart pumps are expensive applications and have to compete with other investments for a health care organization's limited resources. Financial models for the benefits of CPOE are beginning to emerge (Kaushal et al., 2006).

• How to select an individual application, such as CPOE, bar coding, and smart pumps. Tools are needed to evaluate applications in the way they present information to users, their effectiveness at intercepting medication errors, and the quality of the information provided through decision-support tools. Leapfrog has begun to develop a tool to evaluate hospital CPOE systems with decision support (Kilbridge et al., 2006).

• How to implement individual approaches, such as CPOE, bar coding, and smart pumps. Implementation problems with electronic prescribing systems and unintended consequences arising from the implementation of such systems have been well documented (Ash et al., 2004; Han et al., 2005; Berger and Kichak, 2004; Koppel et al., 2005; Fernando et al., 2004). Guidance manuals are needed to help all stakeholders implement these systems successfully. In particular, more research is needed to understand the specific challenges that exist for institutions of different sizes and different staffing models (Kuperman and Gibson, 2003).

• How to link the various individual applications (CPOE, bar coding, and smart pumps) together and with electronic health records and the patient's personal health record. A better understanding is needed of how to ensure that data can pass seamlessly from one application to another, and that the data are interpreted in a consistent way across all applications.

• New approaches to improve the safety of transitions between providers and patient care units, and especially as the patient leaves the hospital. Most current prevention strategies are applied in one particular care setting. Transitions from one provider to another are error prone (Forster et al., 2003). Applications need to be developed that can keep all a patient's providers (inpatient and outpatient prescribers, pharmacists) up to date when any one of the prescribers or the patient changes the patient's medication or the pharmacist learns that the patient has failed to fill a particular prescription.

Nursing Home Care

Although CPOE with clinical decision support has been implemented successfully in many acute care hospitals, there are few descriptions of its use in the long-term care setting (Rochon et al., 2005). Use of the technology in nursing homes poses many challenges, and its effectiveness in preventing medication errors and ADEs in this setting needs to be assessed. The impact of staffing levels on medication errors and preventable ADEs in the nursing home setting also has not been adequately studied, nor have deficiencies in communication between nursing home staff and the clinicians accountable for prescribing medications.

Ambulatory Care

Many approaches to medication safety derive from the inpatient setting, and it is not clear to what extent these approaches are transferable to the ambulatory setting. For example, instruments used to assess the safety climate for the ambulatory setting lag far behind those for the inpatient setting (Nieva and Sorra, 2003). Tools for such assessment for a full range of ambulatory institutions need to be developed. Even the effect of electronic prescribing on medication safety in the ambulatory setting has not been well studied; the same is true of the impact of providing different levels of decision support. Effectiveness studies of the most promising error prevention strategies are needed, with priority given to electronic prescribing with clinical decision support and collaborative care approaches involving physicians, nurses, and pharmacists, and with patient self-education/counseling.

The majority of patient–pharmacy interactions on a day-to-day basis involve prescription refills. There is a need for studies targeting safe practices in this area. Also needing study are the effects of time demands on clinicians in the ambulatory setting on safety in general and on medication safety in particular.

Pediatric Care

Standardization of recommended doses for children is essential to enable providers, researchers, and developers of technological prescribing solutions to speak a common language as to what doses are considered acceptable (that is, not errors) for children (McPhillips et al., 2005a,b). Despite the push for CPOE and electronic prescribing, the lack of uniformity on standard pediatric doses is at least part of the reason for the usual absence of pediatric-specific dosing tables powering most commercially available CPOE tools. Because of the inability to build such dosage rules into computerized prescribing tools, children cannot reap the full benefit of information technology in the medication delivery process.

In the home environment, research is needed on standardization of concentrations and dosing spoons, syringes, and other tools used by parents and guardians, similar to the efforts now under way to standardize and limit the number of concentrations used within institutions.

Most of the research to date on pediatric medication errors has been skewed toward prescribing errors. The committee's review of data from error reporting systems revealed that dispensing and administering are as error prone as prescribing. In contrast with the medication-use process for adults, the steps of dispensing and administering in pediatric populations depend much more heavily on manual compounding of liquid medications and administration to patients who are unable to perform their own medication safety checks. Understanding the unique risks for children in these two steps is critical to determining which interventions will eliminate or mitigate these risks.

Many potential approaches to error reduction are relatively inexpensive and are supported by common sense based on knowledge of human factors. Such approaches include representation of pediatric care on formulary committees, appropriate and competent pharmacy and nursing personnel who are knowledgeable about pediatric medication dosages and regimens, policies on oral orders, and clear and accurate medication labeling.

Psychiatric Care

In Chapter 3, it was noted that no study has been carried out to evaluate the efficacy of any prevention strategy for medication errors in psychiatric care. Nevertheless, there are several promising strategies of relevance to psychiatric care that do not involve automation and thus could be evaluated immediately:

- The use of medication ordering protocols for drugs that have a narrow therapeutic index and/or might be unsafe to initiate or resume without laboratory data (for example, lithium carbonate, clozapine, carbamazepine, valproic acid).
- The use of unit-dose distribution systems in which medications are individually prepackaged and delivered in the exact dose to the point of administration.
- Access to drug information at the time of prescribing through inclusion of a clinical pharmacist in rounds, along with immediate drug database access using personal digital assistants (PDAs).
- Orientation and periodic education of nurses and physicians regarding the prescribing, transcribing, dispensing, and administration processes.
- Better patient education in the use of medications.

A number of computerized interventions also appear to have the potential to decrease medication error rates in the psychiatric inpatient setting. Among these are CPOE, bar coding linked to computerized medication administration records, automated dispensing devices, and pharmacy dispensing robotics (Bates and Gawande, 2003). Outside the hospital, tools that can help patients track what medications they have actually taken may be especially beneficial in the psychiatric population.

Care Transitions

As noted elsewhere in this report, the available data indicate that care transitions between institutions and primary or home care pose a high level of risk (Fernald et al., 2004) because medication regimens are frequently altered at these times. Research is needed on ways to improve communication between these components of the medication-use system. All concerned need to acknowledge the problem and evaluate a variety of approaches to error reduction. Specific areas for research include (1) improved methods for helping patients and providers create and maintain accurate and up-to-date medication lists, (2) a better understanding of the benefits and risks of systems that incentivize or require patients to obtain medications from multiple sources (e.g., local and mail order pharmacies, free samples from prescribers), (3) a better understanding of the impact of the use of formularies on medication safety, (4) an improved understanding of the impact of changes in health insurance coverage leading to interruptions in medication use, (5) a better understanding of the impact of changes in formularies leading to changes in medication use and the disruptions they can cause, and (6) an improved understanding of the impact of payer regulations that mandate frequent refills within tight time frames.

The need for improved information transfer between prescribing clinicians and dispensing pharmacies/pharmacists also needs to be studied. The Continuity of Care Record (CCR) and Regional Health Information Organizations are important initiatives aimed at addressing this problem. The CCR is a standard specification developed jointly by the American Society for Testing Materials (ASTM) International, the Massachusetts Medical Society, the Health Information Management and Systems Society, the American Academy of Family Physicians, the American Academy of Pediatrics, and others (Tessier, 2005) and published in early 2006 (ASTM, 2006). It is intended to foster and improve continuity of patient care, to reduce medical errors, and to ensure at least a minimum standard of health information transportability when a patient is referred or transferred to or otherwise seen by another provider. The next step is for vendors to incorporate the CCR standard in their products.

Regional Health Information Organizations represent state and other regional groups seeking to harmonize the privacy and business rules for health information exchange (DHHS, 2005). More than 100 regional projects are under way, funded by the federal government. Several other projects are being supported by private industry or funded at the state level. The CCR and Regional Health Information Organizations could be highly complementary if appropriately combined, with one providing an improved standard for transmission of data and the other the means for rapid transmission to the point of care. Such developments should be supported and evaluated for their impact on the safety and quality of medication use.

IDENTIFICATION METHODS: DATA TRIGGERS

The IOM's report on patient safety (IOM, 2004) recommended research aimed at developing and evaluating various methods for using data-driven triggers to detect ADEs and other high-risk events (e.g., nosocomial infections, patient falls). The committee endorses this recommendation and believes the focus of such research should be on developing efficient, robust tools for computerized monitoring that would allow all organizations to monitor routinely for ADEs. Ultimately, it may be practical to mandate such monitoring. To this end, research is needed on improving, across all settings, the utility and reliability of computerized detection (e.g., eliminating alert fatigue; see Chapter 6); also needed are testing and validation specific to the site of care (Field et al., 2004).

In the ambulatory setting, medication monitoring, particularly for ADEs, is virtually nonexistent. Research is needed on what data sources are necessary for a robust background monitoring system in the ambulatory environment, such as the systems used for inpatients at Brigham and Women's Hospital in Boston, Massachusetts, and LDS Hospital in Salt Lake City, Utah. Development and testing of such systems would be a major step forward in medication safety in the ambulatory setting, particularly if facilitated by the incorporation of electronic health records and electronic prescribing.

INTERNATIONAL STUDIES

International comparison studies provide valuable benchmarking data concerning safe medication practices. These studies help challenge paradigms and encourage thinking beyond the traditional views concerning just what constitutes safe medication practice. An example of such a study is one undertaken in a hospital in the United States and a hospital in the United Kingdom (Dean et al., 1995). The medication error rate in the U.S. hospital was 6.9 percent, higher than the 3.0 percent rate observed in the U.K. hospital. The committee believes this study was very useful, but acknowledges that such studies are challenging to conduct.

The committee suggests that more international sharing of ideas on medication safety would be highly beneficial and recommends that more international studies be carried out to evaluate different medication systems and their effects on the rates of medication errors and ADEs. An important prerequisite is that researchers carrying out such international studies need to adopt common taxonomies for describing errors. In this context, the World Health Organization is taking a lead role (WHO, 2005). In addition, international studies should use multiple error detection methods.

CROSS-INDUSTRY SAFETY STUDIES

Many industries face safety challenges. Industries such as aviation, nuclear power, and chemical manufacturing have implemented successful safety strategies and continue to achieve advances in this regard. These industries have addressed safety issues of relevance to health care, generally and medication safety in particular, such as introducing a culture of safety, implementing computerized error detection and prevention systems, standardizing procedures, reducing errors at care transitions, and developing human–computer interfaces. It is likely that many of the lessons learned in these industries will be relevant to health care delivery. As a consequence, the committee believes workshops and studies should take place regularly so that safety experts in health care can share experiences with safety experts in other industries.

REPORTING SYSTEMS

The committee endorses the recommendation in the IOM's patient safety report (IOM, 2004) that the Agency for Healthcare Research and Quality develop a standard (or common) event taxonomy for data storage and analysis. Specifically, this event taxonomy should address near misses and ADEs, cover errors of both omission and commission, and include hazardous conditions. The report format should include both standardized data elements and free-text narratives.

The committee views the work of the Joint Commission on Accreditation of Healthcare Organizations (JCAHO) in this area as an important development. JCAHO has taken a leadership role (Chang et al., 2005) by developing a Patient Safety Event Taxonomy (NQF, 2005), which was endorsed by the NQF in August 2005 (see also Chapter 8).

The committee also endorses the recommendation of the IOM's patient safety report that further studies on the cost/benefit of reporting systems be undertaken. In particular, there is a need for in-depth studies of the value of various reporting systems with regard to learning about errors and new problems, gaining knowledge from the reports, communicating guidance, and changing care delivery processes.

REFERENCES

Ash JS, Berg M, Coiera E. 2004. Some unintended consequences of information technology in health care: The nature of patient care information system-related errors. *Journal of the American Medical Informatics Association* 11(2):104–112.

ASTM (American Society for Testing Materials). 2006. *Continuity of Care Record Is Developed by ASTM International Health Care Informatics Committee*. [Online]. Available: http://69.7.224.88/viewnews.aspx?newsID=772 [accessed April 18, 2006].

Bates DW, Gawande AA. 2003. Improving safety with information technology. *New England Journal of Medicine* 348(25):2526–2534.

Bates DW, Spell N, Cullen DJ, Burdick E, Laird N, Petersen LA, Small SD, Sweitzer BJ, Leape L. 1997. The costs of adverse drug events in hospitalized patients. Adverse Drug Events Prevention Study Group. *Journal of the American Medical Association* 277(4):307–311.

Bellingham C. 2004. OTC statin may change pharmacy for ever. *The Pharmaceutical Journal* 273:43.

Berger RG, Kichak JP. 2004. Computerized physician order entry: Helpful or harmful? *Journal of the American Medical Informatics Association* 11(2):100–103.

Bone RC, Balk RA, Cerra FB, Dellinger RP, Fein AM, Knaus WA, Schein RM, Sibbald WJ. 1992. Definitions for sepsis and organ failure and guidelines for the use of innovative therapies in sepsis. The ACCP/SCCM Consensus Conference Committee. American College of Chest Physicians/Society of Critical Care Medicine. *Chest* 101(6):1644–1655.

Calis KA, Young LR. 2004. Clinical analysis of adverse drug reactions: A primer for clinicians. *Hospital Pharmacy* 39(7):697–712.

CDER (Center for Drug Evaluation and Research). 2005. *2004 Report to the Nation: Improving Public Health Through Human Drugs.* Washington, DC: U.S. Department of Health and Human Services.

Chang A, Schyve PM, Croteau DJ, O'Leary DS, Loeb JM. 2005. The JCAHO patient safety event taxonomy: A standardized terminology and classification schema for near misses and adverse events. *International Journal for Quality in Health Care* 17(2):95–105.

Classen DC, Pestotnik SL, Evans RS, Lloyd JF, Burke JP. 1997. Adverse drug events in hospitalized patients. Excess length of stay, extra costs, and attributable mortality. *Journal of the American Medical Association* 277(4):301–306.

D'Arcy PF. 1993. Adverse reactions and interactions with herbal medicines. Part 2. Drug interactions. *Adverse Drug Reactions and Toxicological Reviews* 12:147–162.

Dean BS, Allan EL, Barber ND, Barker KN. 1995. Comparison of medication errors in an American and a British hospital. *American Journal of Health-System Pharmacy* 52(22): 2543–2549.

DHHS (U.S. Department of Health and Human Services). 2005. *Regional Health Information Organizations (RHIOs).* [Online]. Available: http://www.hhs.gov/healthit/rhio.html [accessed October 9, 2005].

Fernald DH, Pace WD, Harris DM, West DR, Main DS, Westfall JM. 2004. Event reporting to a primary care patient safety reporting system: A report from the ASIPS Collaborative. *Annals of Family Medicine* 2(4):327–332.

Fernando B, Savelyich BSP, Avery AJ, Sheikh A, Bainbridge M, Horsfield P, Teasdale S. 2004. Prescribing safety features of general practice computer systems: Evaluation using simulated test cases. *British Medical Journal* 328(7449):1171–1172.

Field TS, Gurwitz JH, Harrold LR, Rothschild JM, Debellis K, Seger AC, Fish LS, Garber L, Kelleher M, Bates DW. 2004. Strategies for detecting adverse drug events among older persons in the ambulatory setting. *Journal of the American Medical Informatics Association* 11(6):492–498.

Field TS, Gilman BH, Subramanian S, Fuller JC, Bates DW, Gurwitz JH. 2005. The costs associated with adverse drug events among older adults in the ambulatory setting. *Medical Care* 43(12):1171–1176.

Forster AJ, Murff HJ, Peterson JF, Gandhi TK, Bates DW. 2003. The incidence and severity of adverse events affecting patients after discharge from the hospital. *Annals of Internal Medicine* 138(3):161–167.

Gandhi TK, Bartel SB, Shulman LN, Verrier D, Burdick E, Cleary A, Rothschild JM, Leape LL, Bates DW. 2005. Medication safety in the ambulatory chemotherapy setting. *Cancer* 104(11):2477–2483.

Goldman RD, Scolnik D. 2004. Underdosing of acetaminophen by parents and emergency department utilization. *Pediatric Emergency Care* 20(2):89–93.

Grasso BC, Genest R, Jordan CW, Bates DW. 2003. Use of chart and record reviews to detect medication errors in a state psychiatric hospital. *Psychiatric Services (Washington, D.C.)* 54(5):677–681.

Gurwitz JH, Field TS, Avorn J, McCormick D, Jain S, Eckler M, Benser M, Edmondson AC, Bates DW. 2000. Incidence and preventability of adverse drug events in nursing homes. *The American Journal of Medicine* 109(2):87–94.

Gurwitz JH, Field TS, Harrold LR, Rothschild J, Debellis K, Seger AC, Cadoret C, Fish LS, Garber L, Kelleher M, Bates DW. 2003. Incidence and preventability of adverse drug events among older persons in the ambulatory setting. *Journal of the American Medical Association* 289(9):1107–1116.

Gurwitz JH, Field TS, Judge J, Rochon P, Harrold LR, Cadoret C, Lee M, White K, LaPrino J, Mainard JF, DeFlorio M, Gavendo L, Auger J, Bates DW. 2005. The incidence of adverse drug events in two large academic long-term care facilities. *The American Journal of Medicine* 118(3):251–258.

Han YY, Carcillo JA, Venkataraman ST, Clark RSB, Watson RS, Nguyen TC, Bayir H, Orr RA. 2005. Unexpected increased mortality after implementation of a commercially sold computerized physician order entry system. *Pediatrics* 116(5):1506–1512.

Herzog, A, Shore, MF, Beale, RR, Padrino, SL, Vogel, AV. 2003. *Patient Safety and Psychiatry: Recommendations to the Board of Trustees of the American Psychiatric Association.* [Online]. Available: www.psych.org/edu/other_res/lib_archives/archives/tfr/tfr200301. pdf [accessed September 30, 2005].

IOM (Institute of Medicine). 2004. *Patient Safety: Achieving a New Standard for Care.* Washington, DC: The National Academies Press.

IOM. 2005. *Complementary and Alternative Medicines in the United States.* Washington, DC: The National Academies Press.

Kaushal R, Jha AK, Franz C, Shetty KD, Jaggi T, Glaser J, Middleton B, Kuperman GJ, Khorasani R, Tanasijevic M, Bates DW. 2006. Return on investment for a computerized physician order entry system. *Journal of the American Medical Informatics Association* 13(3):261–266.

Kilbridge PM, Welebob EM, Classen DC. 2006. Development of the Leapfrog methodology for evaluating hospital implemented inpatient computerized physician order entry systems. *Quality and Safety in Health Care* 15(2):81–84.

Koppel R, Metlay JP, Cohen A, Abaluck B, Localio AR, Kimmel SE, Strom BL. 2005. Role of computerized physician order entry systems in facilitating medication errors. *Journal of the American Medical Association* 293(10):1197–1203.

Kuperman G, Gibson RF. 2003. Computer physician order entry: Benefits, costs, and issues. *Annals of Internal Medicine* 139(1):31–39.

Levy MM, Mitchell PF, Marshall JC, Abraham E, Angus D, Cook D, Cohen J, Opal SM, Vincent JL, Ramsay G. 2003. 2001 SCCM/ESICM/ACCP/ATS/SIS international sepsis definitions conference. *Critical Care Medicine* 31(4):1250–1256.

Li SF, Lacher B, Crain EF. 2000. Acetaminophen and ibuprofen dosing by parents. *Pediatric Emergency Care* 16(6):394–397.

McErlean MA, Bartfield JM, Kennedy DA, Gilman EA, Stram RL, Raccio-Robak N. 2001. Home antipyretic use in children brought to the emergency department. *Pediatric Emergency Care* 17(4):249–251.

McPhillips H, Stille C, Smith D, Pearson J, Stull J, Hecht J, Miller M, Davis R. 2005a. Methodological challenges in describing medication dosing errors in children. In: Henriksen K, Battles J, Marks E, Lewin DI, eds. *Advances in Patient Safety: From Research to Implementation.* Vol. 2, Concepts and Methodology. Rockville, MD: Agency for Healthcare Research and Quality.

McPhillips HA, Stille CJ, Smith D, Hecht J, Pearson J, Stull J, Debellis K, Andrade S, Miller MR, Kaushal R, Gurwitz J, Davis RL. 2005b. Potential medication dosing errors in outpatient pediatrics. *The Journal of Pediatrics* 147(6):761–767.

Mitka M. 2004. Are OTC statins ready for prime time? *Journal of the American Medical Association* 293(3):317–318.

Nieva VF, Sorra J. 2003. Safety culture assessment: A tool for improving patient safety in healthcare organizations. *Quality & Safety in Health Care* 12(Suppl. 2):7–23.

NQF (National Quality Forum). 2003. *Safe Practices for Better Healthcare: A Consensus Report*. Washington, DC: NQF.

NQF. 2005. *National Quality Forum Endorses Voluntary Consensus Standard for Standardizing a Patient Safety Taxonomy*. August 3, 2005. [Online]. Available: http://www.qualityforum.org/news/home.htm [accessed November 26, 2005].

Rochon PA, Field TS, Bates DW, Lee M, Gavendo L, Erramuspe-Mainard J, Judge J, Gurwitz JH. 2005. Computerized physician order entry with clinical decision support in the long-term care setting: Insights from the Baycrest Centre for Geriatric Care. *Journal of the American Geriatrics Society* 53(10):1780–1789.

Senst BL, Achusim LE, Genest RP, Consentino LA, Ford CC, Little JA, Raybon SJ, Bates DW. 2001. Practical approach to determining costs and frequency of adverse drug events in a health care network. *American Journal of Health-System Pharmacy* 58(12):1126–1132.

Tessier C. 2005. *Overview of the Continuity of Care Record*. [Online]. Available: http://www.astm.org/COMMIT/E31_CCR0305.ppt#256,1 [accessed October 9, 2005].

WHO (World Health Organization). 2005. *Project to Develop the International Patient Safety Event Taxonomy: Report of the WHO World Alliance for Patient Safety Drafting Group, Vancouver, October, 2005*. Geneva, Switzerland: WHO.

8

Action Agendas for Oversight, Regulation, and Payment

CHAPTER SUMMARY

Legislation, regulation, accreditation, payment mechanisms, and the media shape the way health care is delivered. This chapter proposes ways for these functions to motivate the adoption of practices and technologies that can reduce medication errors, and to ensure that professionals have the competencies required to deliver medications safely.

Earlier chapters of this report have presented the committee's recommended action agendas for patients (Chapter 4) and health care providers (Chapters 4 and 5). Those two chapters are concerned with the first three of the four levels of the chain of effect framework (Berwick, 2002). This framework characterizes the American health care system as comprising the following four levels: the experience of the patient (level A); the functioning of small units of care delivery ("microsystems") (level B); the functioning of the organizations that house or otherwise support the microsystems (level C); and the environment of policy, payment, regulation, accreditation, and professional education (level D) that shapes the behavior, interests, and opportunities of the organizations at level C. Players at the environmental level include legislators, regulators, accreditors, payers, patient safety organizations,[1] and educators. The following recommendation addresses this environmental layer.

---

[1]Patient safety organizations are regulated through the Patient Safety and Quality Improvement Act of 2005 (P.L. 109-41). Broadly, they are organizations separate from health care

Recommendation 7: Oversight and regulatory organizations and payers should use legislation, regulation, accreditation, and payment mechanisms and the media to motivate the adoption of practices and technologies that can reduce medication errors, as well as to ensure that professionals have the competencies required to deliver medications safely.

• Payers and purchasers should continue to motivate improvement in the medication-use process through explicit financial incentives.

• CMS should evaluate a variety of strategies for delivering medication therapy management.

• Regulators, accreditors, and legislators should set minimum functionality standards for error prevention technologies.

• States should enact legislation consistent with and complementary to the Medicare Modernization Act's electronic prescribing provisions and remove existing barriers to such prescribing.

• All state boards of pharmacy should undertake quality improvement initiatives related to community pharmacy practice.

• Medication error reporting should be promoted more aggressively by all stakeholders (with a single national taxonomy used for data storage and analysis).

• Accreditation bodies responsible for the oversight of professional education should require more training in improving medication management practices and clinical pharmacology.

The remainder of this chapter provides a detailed discussion of this recommendation.

GUIDING PRINCIPLES

In developing the above recommendation, the committee took the view that environmental-level stakeholders—legislators, regulators, accreditors, payers, patient safety organizations, and educational accreditors—should:

• Encourage recognition that the use of drugs should take place in a learning environment in which there will always be more to learn about the balance of the effectiveness and safety of drugs in terms of both their intrinsic properties and the ways in which they can be used.

---

providers that collect, manage, and analyze patient safety data and advocate safety improvements on the basis of an analysis of those data.

• Use laws, accreditation practices, payment mechanisms, and the media to foster the safety and quality of medication use.

MOTIVATION FOR PROCESS IMPROVEMENT

Process improvement is primarily the responsibility of providers who must redesign processes at the microsystem level (see Chapter 5). There are, however, key roles in process improvement for legislators, regulators, accreditors, payers, and patient safety organizations.

There are two separate but linked pathways to quality improvement using the measurement of health care performance (see Figure 8-1) (Berwick et al., 2003). Pathway 1 uses performance measurement for accountability purposes—allowing patients, accreditors, and regulators to know how well a particular unit is performing—and for selection purposes—helping patients, referring clinicians, and purchasers decide which providers to use for the services they wish to purchase. Pathway 2 uses performance measurement to design and implement new processes for delivering higher-quality care. The two pathways are linked through the motivation for process

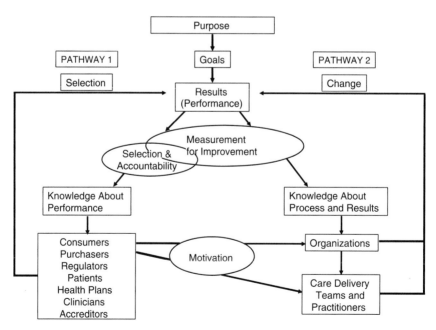

FIGURE 8-1 Two pathways to quality improvement.
SOURCE: Berwick et al., 2003.

improvement (Pathway 2) provided by accountability/selection (Pathway 1). Motivation for process improvement may be influenced by good publicity, higher payments, or access to larger markets.

A number of Pathway 1 motivations relating to medication safety have already been implemented on a trial basis:

• *Public recognition.* Since 1999, the Centers for Medicare and Medicaid Services (CMS) has produced comparative performance reports for Medicare providers. These reports are available online through the CMS website. In Hospital Compare (DHHS, 2005), many of the measures used are medication-related. For heart attack patients, for example, the measures include percent of patients given angiotensin-converting enzyme (ACE) inhibitors, percent given aspirin at arrival, percent given aspirin at discharge, percent given beta-blockers at arrival, percent given beta-blockers at discharge, and percent given thrombolytic medication.

• *Preferred provider status.* The Leapfrog Group (Leapfrog, 2005) is a consortium of buyers of health care. Members have agreed to base their purchase of health care on principles that encourage quality improvement on the part of providers. The Leapfrog Group introduced three safety practices, one of which—the use of computerized provider order entry (CPOE)—directly relates to medication safety; the other two are evidence-based hospital referral and staffing of intensive care units with doctors who have specialized clinical care training. A fourth leap has also been added, consisting of the National Quality Forum's (NQF) 30 safe practices (NQF, 2003), many of which are medication-related.

• *Rewarding investment in information technology.* Bridges to Excellence is an employer-led group aimed at improving the quality of care by recognizing and rewarding health care providers for implementing high-quality care delivery processes (BTE, 2003). For instance, through the Physician Office Link (POL), Bridges to Excellence rewards practices (in specific geographic areas) according to the number of modules implemented from a schedule monitored by the National Committee for Quality Assurance (NCQA, 2004). These include (1) clinical information systems/evidence-based medicine (electronic capabilities for prescriptions and texts, use of electronic systems for prescribing and checking for safety and efficiency, contents of patient information in electronic health records (EHRs), and use of EHRs for decision support), (2) patient education and support, and (3) care management.

• *Pay for performance.* Good performance by hospitals participating in the first year of a joint Premier Inc.–CMS demonstration project (Premier, 2005b) has made hospitals eligible for increased payments of $8.85 million (Premier, 2005a). The initiative covers five conditions (acute myocardial infarction, coronary artery bypass graft, heart failure, community acquired pneumonia, hip and knee replacement) and 34 quality measures, many of which are medication-related (e.g., ACE inhibitors for heart failure, beta-blockers after myocardial infarction).

• *Innovative approaches to improving quality.* Rewarding Results is a joint initiative of The Robert Wood Johnson Foundation and the California HealthCare Foundation, with support from the Commonwealth Fund, administered by the Leapfrog Group (Rewarding Results, 2002). There are seven grantees, including Blue Cross Blue Shield of Michigan, which received a grant to evaluate its hospital incentive program; this program has several elements related to medication safety (BCBS of Michigan, 2002).

Interest in pay for performance is growing. According to a 2004 survey, nearly 100 pay-for-performance initiatives are under way (Baker and Carter, 2005). Many such initiatives, such as Rewarding Results, are currently being evaluated (RWJF, 2005). As yet there is a limited evidence base validating these initiatives. In a 2004 review of the literature sponsored by the Agency for Healthcare Research and Quality (AHRQ), the authors found only nine randomized controlled trials of pay-for-performance initiatives. They concluded there is some evidence supporting the effectiveness of both payment and reputation incentives, but that there is little unequivocal evidence on which to establish quality-based purchasing strategies (Dudley et al., 2004). There are also complex methodological problems to address in evaluating pay-for-performance initiatives. A lengthy editorial in the *Journal of the American Medical Association* has set forth some guidelines for carrying out pay-for-performance research (Dudley, 2005).

Against this backdrop of uncertainties, the committee recommends that payers and purchasers continue to experiment with pay for performance and value-based purchasing to motivate improvement in the medication-use process The Institute of Medicine's (IOM) *Quality Chasm* report drew attention to the disincentives to quality improvement imbedded within current payment approaches (IOM, 2001). The committee believes incentives should be crafted so that the profitability of hospitals, clinics, pharmacies, insurance companies, and manufacturers is aligned with patient safety goals; that is, the incentives should strengthen the business case for quality and safety.

The committee notes that a majority of the pay-for-performance and value-based purchasing initiatives undertaken to date have been for institutional care (for example, hospitals and nursing homes). The committee recommends that such initiatives also be used to foster improvements in the medication-use process in ambulatory care. Such initiatives might incorporate measures from the National Voluntary Consensus Standards for Ambulatory Care, endorsed in late 2005 by the NQF (NQF, 2005b).

The committee recognizes that the successful application of pay-for-performance and value-based purchasing initiatives requires valid and comprehensive patient data. The use of robust EHRs with interoperable data exchange will greatly assist in the implementation of such initiatives.

MEDICATION THERAPY MANAGEMENT

Medication therapy management is a relatively ill-defined set of services aimed at optimizing the outcomes of drug therapy for individual patients. These services can be provided by appropriately qualified health care providers independently or in conjunction with the provision of medications by pharmacists. While the concept of medication therapy management is promising, there is as yet no clear view as to what services should be provided or will be cost-effective.

Experiments with medication therapy management have demonstrated benefits at several levels for diabetes patients. For example, two large self-insured employers in North Carolina compensated pharmacists on a fee-for-service basis for providing advisory services to employees with diabetes mellitus (the Asheville Project). As a result, hemoglobin A1c levels were better controlled, and employers' total mean medical costs decreased by $1,622 per patient to $3,356 per patient per year (Cranor et al., 2003). Both employers have permanently added the benefit to their health plans. Another study examining the impact of pharmacy care services for patients with diabetes also produced good results (Garrett and Bluml, 2005). Over the initial year of the program, patients participating in the study showed significant improvement in clinical indicators and higher rates of self-management. Mean total health costs (including the costs of the medication therapy) were $918 per patient per year less than employers' expected total costs.

Under the new Medicare Part D prescription drug benefit, Medicare beneficiaries who use multiple medications, have multiple chronic conditions, and generate high expenses will be eligible for medication therapy management at no cost. Congress provided the framework for a prescription drug benefit, and CMS is working out the details (Zagaria, 2005). Among other services, medication therapy management may include formulating a medication treatment plan; selecting, initiating, modifying, or administering medication therapy; monitoring and evaluating the patient's response to therapy, including safety and effectiveness; performing comprehensive medication reviews to identify, resolve, and prevent medication-related problems, including adverse drug events (ADEs); providing verbal education and training designed to enhance patient understanding and appropriate use of medications; and coordinating and integrating medication therapy management services within the broader health care–management services being provided to patients (NACDS Foundation, 2005).

The implementation of the Medicare Part D drug benefit offers an opportunity to investigate medication therapy management. The committee recommends that CMS carry out studies on the use of medication therapy management addressing the following issues:

• The specific services that should be provided as part of medication therapy management
• The target populations that would benefit most from these services
• The types of health care personnel that would provide the lowest-cost, highest-value outcomes through these services
• Whether and how medication therapy management should be reimbursed
• How potential savings might be shared between insurers and providers

MINIMUM FUNCTIONALITY STANDARDS FOR INFORMATION TECHNOLOGY

Recent IOM reports have strongly recommended greater use of information technology in the delivery of health care (IOM, 2000, 2001, 2004). A national health information infrastructure—a foundation of systems, technologies, applications, standards, and policies—is required (IOM, 2004). The IOM's report on patient safety (IOM, 2004) called upon the federal government to facilitate the deployment of this infrastructure through the provision of targeted financial support and the ongoing promulgation and maintenance of standards for data needed to improve patient safety. That report also called on health care providers to invest in EHR systems that would enable the provision of safe and effective care and the continuous redesign of care processes to improve patient safety (IOM, 2004).

Less than 1 year after the IOM report *To Err Is Human: Building a Safer Health System* (IOM, 2000) was released, the California legislature enacted Senate Bill 1875, requiring all California hospitals to submit a plan to the Department of Health that would substantially eliminate medication-related errors (SB 1875, 2000). A 2003 analysis of 344 hospital plans revealed that California hospitals were planning on average to implement 2.8 error-reducing technology applications by 2005 (Spurlock et al., 2003). The most frequently cited technology was CPOE (46 percent of hospitals), followed by pharmacy information systems (44 percent), automated dispensing units (38 percent), and electronic medication administration records (31 percent).

In September 2005, an expert panel published estimates of the likely investment by health care providers in EHRs and CPOE systems, based on current trends. The experts projected that in 5 years, 25–38 percent of office practices, 29–41 percent of hospitals, 14 percent of skilled nursing facilities, and 21 percent of home health agencies would have implemented EHRs, and that 21–32 percent of office practices, 26–54 percent of hospitals, and 14 percent of skilled nursing facilities would have implemented CPOE (Kaushal et al., 2005). The committee believes this projected rate of adoption is too slow and that efforts should be made to speed it up.

The committee believes the California legislation discussed above is an important step toward the implementation of technologies for reducing medication errors. The committee believes further that this initiative should be expanded. Accordingly, the committee recommends that regulators, accreditors, and legislators set minimum functionality standards for information technology as conditions of participation, accreditation requirements, and licensing requirements, drawing on existing functionality models for electronic prescribing (to meet the 2010 deadline recommended in Chapter 5), CPOE, and EHRs. Several models exist on which to base these minimum functionality standards:

- The Veterans Health Administration operates one of the largest integrated health information systems in the United States (IOM, 2002). The Veterans Health Information Systems and Technology Architecture (VistA), now known as HealtheVet-VistA, is an EHR system that incorporates CPOE, a clinical ordering and decision-support system providing drug–drug and drug–disease interactions. This system is available as free, public-domain software obtainable under the Freedom of Information Act through e-FOIA at ftp://ftp.va.gov/VistA.[2]

- The Medicare Modernization Act of 2003 mandated that the National Committee on Vital and Health Statistics develop recommendations for uniform standards to enable electronic prescribing in ambulatory care. In a September 2004 letter to the secretary of the Department of Health and Human Services (DHHS), the committee addressed message format standards (NCVHS, 2004); in a March 2005 letter, the committee addressed electronic signatures and other issues (NCVHS, 2005).

- An eHealthInitiative report (eHI, 2004) and several journal articles have outlined functionality standards for electronic prescribing/clinical decision support (Bates et al., 2003; Bell et al., 2004; Teich et al., 2005). The Leapfrog Group, with support from the California Health Care Foundation and The Robert Wood Johnson Foundation, is also active in promoting standards for CPOE (Metzger and Turisco, 2001; Forester et al., 2003), including electronic prescribing in ambulatory care (Classen, 2005).

---

[2]The Healthe Vet-*VistA* system may also be obtained on DVD from the following address: Department of Veterans Affairs, VHA Office of Information Field Office, ATTN: National Help Desk (FOIA Request), 3701 Loop Road East, Building 40, Tuscaloosa, AL 35404.

- The IOM's report on patient safety (IOM, 2004: Appendix E) proposed a set of functionality standards for EHRs in hospitals, nursing homes, and ambulatory care and for the personal health record. These standards were used as input to Health Level 7's Electronic Health Record Functional Model (HL7, 2005).

STATE ELECTRONIC PRESCRIBING LAWS

In November 2001, the California Healthcare Foundation published a report on electronic prescribing that described a patchwork of laws governing the practice; for example, 11 states prohibited electronic prescribing by both in-state and out-of-state providers, and only 4 states allowed it with the exception of certain drug types (e.g., controlled drugs) (Kilbridge and Gladysheva, 2001). Laws in many more states are now favorable to electronic prescribing. By 2004, 43 states allowed prescriber-to-pharmacy electronic medication orders (NABP, 2004). Allowing electronic connectivity is not enough, however; some states require dispense-as-written requirements that cannot be met using electronic technologies.

In November 2005, CMS issued the final rule for electronic prescribing of drugs covered under Medicare Part D. This rule contains a preemption covering state laws that prohibit electronic prescribing; that prohibit the transmission of electronic prescriptions through intermediaries; that require certain language to be used, such as "dispense as written," to indicate whether generic drugs may or may not be substituted; and that require handwritten signatures or other handwriting on prescriptions (FR, 2005). As the rule is currently drafted, the scope of preemption includes electronic prescribing for Part D–eligible individuals (whether or not they are enrolled in a Part D plan) for drugs that may be covered by Part D in at least some circumstances (FR, 2005). Thus the preemption does not cover electronic prescribing for those under 65 and for controlled substances.

The Medicare preemption would create different rules for Medicare and other payers—which would be costly for prescribers, pharmacies, and plans to address and administer—and limit the uptake of electronic prescribing. Hence, states should enact legislation consistent with and complementary to the Medicare Modernization Act's electronic prescribing provisions and remove existing barriers to the practice. The DHHS and the Drug Enforcement Administration are working on ways to enable electronic prescribing to encompass controlled substances, an effort the committee believes to be important.

STATE PHARMACY BOARDS

With a few exceptions, there is currently little or no oversight of community pharmacies related to medication safety. State boards do send surveyors out, but they may or may not be pharmacists. What they look for are issues related to state practice acts; there is no focus on the types of issues that parallel the requirements hospital pharmacies must meet under the National Patient Safety Goals of the Joint Commission on Accreditation of Healthcare Organizations (JCAHO) (JCAHO, 2005) or accreditation requirements for medication management systems (Rich, 2004).

In the community pharmacy setting, there is little understanding of error rates; for example, the committee could find only one study (Flynn et al., 2003) on error rates when medications are refilled. In addition, much greater focus is needed on error prevention strategies. The committee believes state boards should assume a larger role in learning from errors and sharing lessons learned with all pharmacies while avoiding punitive measures in response to reported errors.

A small number of states have developed medication safety initiatives (NABP, 2004). In 2001, in response to medication error rates and medication distribution issues, the Massachusetts Board of Registration in Pharmacy issued a set of best-practice recommendations as standards of professional practice to be considered for implementation as appropriate by all pharmacies (MBRP, 2005b), For example, the first recommendation calls for incident reports to be completed and submitted to the United States Pharmacopeia (USP)–Institute for Safe Medication Practices (ISMP) Medication Errors Reporting Program (MERP). These recommendations were followed up in January 2005 with regulations that require all pharmacies to establish continuous quality improvement programs by the end of 2005 (MBRP, 2005a). To aid in this process, a quality improvement specialist is available to advise individual pharmacies. Based on errors reported by consumers to the board, this specialist can give advice proactively to individual pharmacies and in certain situations visit pharmacies to review progress.

Another important initiative is requiring continuing education on the topic of medication errors. The state board of New York has implemented such a requirement, and Pennsylvania will do so soon. New Mexico is one of a few states that require dispensing errors associated with ADEs to be reported to the board. The New Mexico Board of Pharmacy is also active in providing information about preventing medication errors through its website (NMBP, 2005).

The committee recommends that all state boards of pharmacy implement quality improvement programs. In particular, the committee recommends that each state convene a voluntary panel of pharmacists (including a state board member and representatives of hospitals, the community, and consumers) to review major quality and safety issues associated with medication dispensing. These issues could be derived from reviews of error reports. Information about error prevention measures provided by patient safety organizations could be shared, as well as any reports from state reporting programs, recognizing that much can be learned from efforts in other states and through national programs. The panel should focus on errors that are most serious and most likely to occur, and review all available information on the chosen topics. After consulting with experts and patient safety organizations, as appropriate, the panel should publish its findings in the state newsletter and ask for voluntary compliance with new procedures (although oversight by means of surveying would be better), and perhaps make recommendations to the state board for regulatory changes.

Quality improvement programs might also include approaches similar to those adopted in Massachusetts: requiring all pharmacists and pharmacy technicians to take a few continuing education credits specifically directed at medication error issues, distributing information about good practice and recent examples of hazardous situations through a regular newsletter, and informing patients that complaints regarding medication errors can be directed to state boards.

The funding of a quality improvement program may be difficult for many state pharmacy boards. The committee believes Congress should fund a study on the development and funding of a national medication error prevention effort in community pharmacies, coordinated by state pharmacy boards.

REPORTING PROGRAMS FOR MEDICATION ERRORS/ADVERSE DRUG EVENTS

In Chapter 2, external and internal error reporting programs were discussed briefly, while the committee's recommendations for internal monitoring programs were presented in Chapter 5. This section addresses the committee's recommendations for external reporting programs.

Ways to Encourage Reporting

Generally, rates of reporting of errors and hazardous situations to external programs have been low (Leape, 2002). Although it may take only a few reports to raise awareness about a hazardous condition that requires immediate attention, errors need to be reported and analyzed if improvements in care are to be effected. Accordingly, the committee recommends that medication error and ADE reporting both internally and to external programs be promoted by care providers, accreditation agencies, state professional boards, and the relevant state and federal agencies.

Reporting programs are the primary means of providing early warnings of new types of errors, errors at the interfaces between care providers, and errors in care settings without EHRs (the majority of care settings today) or settings that may never have EHRs (for example, the home). Voluntary reporting to an external program is often the only way providers can effect change outside their organization. Computerized analysis of patient records using a database trigger system (see Chapter 5) will be an important way of identifying many medication errors, but will not eliminate the need for reporting programs.

Legal impediments likely represent one key barrier to external reporting. The signing into law of the Patient Safety and Quality Improvement Act of 2005 (P.L. 109-41), which contains legal liability protections related to reporting, should encourage more reporting. The legislation calls for the establishment of patient safety organizations that will receive confidential patient safety data, including error reports; analyze the data; and disseminate recommendations for ways to reduce the risk of errors. The information provided to patient safety organizations will not be usable as evidence in the event of civil or administrative legal proceedings. Work is currently under way on defining the certification process for patient safety organizations.

Given the sometimes negative attitudes toward reporting of errors, multiple channels of reporting should be encouraged. Some systems will accept the simplest form of reporting, such as a narrative of the event delivered orally or in written form, while others will require a narrative plus structured data items using a computer system. For the latter, a single national taxonomy should be agreed upon and used.

A National Taxonomy: Better Coordination of Reporting Programs

In an institutional setting, reports are often funneled through a patient safety office that provides multiple outputs to local institutions (e.g., hospital systems), state reporting systems, federal systems (e.g., MedWatch), and proprietary programs (e.g., USP MedMarx, University Hospital Consortium Patient Safety Net) as appropriate. A national taxonomy with sufficient granularity would facilitate reporting to multiple programs.

The committee believes better coordination of all reporting systems is needed. Regulation of drugs is done at the federal level through the Food and Drug Administration (FDA), yet many of the reporting systems are implemented at the state level, with great variability in the incidents that must be reported and the data collected for each incident. There is a need for greater uniformity among state-based and other systems so the data can be aggregated to aid in shaping health policy. The use of a national taxonomy by all reporting systems would greatly facilitate such coordination. Using a single taxonomy would also enable databases to merge for datamining purposes. The difficulty of developing a single taxonomy is illustrated by the experience of a nursing faculty member at MD Anderson, who studied 50 different incident reporting systems and found 856 different data fields (Personal communication, Deborah Simmons, October 6, 2005). Further, the development of a consistent taxonomy for patient safety is a critical bottleneck affecting the rapidity with which automated safety surveillance systems can be deployed.

The past few years have seen significant progress toward the establishment of a national taxonomy for patient safety. As noted in Chapter 7, JCAHO has taken a leadership role in the development of such a taxonomy (Chang et al., 2005). The goals of this effort are to promote a national reporting system for adverse events through the use of a standardized patient safety taxonomy and ontology. The Patient Safety Event Taxonomy (PSET) developed by JCAHO (and approved by NQF in August 2005) combines and classifies data from disparate reporting systems to facilitate comparisons across hospitals (NQF, 2005a). The second application developed under the study is the Hospital Incident Reporting Ontology (HIRO), which examines the relationships among the variables collected and classified by the PSET to facilitate data mining and sharing of patient safety data among hospitals. Lessons learned during the study will be disseminated to the health care community (http://wwwcf.nlm.nih.gov/hsr_project/view_ hsrproj_record.cfm?PROGRAM_CAME=search_fields.cfm&NLMUNI QUE_ ID= 20051166&SEARCH_FOR=reporting).

The IOM report on patient safety (IOM, 2004) described the need for a common patient safety reporting format, as well as the minimum data that should be collected in a standard report. The domain areas described include the following:

- The discovery
- The event itself
- A narrative of the event, including contributing factors
- Ancillary information
- Detailed causal analysis
- Lessons learned

Under the Patient Safety and Quality Improvement Act of 2005 (P.L. 109-41), the Secretary of the DHHS may determine common formats for reporting to and among a network of patient safety databases. Consideration should also be given to using the World Health Organization's Draft Guidelines for Adverse Event Reporting and Learning Systems, which are designed to promote an international reporting system (WHO, 2005).

Reporting of Practice-Related Errors

Practice-related reports make up a minority of the reports in MedWatch, an FDA system focused on ADEs. These practice-related error reports are an important resource but are difficult to retrieve for those outside the FDA. A Freedom of Information Act request may be filed, but without knowing the nature of the reports, it is difficult to know what needs to be retrieved. Moreover, the retrieval process may take several months to complete. The committee believes it might be more conducive to learning if practice-related medication errors were reported initially to USP or ISMP-MERP, which would automatically pass all such error reports on to the FDA MedWatch program.

Administrative Databases

Until the widespread implementation of EHRs is realized, the committee believes claims databases should continue to be used for pay-for-performance, accountability reporting, and policy development purposes. The addition of diagnostic test results to administrative data will expand the range of possible quality measurement. For example, it will be possible to use Health Plan Employer Data and Information Set (HEDIS) measures for glycemic control and for achievement of goals for reducing LDL (low-density lipoprotein) cholesterol.

In testimony to the Senate Finance Committee in July 2005 (MedPAC, 2005), MedPAC stated that claims data are an important source for assessing the performance of providers of Medicare services. MedPAC recommended that the information on claims forms be expanded. Measurement of the rate of adverse events in hospitals would require information on the conditions present in the patient on arrival at the hospital. In the ambulatory setting, claims data would be an even better source for quality measures if they could be linked to prescription data from the Medicare Part D program (when available) and laboratory data.

Data from the Part D program also have the potential to be a useful resource for understanding and preventing medication errors, especially for medication use by the elderly and the chronically ill (Platt and Ommaya, 2005). These data will be more valuable still if Medicare drug claims can be linked with diagnosis and procedure claims, as has been proposed by CMS (CMS, 2005). Such linked databases would help provide evidence on the occurrence of ADEs and the costs of such events.

Reporting Back

Reporting programs should provide feedback locally to reporters to the extent possible. Similarly, state- and federally based databases that aggregate and analyze these data should regularly provide feedback to health care practitioners, health care organizations, industry, and policy makers. Providing feedback is often a challenge as there may be only a small number of reported events, the programs may lack the resources to carry out the analyses, and user-friendly reporting formats are difficult to craft. In this regard, in 2005 the National Academy for State Health Policy produced some important guidance on how state adverse event data can be used to improve patient safety (Rosenthal and Booth, 2005).

The ideal reporting system would facilitate widespread access to the databases to speed improvement in the accuracy of medication prescribing, dispensing, and administration processes. An individual health care professional should eventually be able to review errors and effective preventive actions by searching the Internet.

WORKFORCE DEVELOPMENT AND RETOOLING

The training of health care professionals addresses medication safety insufficiently, despite frequent recommendations to increase the emphasis on medication safety in training programs (HRSA, 2000; IOM, 2000, 2003; AAMC, 2003). In an interview coinciding with the fifth anniversary of the release of the IOM's *To Err Is Human* report (IOM, 2000), Timothy Flaherty, MD, chairman of the board of the National Patient Safety Foundation, commented that medical education is an area in which patient safety has seen no dramatic improvements (NPSF, 2004).

A 2000 survey of U.S. internal medicine clerkships and internal medicine residency programs for third-year medical students found that little or none of the curriculum had been dedicated to clinical pharmacology during medical school, and only modest amounts during internal medicine resident training (Rosebraugh et al., 2002). The committee is very concerned about this low level of training in clinical pharmacology given the amount of medication prescribing in clinical practice. A 2001 survey of schools of pharmacy in the United States found that the quality and quantity of instruction in medication errors varied significantly, and that key domains of knowledge were lacking in some programs (Johnson et al., 2002). A small survey of the state members of the National Council of State Boards of Nursing revealed that nursing education programs are required by most states to include generic content on medication administration safety, but only one state (Florida) mandates continuing nursing education specifically focused on medication errors (Personal communication, Kathleen Stevens, EdD, RN, December 6, 2005).

Within individual institutions, considerable variability can be found across the various professional schools. Prior to the introduction of an interprofessional patient safety course at Creighton University (Galt et al., in press), for example, the patient safety materials already included in the curriculum for each of the health professions (nursing, medicine, pharmacy, physical therapy, and dentistry) were narrowly focused and integrated into other courses. Further, despite the recognition that interprofessional collaboration is a major element in the delivery of quality care (IOM, 2001), there is limited interprofessional education related to patient safety (Mitchell et al., 2005).

A number of institutions are beginning to offer courses in medication/patient safety:

• The Faculty Leadership in Interprofessional Education to Promote Patient Safety project created a patient safety–oriented curriculum for the training of health profession faculty leaders (Mitchell et al., 2005).
• Creighton University has an interprofessional patient safety course available for students in business, law, social work, medicine, pharmacy, physical therapy, occupational therapy, nursing, and dentistry (Creighton, 2005).
• The British Pharmacological Society's Clinical Section Committee has developed a core curriculum for the teaching of safe and effective prescribing in U.K. medical schools (Maxwell and Walley, 2003).
• With the help of a grant from AHRQ, a continuing education curriculum in ambulatory care aimed at advancing patient safety and incorporating a medication errors module was developed (Mottur-Pilson, 2005).
• The University of Wisconsin-Madison Center, again with funding from AHRQ, has developed a graduate certificate in patient safety (BT Karsh). The certificate requires five courses (including a mandatory course on medication-use safety), a patient safety practicum, and a series of seminars by guest lecturers.
• Through a grant from AHRQ, the National Patient Safety Foundation partnered with the Medical College of Wisconsin to develop web-based educational patient safety materials for physicians, nurses, and patients (Hendee et al., 2005; NPSF, 2005).

Other sources of educational material are the Centers for Education and Research on Therapeutics, a research program administered by AHRQ in consultation with the FDA and agencies within DHHS. The mission of the Centers for Education and Research on Therapeutics is to conduct research and provide education that will advance the optimal use of drugs, medical devices, and biological products. In early 2006, four more centers, including one devoted to consumer use of medication, were added to the network (CERTS, 2006).

Finally, regarding the use of information technology systems to improve medication safety, a joint American Health Information Management Association/American Medical Informatics Association report has pointed out that no systematic plan exists for training the current health care workforce to use information technology tools to do their jobs (AHIMA/AMIA, 2006). This report called on the health care industry to educate its employees at all levels that information technology is an integral part of health care work. To address this challenge, the American Medical Informatics Association announced its 10-by-10 program, which aims to realize a goal of training 10,000 health care professionals, especially in applied clinical informatics, by the year 2010 (AMIA, 2005).

The committee recommends that the relevant accreditation organizations—the Liaison Committee on Medical Education, Accreditation Council for Graduate Medical Education, Accreditation Council for Continuing Medical Education, Accreditation Council for Pharmacy Education, American Society of Health-System Pharmacists, National League for Nursing Accrediting Commission, and Commission on Collegiate Nursing Education—ensure that the curricula of undergraduate and graduate pharmacy, nursing, and medical schools and continuing education include:

- Appropriate medication safety modules to cover an overview of the system for drug development, regulation, distribution, and use; an understanding of where medication errors can take place; the need to monitor continuously for medication errors; how to recognize medication errors and the tools for identifying such errors; what to do once a medication error has been found; reporting and analysis of medication errors; and ways of improving the safety of the medication-use process.
- Appropriate clinical pharmacology training commensurate with the amount of medication prescribing in clinical practice.
- Training in the delivery of patient-centered care and the use of information technology tools to enable implementation of the recommendations presented in Chapters 4 and 5.

REFERENCES

AAMC (Association of American Medical Colleges). 2003. *Patient Safety and Graduate Medical Education.* Washington, DC: AAMC.

AHIMA/AMIA (American Health Information Management Association/American Medical Informatics Association). 2006. *Building the Work Force for Health Information Transformation.* Chicago, IL: AHIMA and Bethesda, MD: AMIA.

AMIA (American Medical Informatics Association). 2005. *Training Health Care Professionals to Serve as Local Informatics Leaders and Champions,* 2005. [Online]. Available: http://www.amia.org/10x10 [accessed May 7, 2006].

Baker G, Carter B. 2005. *Provider Pay-for-Performance Incentive Programs: 2004 National Study Results.* San Francisco, CA: Med-Vantage.

Bates DW, Kuperman GJ, Wang S, Gandhi T, Kittler A, Volk L, Spurr C, Khorasani R, Tanasijevic M, Middleton B. 2003. Ten commandments for effective clinical decision support: Making the practice of evidence-based medicine a reality. *Journal of the American Medical Informatics Association* 10(6):523–530.

BCBS of Michigan. 2002. *Rewarding Results Grantees: Blue Cross Blue Shield of Michigan.* [Online]. Available: http://www.leapfroggroup.org/RewardingResults/bcbsmi.htm [accessed October 30, 2005].

Bell DS, Cretin S, Marken BS, Landman AB. 2004. A conceptual framework for evaluating outpatient electronic prescribing systems based on their functional capabilities. *Journal of the American Medical Informatics Association* 11(1):60–70.

Berwick DM. 2002. A user's manual for the IOM's "Quality Chasm" report. *Health Affairs (Millwood)* 21(3):80–90.

Berwick DM, James B, Coye MJ. 2003. Connections between quality measurement and improvement. *Medical Care* 41(Suppl. 1):130–138.

BTE (Bridges to Excellence). 2003. *Bridges to Excellence: Rewarding Quality Across the Healthcare System.* [Online]. Available: http://www.bridgestoexcellence.org/bte [accessed October 30, 2005].

CERTS (Centers for Education and Research on Therapeutics). 2006. *AHRQ Expands Therapeutics Education and Research Network to Focus on Critical Issues Facing the Health Care System.* [Online]. Available: http://www.certs.hhs.gov/whats_new/archive/2006/20060425_01.html [accessed May 7, 2006].

Chang A, Schyve PM, Croteau DJ, O'Leary DS, Loeb JM. 2005. The JCAHO patient safety event taxonomy: A standardized terminology and classification schema for near misses and adverse events. *International Journal for Quality in Health Care* 17(2):95–105.

Classen D. 2005. A national standard for medication use. In: *Building a Better Delivery System: A New Engineering/Health Care Partnership*, NAE/IOM. Washington, DC: The National Academies Press.

CMS (Centers for Medicare and Medicaid Services). 2005. *Medicare Prescription Drug Data Strategy: Improving Evidence for Patient Care Through the Medicare Prescription Drug Benefit.* Washington, DC: Department of Health and Human Services.

Cranor CW, Bunting BA, Christensen DB. 2003. The Asheville Project: Long-term clinical and economic outcomes of a community pharmacy diabetes care program. *Journal of the American Pharmaceutical Association* 43(2):173–184.

Creighton. 2005. *Interprofessional IPE 410 Foundations in Patient Safety.* [Online]. Available: http://www.creighton.edu/ipe/ptsafetyspring05.htm [accessed November 2, 2005].

DHHS (U.S. Department of Health and Human Services). 2005. *Hospital Compare.* [Online]. Available: http://www.hospitalcompare.hhs.gov [accessed October 17, 2005].

Dudley RA. 2005. Pay-for-performance research: How to learn what clinicians and policy makers need to know. *Journal of the American Medical Association* 294(14):1821–1823.

Dudley RA, Frolich A, Robinowitz DL, Talavera JA, Broadhead P, Luft HS. 2004. *Strategies to Support Quality-Based Purchasing: A Review of the Evidence.* Rockville, MD: Agency for Healthcare Research and Quality.

eHI (eHealth Initiative). 2004. *Electronic Prescribing: Toward Maximum Value and Rapid Adoption.* Washington, DC: eHI.

Flynn EA, Barker KN, Carnahan BJ. 2003. National observational study of prescription dispensing accuracy and safety in 50 pharmacies. *Journal of the American Pharmaceutical Association* 43(2):191–200.

Forester AJ, Murff HJ, Peterson JF, Gandhi TK, Bates DW. 2003. The incidence and severity of adverse events affecting patients after discharge from the hospital. *Annals of Internal Medicine* 138(3):161–167.

FR (Federal Register). 2005. *Department of Health and Human Services: Centers for Medicare and Medicaid Services: 42 CFR Part 423: Medicare Program; E-Prescribing and Prescription Drug Program; Final Rule.* Washington, DC: National Archives and Records Administration.

Galt KA, O'Brien R, Paschal K, Clark B, Bramble JD, Gleason J, McQuillan R, Graves J, Harris B, Hoidal P, Mahern C, Mu K, Rule A, Scheirton L, Gerardi D, Sonnino R, Bradberry JC. In press. Description and evaluation of an interprofessional patient safety course for health professions and related sciences students. *Journal of Patient Safety.*

Garrett DG, Bluml BM. 2005. Patient self-management program for diabetes: First-year clinical, humanistic, and economic outcomes. *Journal of the American Pharmaceutical Association* 45(2):130–137.

Hendee WR, Keating-Christensen C, Loh YH. 2005. Development of a patient safety web-based education curriculum for physicians, nurses, and patients. *Journal of Patient Safety* 1(2):90–99.

HL7 (Health Level 7). 2005. *HL7 Electronic Health Record (EHR) Technical Committee's Home Page.* [Online]. Available: http://www.hl7.org/ehr [accessed October 16, 2005].

HRSA (Health Resources and Services Administration). 2000. *Collaborative Education to Ensure Patient Safety: Council on Graduate Medical Education and National Advisory Council on Nurse Education and Practice.* Washington, DC: DHHS.

IOM (Institute of Medicine). 2000. *To Err Is Human: Building a Safer Health System.* Washington, DC: National Academy Press.

IOM. 2001. *Crossing the Quality Chasm: A New Health System for the 21st Century.* Washington, DC: National Academy Press.

IOM. 2002. *Leadership by Example: Coordinating Government Roles in Improving Health Care Quality.* Washington, DC: The National Academies Press.

IOM. 2003. *Health Professions Education: A Bridge to Quality.* Washington, DC: The National Academies Press.

IOM. 2004. *Patient Safety: Achieving a New Standard for Care.* Washington, DC: The National Academies Press.

JCAHO (Joint Commission on Accreditation of Healthcare Organizations). 2005. *2006 Critical Access Hospital and Hospital National Patient Safety Goals.* [Online]. Available: http://www.jcipatientsafety.org/show.asp?durki=10293&site=164&return=10289 [accessed August 22, 2005].

Johnson MS, Latif DA, Gordon B. 2002. Medication error instruction in schools of pharmacy curricula: A descriptive study. *American Journal of Pharmaceutical Education* 66:364–371.

Kaushal R, Bates DW, Poon EG, Jha AK, Blumenthal D. 2005. Functional gaps in attaining a national health information network. *Health Affairs (Millwood)* 24(5):1281–1289.

Kilbridge P, Gladysheva K. 2001. *E-Prescribing.* Oakland, CA: California HealthCare Foundation.

Leape LL. 2002. Reporting of adverse events. *New England Journal of Medicine* 347(20): 1633–1638.

Leapfrog. 2005. *The Leapfrog Group Fact Sheet.* [Online]. Available: http://www.leapfrog group.org/about_us/leapfrog-factsheet [accessed October 17, 2005].

Maxwell S, Walley T. 2003. Teaching safe and effective prescribing in UK medical schools: A core curriculum for tomorrow's doctors. *British Journal of Clinical Pharmacology* 55(6): 496–503.

MBRP (Massachusetts Board of Registration in Pharmacy). 2005a. *April Newsletter: Item 5. The Board Adopts New Regulations to Improve Patient Outcomes.* Boston, MA: MBRP.

MBRP. 2005b. *Massachusetts Board of Registration in Pharmacy.* [Online]. Available: http://www. mass.gov/dpl/boards/ph/cmr/24175.htm [accessed January 10, 2006].

MedPAC (Medicare Payment Advisory Commission). 2005. *Testimony: Pay for Performance in Medicare (July 27, 2005). U.S. Senate, Committee on Finance.* [Online]. Available: http://www.medpac.gov/publications/generic_report_display.cfm?report_type_id= 2&sid=2&subid=0 [accessed October 17, 2005].

Metzger J, Turisco F. 2001. *Computerized Physician Order Entry: A Look at the Vendor Marketplace and Getting Started.* Washington, DC: The Leapfrog Group.

Mitchell PH, Robins LS, Schaad D. 2005. Creating a curriculum for training health profession faculty leaders. In: Henrikson K, Battles JB, Marks ES, Lewin DI, eds. *Advances in Patient Safety: From Research to Implementation.* Rockville, MD: Agency for Healthcare Research and Quality.

Mottur-Pilson C. 2005. An ambulatory care curriculum for advancing patient safety. In: Henrikson K, Battles JB, Marks ES, Lewin DI, eds. *Advances in Patient Safety: From Research to Implementation*. Rockville, MD: Agency for Healthcare Research and Quality.

NABP (National Association of Boards of Pharmacy). 2004. *Survey of Pharmacy Law*. Mount Pleasant, IL: NABP.

NACDS Foundation (National Association of Chain Drug Stores Foundation). 2005. *National Association of Chain Drug Stores Foundation: Medication Therapy Management in Community Pharmacy Practice*. [Online]. Available: http://www.nacdsfoundation.org/user-assets/Documents/PDF/MTM%20Model%20final.pdf [accessed November 13, 2005].

NCQA (National Committee for Quality Assurance). 2004. *Bridges to Excellence: Physician Office Link*. [Online]. Available: http://www.ncqa.org/pol [accessed October 17, 2005].

NCVHS (National Committee on Vital and Health Statistics). 2004. *Letter to Secretary Thompson at DHHS, September 2, 2004*. [Online]. Available: http://www.ncvhs.hhs.gov/040902lt2.htm [accessed October 30, 2005].

NCVHS. 2005. *Letter to Secretary Leavitt at DHHS, March 4, 2005*. [Online]. Available: http://www.ncvhs.hhs.gov [accessed October 30, 2005].

NMBP (New Mexico Board of Pharmacy). 2005. *New Mexico Board of Pharmacy: Adverse Drug Events and Medication Errors*. [Online]. Available: http://www.state.nm.us/pharmacy [accessed January 10, 2006].

NPSF (National Patient Safety Foundation). 2004. *Focus on Patient Safety Newsletter. Vol. 7, No. 3. Five Years After To Err Is Human: A Look at the Patient Safety Landscape*. [Online]. Available: http://www.npsf.org/html/Focus.html [accessed October 13, 2005].

NPSF. 2005. *National Patient Safety Foundation: Patient Safety Programs and Opportunities*. [Online]. Available: http://www.npsf.org/html/programs.html [accessed November 2, 2005].

NQF (National Quality Forum). 2003. *Safe Practices for Better Healthcare: A Consensus Report*. Washington, DC: NQF.

NQF. 2005a. *National Quality Forum Endorses Voluntary Consensus Standard for Standardizing a Patient Safety Taxonomy. August 3, 2005*. [Online]. Available: http://www.qualityforum.org/news/home.htm [accessed November 26, 2005].

NQF. 2005b. *NQF Endorses Additional Voluntary Consensus Standards for Standardizing Measures of Physician-Focused Ambulatory Care. October 11, 2005*. [Online]. Available: http://www.qualityforum.org/news/home.htm [accessed November 26, 2005].

Platt R, Ommaya A. 2005. A beneficial side effect of the Medicare drug benefit. *New England Journal of Medicine* 353(26):2742–2743.

Premier. 2005a. *CMS/Premier Pay-for-Performance Model Produces Remarkable Quality Improvements Among Nation's Hospitals*. [Online]. Available: http://www.premierinc.com/all/newsroom/press-releases/05-nov/cms-pay-for-performance-year-one-results.jsp [accessed November 26, 2005].

Premier. 2005b. *HQI Demonstration Overview*. [Online]. Available: http://www.premierinc.com/all/quality/hqi/index.jsp [accessed October 17, 2005].

Rewarding Results. 2002. *Rewarding Results: About the Program*. [Online]. Available: http://www.leapfroggroup.org/RewardingResults/about.htm [accessed October 30, 2005].

Rich DS. 2004. New JCAHO medication management standards for 2004. *American Journal of Health-System Pharmacy* 61(13):1349–1358.

Rosebraugh CJ, Honig PK, Yasuda SU, Pezzullo JC, Woosley RL. 2002. Centers for education and research on therapeutics report: Survey of medication errors education during undergraduate and graduate medical education in the United States. *Clinical Pharmacology and Therapeutics* 71(1):4–10.

Rosenthal J, Booth M. 2005. *Maximizing the Use of State Adverse Event Data to Improve Patient Safety*. Portland, ME: National Academy for State Health Policy.

RWJF (Robert Wood Johnson Foundation). 2005. *Robert Wood Johnson Foundation: Evaluation of the Rewarding Results Program.* [Online]. Available: http://www.rwjf.org/research/researchdetail.jsp?id=2154&ia=142 [accessed October 30, 2005].

SB 1875 (Senate Bill 1975). 2000. *California Senate Bill 1875.* [Online]. Available: http://info.sen.ca.gov/pub/99-00/bill/sen/sb_1851-1900/sb_1875_bill_20000928_chaptered.html [accessed October 30, 2005].

Spurlock B, Nelson M, Paterno J, Tandel S. 2003. *Legislating Medication Safety: The California Experience.* Oakland, CA: California Healthcare Foundation.

Teich JM, Osheroff JA, Pifer EA, Sittig DF, Jenders RA, The CDS Expert Review Panel. 2005. Clinical decision support in electronic prescribing: Recommendations and an action plan: Report of the joint clinical decision support workgroup. *Journal of the American Medical Informatics Association* 12(4):365–376.

WHO (World Health Organization). 2005. *World Alliance for Patient Safety: WHO Draft Guidelines for Adverse Event Reporting and Learning Systems.* Geneva, Switzerland: WHO.

Zagaria ME. 2005. Senior care: Medication therapy management services. *U.S. Pharmacist* 4:35–42.

A

Biographical Sketches of Committee Members

J. Lyle Bootman, Ph.D., Sc.D., *Cochair,* is dean and professor at the University of Arizona College of Pharmacy. He is the founding and executive director of the University of Arizona Center for Health Outcomes and PharmacoEconomic (HOPE) Research, one of the first such centers developed in the world. Dr. Bootman also holds a joint appointment as professor in both the College of Medicine and the College of Public Health. He is former president of the American Pharmaceutical Association. He received his pharmacy education at the University of Arizona and his doctorate at the University of Minnesota. Additionally, he completed a clinical pharmacy residency at the National Institutes of Health. Dr. Bootman has received numerous outstanding achievement awards, most notably from the American Association of Pharmaceutical Scientists and the American Pharmaceutical Association. He has published several books, including the first text introducing the principles of pharmacoeconomics, which is used in more than 35 countries and translated into six languages. His research regarding the outcomes of drug-related morbidity and mortality has received worldwide attention by the professional and public media. Dr. Bootman is a member of the Institute of Medicine (IOM).

Linda R. Cronenwett, Ph.D., M.A., R.N., *Cochair,* is dean and professor of the School of Nursing, University of North Carolina (UNC) at Chapel Hill, and associate chief nursing officer for Academic Affairs at the University of North Carolina Hospitals. She is a member of the board of directors of the Institute for Healthcare Improvement and The Robert Wood Johnson Foundation's Transforming Care at the Bedside National Advisory Committee. Dr. Cronenwett earned her master's degree in nursing from the University of Washington and her undergraduate and doctoral degrees from the University of Michigan. Prior to her appointment as dean, she was Sarah Frances Russell Distinguished Professor of Nursing Systems at UNC-Chapel Hill. Dr. Cronenwett is an elected fellow of the American Academy of Nursing and the National Academies of Practice. She served the scientific community as a member of the Nursing Research Study Section and subsequently as a member of the National Advisory Council for Nursing Research at the National Institutes of Health. She has served on the editorial advisory boards of *Applied Nursing Research*, the *Online Journal of Knowledge Synthesis for Nursing*, the *Journal of Nursing Measurement*, and the *Joint Commission Journal on Quality Improvement*. She has held numerous offices in professional associations, including president of the New Hampshire Nurses Association and chair of the American Nurses Association's Congress of Nursing Practice. She is currently principal investigator for a national initiative, Quality and Safety Education for Nurses, funded by The Robert Wood Johnson Foundation. Through organizational initiatives, she provides leadership for efforts to improve health care education to ensure that future health professionals will be committed to and capable of creating and constantly improving the safety and quality of the health care delivery systems in which they work.

David W. Bates, M.D., M.Sc., is chief of the Division of Internal Medicine at the Brigham and Women's Hospital in Boston, Massachusetts, and a professor at Harvard Medical School and the Harvard School of Public Health, where he is codirector of the Program in Clinical Effectiveness. He is also the medical director of clinical and quality analysis for Partner's Healthcare Systems, where he evaluates the impact of information systems across the Partner's network. Dr. Bates' primary interest has been the use of computer systems to improve care, and he has conducted extensive work on evaluating the incidence and preventability of adverse drug events. At the national level, Dr. Bates is chair of the National Alliance for Primary Care Informatics, and he served as one of two science advisors to the SCRIPT project, which developed medication indicators for the Centers for Medicare and Medicaid Services (CMS). In addition, he serves as an advisor to the Leapfrog Group on computerized order entry and is the editor of the *Journal of Clinical Outcomes Management*. Dr. Bates received his M.D. from The Johns Hopkins University School of Medicine in 1983; in 1990, he received his M.Sc. from the Harvard School of Public Health. Dr. Bates is a practicing, board-certified physician in internal medicine.

Robert M. Califf, M.D., is associate vice chancellor for clinical research; director of the Duke Clinical Research Institute (DCRI); and professor of medicine, Division of Cardiology, at the Duke University Medical Center, Durham, North Carolina. He has served as an editor of landmark textbooks on cardiovascular medicine and has been an author or coauthor of more than 650 peer-reviewed journal articles. Dr. Califf has led the DCRI efforts for many of the best-known clinical trials in cardiovascular disease. He is considered an international leader in the fields of health outcomes, quality of care, and medical economics. Additionally, he has served on the Cardiorenal Advisory Panel of the U.S. Food and Drug Administration (FDA) and the Pharmaceutical Roundtable of the IOM. He also served on the IOM committee that recommended Medicare coverage of clinical trials, and he is director of the coordinating center for the Centers for Education & Research on Therapeutics (CERTs), a public–private partnership among the Agency for Healthcare Research and Quality, the FDA, academia, the medical products industry, and consumer groups. This partnership focuses on research and education that will advance the best use of medical products. Dr. Califf graduated from Duke University in 1973 and from Duke University Medical School in 1978. He performed his internship and residency at the University of California at San Francisco and his fellowship in Cardiology at Duke University. He is board-certified in internal medicine (1984) and cardiology (1986) and is a fellow of the American College of Cardiology (1988).

H. Eric Cannon, Pharm.D., is director of pharmacy services and health and wellness at IHC Health Plans, a division of Intermountain Health Care in Salt Lake City, Utah. IHC is an integrated health care system with 20 hospitals, 68 physician clinics and surgery centers, and more than 450 employed community-based physicians. Dr. Cannon has worked in pharmacy for the past 15 years. He received his doctor of pharmacy degree from Idaho State University. He has pharmacy experience in the hospital, retail, long-term care, and home health areas. Dr. Cannon is a member of the Academy of Managed Care Pharmacy and currently serves on the legislative committee, which he will chair in the coming year. At IHC Health Plans, he works to develop, implement, and administer programs to control the cost and utilization of pharmaceuticals within the IHC system. He makes frequent presentations to employers, brokers, and health care providers on pharmaceutical trends and pharmaceutical management techniques. Dr. Cannon has responsibility for the management and administration of pharmaceuticals used by IHC's members. As cochair of IHC's Corporate Pharmacy and Therapeutics Committee, he helps promote physician/pharmacy education and interaction programs, as well as formulary development and maintenance. Through IHC Health Plans, he is working to incorporate outcomes-based pharmacoeconomic research into the formulary process. Recently, Dr. Cannon helped establish Utah AWARE, an alliance of health care providers, payers, and the pharmaceutical industry in the state of Utah that is working to educate the community about appropriate antibiotic use. He is actively involved in Intermountain's efforts in clinical integration, disease management, and research. In addition to his responsibilities for pharmacy, Dr. Cannon oversees all health and wellness programs for the plan. He is currently working with employers to implement health management designed to improve employee productivity and decrease absenteeism.

Rebecca W. Chater, R.Ph., M.P.H., is director of clinical services, Kerr Drug, Inc./KDI Clinical Services. She is a national leader in community pharmacy practice innovation. She earned both her B.S. in pharmacy and master's in public health from UNC-Chapel Hill. A past faculty member of the UNC School of Pharmacy, she is president of the North Carolina Board of Pharmacy and a former trustee of the American Pharmacists Association. She has served in several leadership capacities with the National Association of Boards of Pharmacy. She is the 2005 recipient of the North Carolina Association of Pharmacists Innovative Pharmacy Practice Award. Ms. Chater has served on key national committees to develop a consensus definition of medication therapy management (MTM), design a model framework for MTM delivery, and collaborate with the American Medical Association to successfully establish Current Procedural Terminology billing codes specific to pharmacist services. Additionally, she was concept originator and project manager for Kerr's new Community Healthcare Center, which anchors clinical community pharmacy services as central to an interdisciplinary health care practice. Ms. Chater has more than 100 presentations and publications to her credit and has been invited to lend her expertise to more than 30 advisory boards. She is a fellow of both the American Pharmacists Association and of the Wharton School of Business.

Michael R. Cohen, Sc.D., is president of the Institute for Safe Medication Practices (ISMP), an independent nonprofit agency that reviews medication error reports submitted by practitioners to the national medication errors reporting programs operated by the U.S. Pharmacopeia (USP) and the Food and Drug Administration (FDA). ISMP also provides expert analysis of medication-related events for the Patient Safety Authority of the Commonwealth of Pennsylvania, which operates the Pennsylvania Patient Safety Reporting System. ISMP regularly provides drug safety alerts to an estimated 3.5 million U.S. and international readers through various professional journals; newsletters; websites; and four ISMP *Medication Safety*

Alert! publications tailored for consumers, acute care, nurses, and community/ambulatory care providers. Dr. Cohen serves as associate editor of the *Journal of Hospital Pharmacy* and is on the editorial boards of the *Journal of Intravenous Nurse Society*, *Journal of Patient Safety*, *Nursing 2006*, and *Healthcare Risk Control* (ECRI, Plymouth Meeting, Pennsylvania). He also is a member of the Sentinel Event Advisory Group for the Joint Commision on Accreditation of Healthcare Organizations (JCAHO), and a member of the FDA's Drug Safety and Risk Management Advisory Panel. Dr. Cohen is author of the book *Medication Errors* (APhA, 2006).

James B. Conway, M.S., is senior fellow at the Institute for Healthcare Improvement, Cambrige, Massachusetts, and senior consultant at the Dana-Farber Cancer Institute, Boston, Massachusetts. Previously he served as executive vice president and chief operating officer of the Dana-Farber Cancer Institute from 1995 to 2005. He is also board chairman and president of the Healthcare Dimensions Hospice. Prior to joining Dana-Farber, he had a 27-year career at Children's Hospital, Boston, as radiology administrator, assistant vice president of finance, and assistant hospital director for patient care services. He holds a master of science degree from Lesley College, Cambridge, Massachusetts, and is adjunct lecturer on health care management in the Department of Health Policy and Management at Harvard School of Public Health. A diplomat of the American College of Healthcare Executives, he received the college's 1999 Massachusetts Regents Award as Healthcare Executive of the Year and the first Individual Leadership Award in Patient Safety from JCAHO and the National Committee for Quality Assurance (NCQA). He serves as a member and vice-chairman of the JCAHO Sentinel Events Advisory Committee, advisor to the Massachusetts Coalition for the Prevention of Medical Errors, and distinguished advisor to the National Patient Safety Foundation. He is also a member of the Clinical Issues Advisory Council of the Massachusetts Hospital Association; a member of the Medically Induced Trauma Support Services Board of Directors; a member of the executive committee of the Medical, Academic and Scientific Community Organization; and a long-time member of the board of the Ronald McDonald House in Boston.

R. Scott Evans, Ph.D., M.S., is a senior medical informaticist in the Department of Medical Informatics at LDS Hospital and Intermountain Health Care, director of research in the Department of Medical Informatics at LDS Hospital, and research professor in the Department of Medical Informatics and adjunct research professor in the Department of Medicine at the University of Utah, Salt Lake City, Utah. Dr. Evans received his bachelor of science degree in zoology and master of science degree in microbiology/parasitology from Brigham Young University. He received his Ph.D. in medical biophysics and computing from the University of Utah. He is a member of the American Medical Informatics Association and a fellow in the American College of Medical Informatics. He is on the editorial board of the *Journal of the American Medical Informatics Association* and a reviewer for a number of peer-reviewed journals in medicine and informatics. In 1993 he received the Priscilla M. Mayden Award for outstanding contributions in the field of medical informatics, and in 1997 he received the Oslers Cloak award for excellence in caring and curing from Intermountain Health Care. His major experience and interests have been in the design, development, and evaluation of computerized tools for the selection and management of anti-infective agents, computer methods to identify and reduce adverse drug events and adverse medical device events, computerized methods to identify patients needing isolation, computerized methods to identify and reduce hospital-acquired infections, and use of medical device interfaces to improve patient safety. A number of these computerized tools are clinically operational at several Intermountain Health Care hospitals.

Elizabeth A. Flynn, Ph.D., R.Ph., is associate research professor at the Center for Pharmacy Operations and Designs at Auburn University. Her specialties are the application of ergonomic design principles to prevent errors and evaluation of technology for effects on medication errors and efficiency. Among her publications are "Fundamentals of medication error research" and "National observational study of prescription dispensing accuracy and safety in 50 pharmacies." Dr. Flynn has been a coinvestigator on research for automation companies in community and hospital pharmacy settings, and has conducted or overseen observation studies in more than 100 sites in the United States, France, the United Kingdom, and Italy. As a member of the Graduate Faculty at Auburn, she currently serves on two graduate student committees that involve medication error research. Dr. Flynn has been an investigator on research contracts totaling over $2 million. She holds a bachelor of science in pharmacy degree from the University of Florida, a master of science degree from the University of North Carolina, and a Ph.D. from Auburn University. She completed a residency at North Carolina Memorial Hospital. She received a 1999 Cheers Award from ISMP for contributions to error prevention and the 2001 Dorothy Dillon Memorial Award from the New Mexico Society of Health-System Pharmacists. Dr. Flynn is a member of the USP's Safe Medication Use Expert Committee (2005–2010) and the Medication Error and Technologies Analysis Network in the United Kingdom.

Jerry H. Gurwitz, M.D., is a nationally recognized expert in geriatric medicine and the use of drug therapy in the elderly. He holds the Dr. John Meyers Endowed Chair in Primary Care Medicine at the University of

Massachusetts Medical School, where he is chief of the Division of Geriatric Medicine and professor of medicine and family medicine/community health. He also serves as executive director of the Meyers Primary Care Institute, a joint initiative of the University of Massachusetts Medical School, Fallon Foundation, and Fallon Community Health Plan, focused on promoting primary care research and education. He received his bachelor's degree from Dartmouth College and his M.D. degree from the University of Massachusetts Medical School. Dr. Gurwitz has published numerous original articles, reviews, commentaries, and book chapters on the optimal use of drug therapy in elderly patients. He has been the recipient of the William B. Abrams Award in Geriatric Clinical Pharmacology from the American Society for Clinical Pharmacology and Therapeutics and the George F. Archambault Award from the American Society of Consultant Pharmacists. Dr. Gurwitz's most recent research efforts relate to developing and testing interventions to reduce the risk of medication errors that lead to adverse drug events in the elderly.

Charles B. Inlander is former president of the nonprofit People's Medical Society, founded in early 1983. He guided the People's Medical Society to its status as one of the most influential consumer health advocacy organizations in the United States. Mr. Inlander is a faculty lecturer at the Yale University School of Medicine; an adjunct faculty member at the Chicago-Kent College of Law; and a fellow of the Institute for Science, Law and Technology at the Illinois Institute of Technology. He is a health commentator on Public Radio International's Marketplace, heard throughout the country on public radio stations. He is a founder of the Civil Justice Foundation and serves or has served on the board of directors of Consumers for Civil Justice, the National League for Nursing, the Pennsylvania League for Nursing, and the Lehigh Valley Business Conference on Health Care. He is on the advisory boards of the Citizen Advocacy Center, the Primary Care Management Association, the American Academy of Family Physicians, Health Market, and Bottom Line/Personal Publications. He was a columnist for *Nursing Economics* and a contributing editor for *Medical Self-Care* magazine. He has authored or coauthored more than 20 best-selling consumer health books. His articles regularly appear in such publications as *The New York Times, Glamour,* and *Boardroom.* Prior to joining the People's Medical Society, Mr. Inlander established a national reputation as an advocate for the rights of handicapped citizens. He is a graduate of American University.

Kevin B. Johnson, M.D., M.S., is associate professor and vice-chair of biomedical informatics, with a joint appointment in the Department of Pediatrics, at Vanderbilt University Medical School. He received his M.D.

from The Johns Hopkins University School of Medicine and his master of science degree in medical informatics from Stanford University. He served as a pediatric chief resident at Johns Hopkins. He was a member of the faculty in both pediatrics and biomedical information sciences at Johns Hopkins until 2002. He is a practicing, board-certified physician in pediatrics. His research areas are clinical information systems development; the uses of advanced computer technologies, including the World Wide Web, personal digital assistants, and pen-based computers, in medicine; and electronic prescription writing tools. Dr. Johnson has served on the editorial boards of the Ambulatory Pediatrics Association as well as the *Journal of the American Informatics Association* (JAMIA), for which he is an assistant editor. He recently was appointed director of JAMIA's student editorial board. He has been an active participant in the informatics efforts of many national organizations, including the American Medical Informatics Association, the American Board of Pediatrics, the Medical Informatics Special Interest Group of the Ambulatory Pediatrics Association, the American Academy of Pediatrics' Steering Committee on Clinical Information Technologies, and the IOM's Patient Safety Data Standards subcommittee.

Wilson D. Pace, M.D., is professor of family medicine and Green-Edelman Chair for Practice-based Research at the University of Colorado. He is director of the American Academy of Family Physicians (AAFP) National Research Network. He also directs SNOCAP, a consortium of practice-based research networks within the University of Colorado. Dr. Pace's research has focused on practice reorganization and patient safety. He leads a patient safety consortium in Colorado focused on improving care delivery in primary care offices, as well as overseeing the AAFP Developmental Center for Evaluation and Research in Patient Safety in Primary Care. He serves in an advisory capacity to a number of clinical and research health information technology projects. Dr. Pace received his M.D. degree from the University of California, Irvine in 1979. He is a board-certified practicing family physician with a Certificate of Added Qualifications in geriatrics.

Kathleen R. Stevens, Ed.D., M.S., R.N., FAAN, is professor of nursing at The University of Texas Health Science Center at San Antonio, Texas. She is also founding director of the Academic Center for Evidence-based Practice, where she works to advance evidence-based quality improvement through research, education, and practice. She is an investigator with the Veterans Evidence-based Research, Dissemination, and Implementation Center for the Veterans Health Administration, with emphasis on systematic reviews and organizational change for evidence-based quality improvement. Her research includes comparison of evidence-based and traditional interventions in reducing health risk behavior, as well as investigations of evidence-based practice processes. She serves as an advisor to hospitals seeking magnet recognition status and faculty updating education programs on the topic of evidence-based quality improvement. Dr. Stevens initiated the Summer Institute on Evidence-based Practice, a national interdisciplinary conference receiving funding from the Agency for Healthcare Research and Quality (AHRQ). At the national level, Dr. Stevens is an elected officer on the board of governors of the National League for Nursing, a leading nursing education organization that sets standards for faculty and nursing education programs. She received her bachelor of science degree in nursing from Northwestern State University of Louisiana, her master of science degree in maternal and child health from Texas Woman's University, and her doctorate in health science research and education from the Baylor College of Medicine/University of Houston program, and is a fellow in the American Academy of Nursing.

Edward Westrick, M.D., Ph.D., M.S., is vice president of medical management for UMass Memorial Health Care, where he develops clinical performance improvement interventions for a large managed care network and medical center. During the last 10 years Dr. Westrick has worked with multiple Quality Improvement Organizations in Medicare's Health Care Quality Improvement Program and served in the leadership of the American Health Quality Association. He frequently serves on expert panels and boards for such national organizations as the National Quality Forum (NQF), USP, NCQA, JCAHO, CMS, the American Health Care Association (AHCA), the Department of Veterans Affairs (VA), the Medicare Payment Advisory Commission (MedPAC), American Pharmaceutical Association (APhA), and RAND. His particular areas of expertise include performance measurement and medication management. He previously directed the SCRIPT Project on behalf of the Coalition for Quality in Medication Use. He serves on the faculties of the University of Rhode Island and Brown University Medical School and the medical staff of Eleanor Slater Hospital. His educational history includes his internship and residency (internal medicine) from Brown University, M.D. from New Jersey Medical School, Ph.D. from the University of Rhode Island (pharmacoepidemiology and pharmacoeconomics), master of science degree from Rutgers University (psychology), and bachelor of arts degree from the University of Pennsylvania (psychology).

Albert W. Wu, M.D., M.P.H., is professor of health policy and management at the Johns Hopkins Bloomberg School of Public Health, with joint appointments in Epidemiology and International Health and in Medicine and Surgery in the School of Medicine. He received bachelor of arts and M.D. degrees from Cornell University, and completed internal medicine residency training at the Mount Sinai Hospital in New York and the University of California at San Diego. He was a Robert Wood Johnson Clinical Scholar at the University of California at San Francisco and received a master of public health degree from the University of California at Berkeley. His research and teaching focus on measuring health and patient outcomes and using the measures to assess treatments and quality of care. He has studied the handling and impact of medical errors since 1988. He is an authority on the development and use of patient-reported outcome assessments for HIV/AIDS, as well as other chronic diseases and critical illnesses. Dr. Wu is past president of the International Society for Quality of Life Research. He was senior associate editor of the *Journal of General Internal Medicine* and is associate editor of *Quality of Life Research*, the *Journal of Patient Safety*, and *AHRQ Web M&M*. He was co–principal investigator for an AHRQ-funded grant that developed a web-based incident reporting system for intensive care units. He is principal investigator on a National Cancer Institute grant to develop a web-based mechanism for capturing patient-reported data for outpatient practice. He is principal investigator of the AHRQ-funded Johns Hopkins DEcIDE center for the conduct of rapid, policy-relevant studies of comparative effectiveness. He is studying video vignettes of disclosure to patients and their families, and recently developed an educational video for practitioners titled "Removing Insult from Injury: Disclosing Adverse Events." He is author of over 200 peer-reviewed publications; leads courses in the Bloomberg School of Public Health on patient-reported outcomes, quality of care, and patient safety; and is an active clinician in general internal medicine and treatment of HIV.

B

Glossary of Terms and Acronyms

TERMS

ACE inhibitor. Angiotensin-converting enzyme inhibitor.

Adverse drug event. Any injury due to medication (Bates et al., 1995b).

Adverse event. An event that results in unintended harm to the patient due to an act of commission or omission rather than the underlying disease or condition of the patient (IOM, 2004).

Ambulatory care. For the purposes of this study, care given in (1) the ambulatory clinic, (2) the community pharmacy, (3) the home care setting, (4) the self-care setting, or (5) the school setting.

Biologics (including vaccines, blood, and blood products). A subset of drug products. Biologics are distinguished from other drugs by their manufacturing process—biological as opposed to chemical.

Clinician. An individual who uses a recognized scientific knowledge base and has the authority to deliver health care services to patients (IOM, 1996). The term encompasses prescribers, nurses, and pharmacists.

Dietary supplement. A product (other than tobacco) intended to supplement the diet that bears or contains one or more of the following dietary ingredients: a vitamin; a mineral; an herb or other botanical; an amino acid; a dietary substance for use by man to supplement the diet by increasing the dietary intake; or a concentrate, metabolite, constituent, extract or combination of any ingredient described above (Dietary Supplement Health and Education Act of 1994 [P.L. 103-147]).

Drug. A substance that is recognized by an official pharmacopoeia or formulary; intended for use in the diagnosis, cure, mitigation, treatment, or prevention of disease; intended to affect the structure or any function of the body (other than food); intended for use as a component of a medicine but not a device or a component, or a part or accessory of a device (FDA, 2004). Drugs are divided into those that require a prescription and those that do not. Nonprescription drugs are usually called "over-the-counter" (OTC) drugs (see below).

Error. The failure of a planned action to be completed as intended (i.e., error of execution) or the use of a wrong plan to achieve an aim (i.e., error of planning). An error may be an act of commission or an act of omission (IOM, 2004).

Formulary. A schedule of prescription drugs that will be paid for by a health insurance plan and dispensed through participating pharmacies. A formulary can be an important safety tool since it can eliminate (for example, in hospitals) the use of drug products considered to be unsafe.

Hand-off. The process of moving patients and their information from one provider or site to another.

Health care professional. See *clinician.*

Managed Care Organization. A health care provider that attempts to manage the access, cost, and quality of health care.

Medication. See *drug.*

Medication error. Any error occurring in the medication-use process (Bates et al., 1995a).

Medication therapy management. A service or group of services that optimize therapeutic outcomes for individual patients to help ensure that the goals of drug therapy are achieved. These services can be provided in conjunction with or independently of the provision of a medication product by pharmacists or other qualified health care providers.

Nonformulary drug. A medication that has a preferred alternative listed in the drug formulary.

Off-label use. The Food and Drug Administration (FDA) permits the prescribing of approved medications for other than their intended indications. This practice is known as off-label use.

Orphan drug. A product that is used in the diagnosis or treatment of diseases or conditions that are considered rare in the United States.

OTC ("over-the-counter") drug. A drug sold without a prescription. The product's potential for misuse and abuse is low, consumers are successfully able to use it for self-diagnosable conditions, it can be adequately labeled for ease and accuracy of use, and oversight by health practitioners is not needed to ensure its safe and effective use (FDA, 2005).

Potential adverse drug event (ADE). An event in which an error occurred but did not cause injury (for example, the error was intercepted before the patient was affected, or the patient received a wrong dose, but no harm occurred) (Gandhi et al., 2000).

Practicing clinician. See *clinician*.

Practitioner. See *clinician*.

Preventable adverse drug event (ADE). An adverse drug event arising because of an error.

Primary care. The provision health care services by clinicians who are accountable for addressing a large majority of a patient's health care needs, developing a sustained partnership with patients, and practicing in the context of family and community (IOM, 1996).

Provider. See *clinician*.

Reconciliation. Comparison of the medications a person is taking in one care setting with those being provided in another setting.

ACRONYMS

AADA	Abbreviated Antibiotic Drug Application
AAFP	American Academy of Family Physicians
AAMC	Association of American Medical Colleges
ACE	angiotensin converting enzyme
ACGME	Accreditation Council on Graduate Medical Education
ADE	adverse drug event
ADWE	adverse drug withdrawal event
AFB	American Foundation for the Blind
AGS	American Geriatrics Society
AHA	American Hospital Association
AHCA	American Health Care Association
AHRQ	Agency for Healthcare Research and Quality
ALLHAT	Antihypertensive and Lipid-Lowering Treatment to Prevent Heart Attack Trial
AMA	American Medical Association
ANDA	Abbreviated New Drug Application
ANSI	American National Standards Institute
APA	American Psychiatric Association
ASHP	American Society of Health-System Pharmacists
ASTM	American Society for Testing and Materials
BLA	Biologic Licensing Application
BTE	Bridges to Excellence
CC	Cochrane Collaboration
CCR	Continuity of Care Record
CDC	Centers for Disease Control and Prevention
CDER	Center for Drug Evaluation and Research, Food and Drug Administration

CDSS	clinical decision support system
CERTS	Centers for Education and Research on Therapeutics
CGMP	Current Good Manufacturing Practices
CME	continuing medical education
CMS	Centers for Medicare and Medicaid Services
CMWF	The Commonwealth Fund
CoSI	Commission for Systemic Interoperability
COX-2	cyclooxygenase-2
CPOE	computerized provider (physician) order entry
CTFPHC	Canadian Task Force on Preventive Health Care

DCRI	Duke Clinical Research Institute
DDMAC	Division of Drug Marketing, Advertising and Communications, Food and Drug Administration
DHA	Australian Department of Health and Ageing
DHHS	Department of Health and Human Services
dl	deciliter
DMETS	Division of Medication Errors and Technical Support, Food and Drug Administration
DTC	direct-to-consumer

EAN/UCC	European Article Number/Uniform Code Council
eHI	eHealth Initiative
EHR	electronic health record

FACCT	Foundation for Accountability
FDA	U.S. Food and Drug Administration
FMEA	failure modes and effects analysis
FPIN	Family Physicians Inquiries Network
FR	*Federal Register*

GAO	U.S. Government Accountability Office
GMP	Good Manufacturing Practices
GRAM	Geriatric Risk Assessment MedGuide

H_2	histamine-2
HEDIS	Health Plan Employer Data and Information Set
HHS	(Department of) Health and Human Services
HI	Harris Interactive
HIBCC	Health Industry Business Communications Council
HIRO	Hospital Incident Reporting Ontology
HL7	Health Level 7

HMO	health maintenance organization
HOPE	Health Outcomes and PharmacoEconomic
HPA	Health Policy Alternatives, Inc.
HRSA	Health Resources and Services Administration
ICU	intensive care unit
IHI	Institute for Healthcare Improvement
IM	intramuscularly
IND	Investigational New Drug Application
INR	international normalized ratio
IOM	Institute of Medicine
ISMP	Institute for Safe Medication Practices
IV	intravenous
JAMIA	*Journal of the American Informatics Association*
JCAHO	Joint Commission on Accreditation of Healthcare Organizations
JFP	*Journal of Family Practice*
JKF	Josie King Foundation
KFF	Kaiser Family Foundation
kg	kilogram
LDL	low-density lipoprotein
m^2	square meter
MAO	monamine oxidase
MAR	medication administration record
MBRP	Massachusetts Board of Registration in Pharmacy
MCPME	Massachusetts Coalition for the Prevention of Medical Errors
MDS	Minimum Data Set
MERP	Medication Error Reporting Program
mg	milligrams
MHA	Massachusetts Hospital Association
ml	milliliters
MMA	Medicare Prescription Drug Improvement and Modernization Act of 2003 (P.L. 108-173)
MoA	mechanism(s) of action
NABP	National Association of Boards of Pharmacy
NACDS	National Association of Chain Drug Stores

NCCAM	National Center for Complementary and Alternative Medicine
NCCMERP	National Coordinating Council for Medication Error Reporting and Prevention
NCHM	National Center for Health Marketing
NCHS	National Center for Health Statistics
NCPDP	National Council for Prescription Drug Programs
NCPIE	National Council on Patient Information and Education
NCQA	National Committee for Quality Assurance
NCVHS	National Committee on Vital and Health Statistics
NDA	New Drug Application
NDF-RT	National Drug File Reference Terminology
NEISS-CADES	National Electronic Injury Surveillance System-Cooperative Adverse Drug Event Surveillance
NHS	National Health Service
NICHQ	National Initiative for Children's Healthcare Quality
NIH	National Institutes of Health
NIHCMREF	National Institute for Health Care Management and Research and Educational Foundation
NIMH	National Institute of Mental Health
NLM	National Library of Medicine
NMBP	New Mexico Board of Pharmacy
NME	new molecular entity
NPSF	National Patient Safety Foundation
NQF	National Quality Forum
NRC	National Research Council
NSAID	nonsteroidal anti-inflammatory drug
OBRA	Omnibus Budget Reconciliation Act
OIG	Office of Inspector General
OSCAR	Online Survey Certification and Reporting
OTC	over-the-counter
PACE	Program of All-Inclusive Care for the Elederly
PBM	Pharmacy Benefits Manager
PCA	patient-controlled analgesia
PCM	pharmaceutical case management
PCSEPMBBR	President's Commission for the Study of Ethical Problems in Medicine and Biomedical and Behavioral Research
PD	pharmacodynamics
PDA	personal digital assistant
PHR	personal health record
PhRMA	Pharmaceutical Research and Manufacturers of America

PICC   peripherally inserted central catheter
PK   pharmacokinetics
PMS   Pathways for Medication Safety
POCA   Phonetic Orthographic Computer Analysis
POL   Physician Office Link
PPAG   Pediatric Pharmacy Advocacy Group
PSET   Patient Safety Event Taxonomy
PSI   Premier Safety Institute

QSHC   Quality and Safety in Healthcare

R&D   research and development
RFID   radio frequency identification
RHIO   Regional Health Information Organization
RoA   route of administration
RSW   Roper Starch Worldwide
RWJF   The Robert Wood Johnson Foundation

SAGE   Systematic Assessment of Geriatric drug use via
                  Epidemiology
SPL   Structured Product Label

TGA   Therapeutic Goods Administration

UNC   University of North Carolina
USAN   United States Adopted Name Council
USP   U.S. Pharmacopeia
USP-ISMP   United States Pharmacopeia-Institute for Safe Medication
  MERP   Practices Medication Errors Reporting Program

VA   (Department of) Veterans Affairs
VAERS   Vaccine Adverse Event Reporting System
VHA   Veterans Health Administration
VistA   Veterans Health Information Systems and Technology
                  Architecture
VSD   Vaccine Safety Datalink

WHI   Women's Health Initiative
WHO   World Health Organization

REFERENCES

Bates DW, Boyle DL, Vander Vliet MB, Schneider J, Leape L. 1995a. Relationship between medication errors and adverse drug events. *Journal of General Internal Medicine* 10(4): 100–205.

Bates DW, Cullen DJ, Laird N, Petersen LA, Small SD, Servi D, Laffel G, Sweitzer BJ, Shea BF, Hallisey R, Vander Vliet M, Nemeskal R, Leape LL. 1995b. Incidence of adverse drug events and potential adverse drug events. Implications for prevention. ADE Prevention Study Group. *Journal of the American Medical Association* 274:29–34.

FDA (U.S. Food and Drug Administration). 2004. *Drugs @ FDA: Glossary of Terms.* [Online]. Available: http://www.fda.gov/cder/drugsatfda/glossary.htm [accessed June 7, 2005].

FDA. 2005. *Office of Nonprescription Drugs.* [Online]. Available: http://www.fda.gov/cder/offices/otc/default.htm [accessed June 7, 2005].

Gandhi TK, Seger DL, Bates DW. 2000. Identifying drug safety issues: From research to practice. *International Journal for Quality in Health Care* 12(1):69–76.

IOM (Institute of Medicine). 1996. *Primary Care: America's Health in a New Era.* Washington, DC: National Academy Press.

IOM. 2004. *Patient Safety: Achieving a New Standard for Care.* Washington, DC: The National Academies Press.

C

Medication Errors: Incidence Rates

This appendix reviews estimates of the rates of medication errors and adverse drug events (ADEs) in three care settings (hospital, nursing home, and ambulatory care) and in pediatric and psychiatric care. Where possible, error rates for the five stages of the medication-use system and at the interface between care settings are documented separately.

INCIDENCE OF MEDICATION ERRORS IN HOSPITAL CARE

Selection and Procurement of the Drug by the Pharmacy

No studies were identified that specifically identified medication errors of this type. It is possible that these types of errors were included in studies of general medication error rates.

Prescription and Selection of the Drug for the Patient: Errors of Commission

Rates of prescribing errors (for example, dosing errors, prescribing medications to which the patient was allergic, prescribing inappropriate dosage forms) vary considerably from study to study and are quoted in several different ways—errors per 1,000 admissions, errors per 1,000 orders, errors per 100 opportunities for error, and preventable ADEs per 1,000 admissions (see Table C-1):

TABLE C-1 Hospital Care: Prescription and Selection Errors of Commission

Error rates	**Per 1,000 admissions—detection method** 12.3 (Lesar, 2002a)—pharmacist review of written orders 29 (Winterstein et al., 2004)—prompted reporting 52.9 (Lesar et al., 1997)—pharmacist review of written orders 190 (LaPointe and Jollis, 2003)—clinical pharmacist directly participating in clinical care 1,400 (Bates et al., 1995a)—prompted reporting, chart review, review of medication orders **Per 1,000 orders—detection methods** 0.61 (Lesar, 2002a)—pharmacist review of written orders 2.87 (Lesar et al., 1997)—pharmacist review of written orders 3.13 (Lesar et al., 1990)—pharmacist review of written orders 53 (Bates et al., 1995a)—prompted reporting, chart review, review of medication orders **Per 100 opportunities for error—detection method** 1.5 (Dean et al., 2002)—pharmacist review of written orders 6.2 (Bobb et al., 2004)—pharmacist review of written orders 6.7 (Lisby et al., 2005)—direct observation, unannounced control visits, chart review 9.9 (van den Bemt et al., 2002)—pharmacist review of written orders
Preventable ADEs rates	**Per 1,000 admissions—detection method** 3.7 (Hardmeier et al., 2004)—chart review 3.9 (Bates et al., 1995b)—prompted reporting, chart review 84.1 (Nebeker et al., 2005)—review of electronic record

- Prescribing errors totaled 12.3 to 1,400.0 per 1,000 patient admissions: (1) 12.3 in a study of 32,683 admissions in a tertiary care hospital in New York State (Lesar, 2002a); (2) 29 in a study of about 6,000 patients in a tertiary care hospital in Florida (Winterstein et al., 2004); (3) 52.9 in a study of 211,635 admissions in a tertiary care hospital in New York State (Lesar et al., 1997); (4) 190.0 in a study of 24,538 patients in a tertiary care hospital in North Carolina (LaPointe and Jollis, 2003); and (5) 1,400 in a study of 379 patients in an urban tertiary care hospital in Massachusetts (Bates et al., 1995a).

- Prescribing errors occurred per order at rates ranging from 0.6 to 53 per 1,000 orders (Lesar et al., 1990; Bates et al., 1995a; Lesar et al., 1997; Lesar, 2002a).

- Errors per 100 opportunities for error ranged from 1.5 to 9.9 (van den Bemt et al., 2002; Dean et al., 2002; Bobb et al., 2004; Lisby et al., 2005).

In the subset of studies that evaluated preventable ADEs, prescription errors associated with patient injuries ranged from 3.7 to 84.1 per 1,000 admissions (Bates et al., 1995b; Hardmeier et al., 2004; Nebeker et al., 2005).

Preparation and Dispensing of the Drug

Preparation and dispensing errors occurred at a rate of 2.6 per 1,000 admissions in a tertiary care hospital in Florida (Winterstein et al., 2004) (see Table C-2).

Two studies focused exclusively on intravenous (IV) medications. One study, at one U.K. and two German hospitals, found a rate of preparation errors of 26 percent per observed preparation (88 preparation errors out of 337 observations) (Wirtz et al., 2003). The other study, at a tertiary and a community hospital in the United Kingdom, found a rate of preparation errors of 49 percent per observed preparation (212 preparation and administration errors out of 430 doses) (Taxis and Barber, 2003).

Preparation and dispensing errors were associated with preventable ADEs at rates of 0.6 per 1,000 admissions in a Swiss study of 6,383 patients (Hardmeier et al., 2004); 1.1 per 1,000 admissions in a study of 4,031 patients at two tertiary hospitals in Boston, Massachusetts (Bates et al., 1995b); and 1.6 per 1,000 admissions in a study of 937 admissions at a tertiary hospital in Salt Lake City, Utah (Nebeker et al., 2005).

Administration of the Drug

As with prescribing error rates, rates of administration errors varied widely in medical and surgical units (See Table C-3). Rates per opportunity

TABLE C-2 Hospital Care: Preparation and Dispensing Errors

Error rates: general medications	**Per 1,000 admissions—detection method** 2.6 (Winterstein et al., 2004)—prompted reports
Error rates: intravenous (IV) medications	**Per preparation—detection method** 26 percent (Wirtz et al., 2003) (U.K. and German study)—direct observation 49 percent (Taxis and Barber, 2003) (U.K. study)—direct observation
Preventable ADEs	**Per 1,000 admissions—detection method** 0.6 (Hardmeier et al., 2004) (Swiss study)—chart review 1.1 (Bates et al., 1995b)—prompted reporting, chart review 1.4 (Nebeker et al., 2005)—review of electronic medical record

TABLE C-3 Hospital Care: Administration Errors

Error rates: general medications	**Per 100 opportunities/doses—detection method** 2.4 (Taxis et al., 1999) (German part, unit dose system)—direct observation 3 (Dean et al., 1995) (U.K. part)—direct observation 5.1 (Taxis et al., 1999) (German part, traditional system)—direct observation 6.7 (Lisby et al., 2005) (Danish study)—direct observation 6.9 (Dean et al., 1995) (U.S. part)—direct observation 8 (Taxis et al., 1999) (U.K. part)—direct observation 10.8 (Barker et al., 2002)—direct observation 14.9 (Tissot et al., 2003) (French study)—direct observation
Error rates: general medications	**Per 1,000 admissions—detection method** 5.8 (Winterstein et al., 2004)—prompted reports
Error rates in intensive care units (ICUs)	**Per opportunity/dose—detection method** 3.3 percent (Calabrese et al., 2001)—direct observation 6.6 percent (Tissot et al., 1999)—direct observation
Error rates: IV medications only	**Per opportunity/dose—detection method** 34 percent (Wirtz et al., 2003) (U.K. and German study)—direct observation 49 percent (Taxis and Barber, 2003) (U.K. study) (includes both preparation and administration)—direct observation
Preventable ADEs	**Per 1,000 admissions—detection method** 2.1 (Bates et al., 1995b)—prompted reporting, chart review 17.9 (Nebeker et al., 2005)—review of electronic medical record

for error or dose ranged from 2.4 to 14.9 percent: (1) 2.4 percent in a German hospital using a unit dose system (1,318 opportunities for error) (Taxis et al., 1999); (2) 3 percent in a U.K. tertiary hospital (2,756 opportunities for error) (Dean et al., 1995); (3) 5.1 percent in a German hospital using a traditional system (973 opportunities for error) (Taxis et al., 1999); (4) 6.7 percent in a Danish tertiary hospital (2,467 opportunities for error) (Lisby et al., 2005); (5) 6.9 percent in a U.S. tertiary hospital (919 opportunities for error) (Dean et al., 1995); (6) 8 percent in a U.K. hospital using a ward pharmacy system (842 opportunities for error) (Taxis et al., 1999); (7) 10 percent (excluding wrong time errors) in 24 hospitals in Georgia and Colorado (2,765 medication doses) (Barker et al., 2002); and (8) 11 percent (excluding wrong-time errors) (Tissot et al., 2003) in a French tertiary hospital (523 opportunities for error).

Another study, in a tertiary hospital in Florida, involving about 6,000 patients (the authors could not report precisely the number of patients involved), found an administration error rate of 5.8 per 1,000 admissions (Winterstein et al., 2004).

Similar rates to those above have been observed in intensive care unit (ICU) studies. In a study focusing on high-alert medications administered in ICUs in five U.S. tertiary care teaching hospitals, an administration error rate of 3.3 percent was found (5,744 observations) (Calabrese et al., 2001). In another study, carried out in a medical ICU in a French hospital, an administration error rate of 6.6 percent was observed (2,009 medication administration interventions by nurses) (Tissot et al., 1999).

Higher rates were seen in studies that focused exclusively on IV medications—34 percent (93 errors out of 278 observed administrations) (Wirtz et al., 2003) and 49 percent (212 preparation and administration errors out of 430 doses) (Taxis and Barber, 2003).

Two studies looking at preventable ADEs occurring during the administration stage found rates of 2.1 per 1,000 admissions (in a study of 4,031 patients at two tertiary hospitals in Boston, Massachusetts [Bates et al., 1995b]) and 17.9 per 1,000 admissions (in a study of 937 admissions at a tertiary hospital in Salt Lake City, Utah [Bates et al., 1995b; Nebeker et al., 2005]).

Monitoring of the Patient for Effect

Rates of preventable ADEs resulting from errors in the monitoring of patients were reported in two studies as 0.6 per 1,000 admissions (Hardmeier et al., 2004) and 32 per 1,000 admissions (Hardmeier et al., 2004; Nebeker et al., 2005). (See Table C-4).

ADEs during Hospitalization

Five major studies examined the incidence of ADEs occurring during hospitalization (see Table C-5). Using hospital admissions during the period 1990–1993, investigators at LDS Hospital, Salt Lake City, Utah, found that 2,227 out of 91,574 patients experienced ADEs during hospitalization, a rate of 2.43 ADEs per 100 admissions (Classen et al., 1997). Almost 50 percent of the identified ADEs were thought to be preventable. Extrapolat-

TABLE C-4 Hospital Care: Monitoring Errors

Preventable ADEs	Per 1,000 admissions—detection method
	0.6 (Hardmeier et al., 2004) (Swiss study)—chart review
	32 (Nebeker et al., 2005)—review of electronic medical record

TABLE C-5 Hospital Care: ADE Incidence During Hospitalization

Study	ADEs per 100 Admissions	ADEs per 1,000 Patient-Days	Proportion of ADEs Preventable
Classen et al., 1997	2.4	Not given	About 50 percent (out of 2,227 ADEs in study)
Senst et al., 2001	4.2	Not given	15 percent (out of 74 ADEs in the study
Bates et al., 1995b	6.5	11.5	28 percent (out of 247 ADEs in study)
Jha et al., 1998	Not given	21	27 percent (out of 617 ADEs in study)
Nebeker et al., 2005	52	70	27 percent (out of 483 ADEs in study)

ing these figures nationally and assuming 32 million admissions annually, the authors concluded that 770,000 hospital patients in America would experience an ADE annually.

Another study, conducted at two tertiary care hospitals in Boston, involved 4,031 adult admissions. Carried out in 1993 under the Adverse Drug Events Prevention Study, this study found an overall ADE rate of 6.5 per 100 nonobstetric admissions (or 11.5 ADEs per 1,000 patient-days); of these, 28 percent were judged preventable (Bates et al., 1995b). Of the ADEs, 1 percent were fatal (none preventable), 12 percent life-threatening, 30 percent serious, and 57 percent significant. Of the life-threatening and serious ADEs, 42 percent were judged preventable. Assuming an ADE rate of 6.5 per 100 nonobstetric admissions and 25 million nonobstetric admissions to short-term hospitals annually, the authors estimated an annual rate of 1.6 million ADEs in U.S. hospitals.

A third study, utilizing data on ADEs collected in the summer of 1998 from a four-hospital academic medical network, estimated the ADE rate during hospitalization to be 4.2 per 100 admissions (Senst et al., 2001). Fifteen percent of these ADEs were judged preventable.

At a tertiary hospital in Boston, in a study carried out from October 1994 to May 1995, 617 ADEs were observed, 166 of which were judged preventable (Jha et al., 1998). After adjustment for the sampling scheme, the ADE rate was estimated to be 21 per 1,000 patient-days.

Much higher ADE rates were observed in the most recent study, involving a highly computerized hospital that had implemented electronic health records (Nebeker et al., 2005). Computerized order checking was fully functional for allergies, many drug–drug interactions, and limited drug–disease interactions. The system did not, however, feature sophisticated decision-support algorithms. Among 937 hospital admissions, 483 clinically significant inpatients ADEs were identified—52 per 100 admissions, or 70 per 1,000 patient-days. Medication errors contributed to 27 percent of the ADEs. Of all the ADEs, 9 percent resulted in serious harm, 22 percent in additional monitoring and interventions, 32 percent in interventions alone, and 11 percent in monitoring alone; 27 percent should have resulted in additional interventions or monitoring.

Three smaller studies found similar ADE rates. A 37-day study at a Boston tertiary hospital found 27 ADEs (15 considered preventable), for a rate of 6.4 ADEs per 100 admissions or 9.1 ADEs per 1,000 patient-days (Bates et al., 1993). Another small study at the same hospital found 25 ADEs (5 considered preventable), for a rate of 6.6 ADEs per 100 admissions or 14.7 ADEs per 1,000 patient-days (Bates et al., 1995a). In a study of 157 hospitalized patients aged 70 and older, 28 probable ADEs were observed, for a rate of 17.8 ADEs per 100 admissions (Gray et al., 1998). Just over half the ADEs were considered preventable.

Prescription and Selection of the Drug for the Patient: Errors of Omission

Errors of omission occur when a medication necessary for the appropriate care of hospitalized individuals is not prescribed. After reviewing the published literature on medication errors of omission within acute care, the committee identified three broad categories of studies: studies on treatment of acute coronary syndromes, on antibiotic prophylaxis, and on thrombosis prophylaxis (see Table C-6).

TABLE C-6 Hospital Care: Prescription and Selection Errors of Omission

Patients discharged with diagnosis of acute myocardial infarction	Percentage of patients given aspirin within 24 hours of hospitalization 84.9 (Roe et al., 2005) (NSTEMI) 88 (Roe et al., 2005) (STEMI) 92.4 (Granger et al., 2005) 93 (Sanborn et al., 2004) Percentage of patients prescribed aspirin at discharge 53 (Krumholz et al., 2003) 76.8 (Petersen et al., 2001) 83.8 (Roe et al., 2005) (NSTEMI) 84.8 (Petersen et al., 2003) 85.6 (Alexander et al., 1998) 88.9 (Roe et al., 2005) (STEMI) 93.4 (Granger et al., 2005)

continued

TABLE C-6 continued

Percentage of patients given beta-blockers within 24 hours of
hospitalization
66 (Sanborn et al., 2004)
72.2 (Roe et al., 2005) (NSTEMI)
77.8 (Roe et al., 2005) (STEMI)
78 (Granger et al., 2005)

Percentage of patients prescribed beta-blockers at discharge
53 (Krumholz et al., 2003)
56.1 (Petersen et al., 2001)
59.1 (Alexander et al., 1998)
67.3 (Petersen et al., 2003)
78.3 (Roe et al., 2005) (NSTEMI)
78.9 (Granger et al., 2005)
83.4 (Roe et al., 2005) (STEMI)

Percentage of patients prescribed angiotensin-converting enzyme
(ACE) inhibitors at discharge
51.2 (Roe et al., 2005) (NSTEMI)
51.7 (Alexander et al., 1998)
58 (Roe et al., 2005) (78) (STEMI)
58.5 (Petersen et al., 2001)
67.6 (Petersen et al., 2003)
73.1 (Granger et al., 2005)

Rates of antibiotic prophylaxis within surgical studies	**Percentage of procedures in which patients prescribed antibiotics** 70 (Vaisbrud et al., 1999) 74 (Heineck et al., 1999) 92 (Gupta et al., 2003) 95 (Bedouch et al., 2004) 97 (van Kasteren et al., 2003) 97.5 (Quenon et al., 2004)
Rates of thromboembolic prophylaxis within surgical studies	**Percentage of procedures in which thromboembolic prophylaxis carried out** 5 at high risk, 23.0 at medium risk (Ahmad et al., 2002) 22 (Aujesky et al., 2002) 29 (Scott et al., 2003) 31.5 at the highest risk, 81 at high risk, 93 at moderate risk (Tan and Tan, 2004) 46.4 (Ageno et al., 2002) 49.4 (Chopard et al., 2005) 71 (Learhinan and Alderman, 2003) 81 (Freeman et al., 2002) 90 (Campbell et al., 2001)

NOTE: STEMI = acute ST-segment elevation myocardial infarction; NSTEMI = non-STEMI.

Acute Coronary Syndromes

The committee reviewed seven studies on quality of care for acute myocardial infarction. Six of these studies determined prescription rates for indicated medications at discharge (Alexander et al., 1998; Petersen et al., 2001; Krumholz et al., 2003; Petersen et al., 2003; Roe et al., 2005; Granger et al., 2005). For patients discharged with a diagnosis of acute myocardial infarction, aspirin was prescribed to 53 to 93.4 percent of ideal candidates (those with no known contraindication). Beta-blockers were prescribed to 53 to 83.4 percent of ideal candidates, and angiotensin converting enzyme (ACE) inhibitors to 58.5 to 83.4 percent of ideal candidates. Three studies described rates of aspirin and beta-blocker use within the first 24 hours of hospitalization (Sanborn et al., 2004; Roe et al., 2005; Granger et al., 2005). Within the first 24 hours of hospitalization for a myocardial infarction, 66 to 78 percent of patients had received beta-blockers and 84.9 to 93 percent aspirin.

Antibiotic Prophylaxis

The committee identified six studies that described rates of antibiotic prophylaxis for surgical procedures (Heineck et al., 1999; Vaisbrud et al., 1999; van Kasteren et al., 2003; Gupta et al., 2003; Bedouch et al., 2004; Quenon et al., 2004). Rates of antibiotic prophylaxis ranged from 70 to 98 percent within the surgical studies. Although the rates of prescribing any antibiotic were high, antibiotic prophylaxis for surgical procedures requires that the appropriate antibiotic be selected, that the appropriate dose be prescribed, that the drug be administered at the appropriate time, and that the duration of therapy be correct. Absolute compliance with all of these elements of drug therapy was much lower—as low 3 percent in one study (Gupta et al., 2003).

Thrombosis Prophylaxis

The committee identified nine studies that determined rates of thromboembolic prophylaxis in at-risk hospitalized patients (Campbell et al., 2001; Ageno et al., 2002; Ahmad et al., 2002; Aujesky et al., 2002; Freeman et al., 2002; Learhinan and Alderman, 2003; Scott et al., 2003; Tan and Tan, 2004; Chopard et al., 2005). Thromboembolic prophylaxis includes both mechanical means, such as lower-extremity compression hose, and pharmacological means, such as subcutaneous heparin. Because medications are recommended in individuals at high risk for thrombosis, the committee included these studies.

Rates of thromboembolic prophylaxis varied widely—from 5 to 81 percent. Rates of appropriate thromboembolic prophylaxis tended to be higher in surgical patients and in those at lower risk for thrombosis. One study also noted that thromboembolic prophylaxis was prescribed inappropriately in 38 percent of patients without risk factors for thrombosis (Aujesky et al., 2002).

INCIDENCE OF MEDICATION ERRORS IN NURSING HOMES

Studies on the incidence of medication errors and ADEs in nursing homes use a number of different definitions, measures, and metrics. Hence, as with hospital studies, it is difficult to compare the results across studies.

Drug Procurement and Dispensing

Drug procurement and dispensing in the nursing home differ from hospital practice because the pharmacy is generally offsite. Handler and colleagues (2004) identified several aspects of drug delivery: (1) issues of packaging (e.g., patient-specific unit-dose packaging, patient-specific blister packages, 7-day strips of medication, color-coded drug administration devices, or medication bottles similar to usual community practice); (2) access to urgent medications, such as stock drugs in an emergency box; and (3) drug delivery when medications are added or changed, which may require hours to days (Handler et al., 2004). There is minimal research on how the approaches to addressing these issues affect medication safety.

When several pharmacies provide medications to a single nursing facility, staff must learn to use numerous systems, a practice that violates the fundamental safety principle of standardization. An evaluation of the medication-use system in one nursing home found that the facility's 72 patients were served by seven pharmacies, and the consultant pharmacist had no relationship with any of them (Cooper, 1987). The charge nurse verifying refill needs required 8–12 hours per 100 beds per month. Qualitative data underscore the issues of time and error associated with this refill process (Vogelsmeier et al., 2005). Gupta and colleagues (1996a,b) noted that only 8.4 percent of the 19,932 Medicaid patients they studied used a single pharmacy, and the number of pharmacies used was associated with mortality rates (Gupta et al., 1996a,b).

Administration Errors

The committee identified a few studies that measured the incidence of medication administration errors in nursing homes (see Table C-7). A well-known early study using direct observation of medication administration in

TABLE C-7 Nursing Home: Administration Errors

Error rates	Per 100 opportunities/doses—detection method
	6 (Cooper et al., 1994)—direct observation
	12.2 (Barker et al., 1982)—direct observation
	14.7 (Barker et al., 2002)—direct observation
	20 (Baldwin, 1992)—direct observation

58 nursing homes identified a mean error rate of 12.2 percent (range 0–59 percent over the 58 nursing homes), where an error was defined as a dose administered or omitted that deviates from the physician's orders (Barker et al., 1982). The direct observation procedure used in this study detects primarily errors in transcribing and administration. If out-of-date and unsigned orders were excluded, the error rate was 8 percent. The most common error types were unauthorized drug (44.8 percent) and omission (41.5 percent), followed by wrong dose (11 percent), wrong route (2 percent), and wrong form (0.4 percent). Most of the errors involving unauthorized drugs were due to out-of-date orders. Wrong-time errors were not recorded in this study. Because an error is defined as a discrepancy between the drug ordered and the drug received, errors detected by observation may be due to transcription or administration error, but observational studies do not distinguish the phase in which the error originates.

In a 2-year study apparently using observation in one nursing home, Cooper (1987) also concluded that omissions were the most common type of administration error (65 percent of errors). Many of the omissions were caused by patient refusal or sleeping, but the charting often implied that the drug had been administered.

A later study of error rates in skilled nursing facilities and hospitals found an average rate of 21.6 percent in 12 skilled nursing facilities in Georgia and Colorado, using the same direct observation method of error detection and defining an error as a discrepancy between the dose ordered and the dose received. The range of error rates across the 12 nursing facilities was 5.7 to 49.5 percent. The average error rate was not statistically different from the 14.4 percent rate for hospitals (Barker et al., 2002). Excluding wrong-time errors, the rate was 14.7 percent for skilled nursing facilities and 9.9 percent for hospitals. About 7 percent of the errors were judged by a physician panel to be potential ADEs. The rank order of error types was wrong time (9.9 percent of doses, 45.4 percent of errors), omission (7 percent of doses, 32.4 percent of errors), and wrong dose (3.1 percent of doses, 14.2 percent of errors).

Using similar observational methods, Baldwin (1992) detected a 20 percent medication administration error rate in a study of 733 residents of 35 domiciliary homes in North Carolina (error rate range 3–44 percent across the 35 homes). Using observation of 300 doses, Cooper and colleagues (1994) found a 6 percent administration error rate in one 300-bed nursing home during the baseline evaluation, using observation of 300 doses prior to implementation of an automated system.

Wrong-time error is a significant problem in residential care settings. An error rate of 27 percent in assisted-living settings was reduced to 15 percent when a 4-hour interval (as opposed to a 2-hour interval) around the scheduled time was used to designate on-time administration (Young et al., 2005). Four types of error were observed: wrong time (43 percent of errors), wrong dose (30 percent), omitted dose (10 percent), and unauthorized drug (10 percent). Wrong-time errors were even more prevalent in nursing homes, where the error rate decreased from 35.6 to 6.7 percent when wrong-time errors were excluded (Scott-Cawiezell et al., 2005).

Transcription and Documentation

Errors identified by observation of drug administration, which detects errors in transcription as well as administration, are described in the section below on administration. A study of discrepancies in medication orders on documents (medication administration record, hospital summary, and discharge orders) accompanying 20 newly admitted residents at the time of transfer from a Veterans Administration hospital to a Veterans Administration nursing home revealed at least one medication discrepancy for every subject (Siple and Joseph, 1992). Discrepancies were found in medication name, medication dose, omitted or added medications, and instructions for use. Investigators attributed 75 percent of the discrepancies to error and 25 percent to intentional changes.

Monitoring

Although the committee could identify no studies focused specifically on monitoring errors, Gurwitz and colleagues (2005) pointed out that the high rate of preventable ADEs (4.1 per 100 patient months) identified in their cohort study of long-term residents of two academic nursing homes argued for a special focus on ordering and monitoring. Errors occurred at the monitoring stage in 80 percent of the preventable ADEs. The most common monitoring errors were inadequate monitoring and failure to act on monitoring.

Comparison of Error Rates Across Stages of the Medication-Use Process

Few studies directly compare error rates across the stages of the medication-use process. In such a comparison, the method of error detection will substantially influence the estimate of error rates. Flynn and colleagues (2002) collected parallel data on 2,557 doses using direct observation, chart review, and voluntary incident reporting. Rates of error detected by the three methods across all study sites (including 24 hospitals and 12 nursing homes) were 17.8 percent, 0.1 percent, and 0.003 percent, respectively.

Three studies investigated error rates by stage of the medication-use process. Using a cohort design involving chart review and stimulated reporting, Gurwitz and colleagues (2000) detected most errors in the prescribing and monitoring stages. Among the 464 preventable ADEs identified in the study, errors occurred most often in the prescribing stage (315 errors, 68 percent of ADEs) and the monitoring stage (325 errors, 70 percent of ADEs). Errors were rare in the documentation/transcription, dispensing, and administration stages.

Similar results were found in a later study by the same research team using similar chart review methods (Gurwitz et al., 2005). Errors associated with the 338 preventable ADEs were more likely to occur at the prescribing (59 percent of ADEs) and monitoring (80 percent of ADEs) stages. Errors were less common at the dispensing and administration stages. Forty-six percent of preventable ADEs involved errors at two stages of the medication-use process, and 5 percent involved errors at three stages.

Handler and colleagues (2004) analyzed incident reports at one long-term care facility; they found an average of 4.7 reports per month, while residents averaged 11.2 medications per day. A process analysis indicated that the same stages of medication use occur in the nursing home and hospital settings. Consistent with hospital reporting, most incident reports in this study were filed by nurses; 68 percent of reported errors occurred at the administration stage, 20.4 percent at the dispensing stage, and 11.6 percent at both the administration and dispensing stages.

Incidence of ADEs in Nursing Homes

Retrospective Studies

Gurwitz and colleagues (1994) published a retrospective review of incident reports from one 703-bed academic nursing home for 1 year to identify adverse and unexpected events. After falls, medication-related events (n = 180) were most common, at 26 per 100 beds. Errors in dosing (72.2 percent of reports) were more common than adverse drug reactions (26.7 percent). A more recent study based on incident reports during 21 months at a single 126-bed long-term care facility identified 98 errors, but no denominator was used to compute error rates (Handler et al., 2004). Authors of both of these studies acknowledged that the findings under-represented the incidence of ADEs because of the limitations of the voluntary reporting of incidents.

Another retrospective review examined available medical charts for 175 admissions to one academic nursing home in the Veterans Administration system during an 18-month period, defining ADEs using a standardized protocol based on the Naranjo protocol (Gerety et al., 1993). A total of 201 ADEs occurred in 95 of the 175 admissions. On average, 1.2 ADEs occurred per resident (0.44 per patient month). Most ADEs were classified as minor, although 22.3 percent were rated serious, including one death. Limitations of this retrospective methodology for estimating error rates were potential misclassification of events (only 38 percent of ADEs were definitely or probably attributable to the medications) and the failure to identify the preventability of the ADEs (see Table C-8).

Prospective Studies

A prospective study of two Georgia nursing facilities over a 4-year period using monthly drug regimen review identified 444 adverse drug reactions (defined as unwanted consequences of drug therapy) in 74 percent of the 332 residents in the study (Cooper, 1999). There were 64 drug-associated hospitalizations in 52 of the 332 residents (15.7 percent).

Two studies from the same group of investigators used a prospective cohort design. The first (Gurwitz et al., 2000) examined the incidence and preventability of ADEs over a 12-month period in long-term residents of 18 nursing homes served by one pharmacy provider in Massachusetts. Data on ADEs (defined as an injury resulting from the use of a drug) for this cohort study were collected by chart review and simulated reporting, and preventability was judged by two physician reviewers. The overall ADE rate was 1.89 per 100 resident months, with a preventable ADE rate of 0.96 per 100 resident months. More severe ADEs were more likely to be preventable (risk ratio = 2.1, p <0.001).

TABLE C-8 Nursing Homes: ADE Incidence

Study	ADEs per Patient-Month	ADEs per 100 Admissions	Proportion of ADEs Preventable
Gurwitz et al., 2000	0.02	Not given	51 percent (out of 546 ADEs in study)
Gurwitz et al., 2005	0.1	Not given	42 percent (out of 815 ADEs in study)
Gerety et al., 1993	0.44	115	Not given (201 ADEs in study)
Cooper, 1999	Not given	134	Not given (444 ADEs in study)

The same group (Gurwitz et al., 2005) used the above methodology enhanced by the continuous presence of pharmacist investigators and computerized alerts to identify the incidence of ADEs in two academic nursing homes in Connecticut and Ontario, Canada. The study found a rate of 9.6 ADEs per 100 resident-months, with a rate of 4.1 preventable ADEs per 100 resident-months. Overall, 42 percent of ADEs were deemed preventable, while 61 percent of serious, life-threatening, or fatal ADE were judged preventable. While the five-fold increase in ADE rates in this study was attributed to improved detection, the investigators concluded that these rates probably underestimated the ADE incidence since they were based on chart review rather than direct examination of the residents (see Table C-8).

If the findings of these two well-designed studies are applied to all U.S. nursing homes, between 24 and 120 ADEs occur annually in the average nursing home (bed size 105). Between 350,000 and 1.9 million ADEs occur each year among the 1.6 million U.S. nursing home residents, about 40–50 percent of which are preventable. Of the estimated 20,000–86,000 fatal or life-threatening ADEs, about 70–80 percent are preventable.

Adverse Drug Withdrawal Events (ADWEs)

While many investigators have noted that discontinuation of drugs can cause adverse events in nursing home patients (Gurwitz et al., 2000, 2005), only a few researchers have investigated these events separately from other ADEs. Gerety and colleagues introduced the concept of the ADWE into nursing home research in their retrospective chart review of nursing home admissions. Among 62 of 175 residents, 94 ADWEs occurred—a mean rate of 0.54 per resident and 0.32 per patient-month. A more recent study (Boockvar et al., 2004) evaluated adverse events due to drug discontinuations at the time of transfer of 87 residents between four nursing homes in New York and either of two academic hospitals. Medications were altered in 86 percent of the 122 hospital admissions, with a mean of 3.1 alterations per admission and 1.4 medication changes at discharge, excluding new medications. ADEs occurred in 20 percent of bidirectional transfers—50 percent involving medication discontinuation and 36 percent dosage changes. The time from change to ADE occurrence averaged 14 days, so most ADEs occurred on return to the nursing home. Although it was not determined whether the changes at transfer were accidental, this study addressed the problem that generated the 2005 Joint Commission on Accreditation of Healthcare Organizations (JCAHO) goal on medication regimen reconciliation.

Two other studies addressed ADWEs involving psychotropic medications, including benzodiazepines, with no evidence of negative effects on behavior or perception of carefully controlled tapered withdrawal (Cohen-

Mansfield et al., 1999) or more haphazard withdrawal or substitution (Zullich et al., 1993).

Underutilization of Medications

A few studies have considered underutilization of medications in long-term care, that is, failure to prescribe or administer medications for which there is an evidence base for reduction of morbidity and mortality and a best-practice designation (see Table C-9). Economic restrictions on medication acquisition could be a factor in the underutilization rates quoted below.

A retrospective study of 2,014 residents over age 65 from a stratified random sample of 193 assisted-living facilities in four U.S. states demonstrated that underutilization of medications was common (Sloane et al., 2004). Of 328 residents with congestive heart failure, 62 percent were not receiving an ACE inhibitor; of 172 subjects with a history of myocardial infarction, 60.5 percent were not receiving aspirin, and 76 percent were not receiving beta-blockers; of 435 residents with a history of stroke, 37.5 percent were not receiving an anticoagulant or antiplatelet product; and of 315 residents with osteoporosis, 61 percent were not receiving calcium supplementation, and 51 percent were not receiving any treatment.

In another retrospective review of the records of 2,587 nursing home residents, only 53 percent of ideal candidates with atrial fibrillation were receiving warfarin. The therapeutic international normalized ratio (INR) range was maintained only 51 percent of the time (McCormick et al., 2001).

In a Dutch study (van Dijk et al., 2003), the most common prescribing problem was omission of a gastroprotective drug, which occurred in 85 percent of residents taking nonsteroidal anti-inflammatory drugs (NSAIDs). Using judgments of an expert review panel, Ruths and colleagues identified underuse of beneficial therapy in 13 percent of residents in 23 nursing homes in Norway (Ruths et al., 2003).

Studies using the SAGE (Systematic Assessment of Geriatric drug use via Epidemiology) database that linked information from the Minimum Data Set (MDS) and nursing home drug utilization data showed that only 25 percent of 86,094 nursing home residents with congestive heart failure were prescribed an ACE inhibitor (Gambassi et al., 2000). Another study using SAGE data showed that only 55 percent of residents identified as depressed based on the MDS received antidepressants, and 35 percent of those received less than the manufacturer's recommended dose (Brown et al., 2002), although underdosing may be appropriate for more frail elderly adults.

Inadequate pain management is a well-documented example of underutilization of medication, with 45–80 percent of nursing home residents

TABLE C-9 Nursing Home Care: Prescription Errors of Omission

Residents 65+ with congestive heart failure	**Percentage of residents receiving ACE inhibitors** 38 (Sloane et al., 2004) (for resident 65+)
Residents with congestive heart failure	**Percentage of residents prescribed ACE inhibitors** 25 (Gambassi et al., 2000)
Residents 65+ with history of myocardial infarction	**Percentage of residents receiving aspirin** 40 (Sloane et al., 2004)
Residents 65+ with history of myocardial infarction	**Percentage of residents receiving beta-blockers** 24 (Sloane et al., 2004)
Residents 65+ with history of stroke	**Percentage of residents receiving anticoagulant or antiplatelet product** 63 (Sloane et al., 2004)
Residents 65+ with osteoporosis	**Percentage of residents receiving calcium supplementation** 39 (Sloane et al., 2004)
Residents 65+ with osteoporosis	**Percentage of residents receiving any treatment** 49 (Sloane et al., 2004)
Residents with atrial fibrillation	**Percentage of residents receiving warfarin** 53 (McCormick et al., 2001)
Residents taking nonsteroidal anti-flammatory drugs (NSAIDs)	**Percentage of residents receiving gastroprotective drugs** 15 (van Dijk et al., 2003)
Residents with depression	**Percentage of residents receiving antidepressants** 55 (Brown et al., 2002)
Residents with pain	**Percentage of residents having unrelieved pain** 45–80 (AGS, 2002) **Percentage of residents receiving no analgesics** ~25 percent (Bernabei et al., 1998; Won et al., 1999, 2004) **Percentage of residents receiving optimal pain management** 66 percent (Hutt et al., 2006).

having unrelieved pain (AGS, 2002). Cross-sectional studies using the SAGE database or MDS data have indicated that 26 percent of nursing home residents overall and 30 percent of those with a cancer diagnosis have daily pain, and approximately 25 percent of these individuals receive no analgesics (Bernabei et al., 1998; Won et al., 1999, 2004). Using a scale developed to quantify the appropriateness of pain management in nursing homes, Hutt and colleagues (2006) calculated a mean score of 66 percent of optimal pain management in residents of 12 nursing homes in Colorado (Hutt et al., 2006). Fewer than half of the residents with predictably recurrent pain had prescriptions for scheduled pain medication, and only 40 percent with neuropathic pain were on an appropriate analgesic adjuvant.

Overuse of H_2 Blockers

Overutilization of medication, another indicator of inappropriate prescribing, was demonstrated in a retrospective chart review of the use of histamine-2 (H_2) receptor blocker therapy among 711 residents in one academic nursing home (Gurwitz et al., 1992). H_2 blocker therapy was used for unsubstantiated indications in 41 percent of the 110 residents receiving this category of drugs.

INCIDENCE OF MEDICATION ERRORS IN AMBULATORY CARE

For the purposes of this study, the committee examined medication error rates in six different settings within the ambulatory care domain: (1) the interface between care settings, for example, from hospital care to outpatient clinic; (2) the ambulatory clinic; (3) the community or mail order pharmacy; (4) the home care setting; (5) the self-care setting; and (6) the school setting.

Interface Between Care Settings

It is believed that medication errors and ADEs occur frequently in the interfaces between care settings, particularly after hospital discharge, yet the committee could find only two studies estimating error rates for such transitions (see Table C-10). In one study, a total of 42 (49 percent) patients who were discharged from the hospital and received continuing care from their primary care physicians experienced at least one medication error within 2 months of hospital discharge (Moore et al., 2003). In the other study, 45 (11 percent) of the 400 patients discharged from a general medicine service

TABLE C-10 Errors Across the Interfaces of Care

Hospital to clinic	Medication errors per patient—detection method 49 percent (Moore et al., 2003)—comparison of inpatient and outpatient records
Hospital to home	Preventable ADEs per patient—detection method 3 percent (Forster et al., 2005)—record review and patient interview

experienced an ADE: 32 patients had significant injuries, 6 had serious injuries, and 7 had life-threatening injuries; 27 percent of the ADEs were considered preventable, and 33 percent ameliorable (Forster et al., 2005).

The Ambulatory Clinic

Most studies on medication errors in ambulatory care have focused on prescribing errors (see Table C-11).

TABLE C-11 Ambulatory Clinic: Prescribing Errors

Prescription writing errors	Percentage of prescriptions containing at least one prescription writing error—detection method 21 (Shaughnessy and Nickel, 1989)—prescription review
Errors in an ambulatory hemodialysis unit	Percentage of patients with prescribing errors—detection method 97.7 (Manley et al., 2003b)—chart review Medication-related problems per patient per month—detection method 0.45 (Manley et al., 2003a)—pharmacist review of medication orders
Potential drug–drug interactions	Percentage of patients with two or more prescriptions with potential drug–drug interactions—detection method 6.2–6.7 (Solberg et al., 2004)—review of administration data 0.74 (Zhan et al., 2005)—review of administration data
Potential drug–disease interactions	Percentage of patients with two or more prescriptions with potential drug–disease interactions—detection method 2.58 (Zhan et al., 2005)—review of administration data
Dispensing of samples	Percentage of labels with usual dosage not present—detection method 12 (Dill and Generali, 2000)—review of samples
Dispensing of samples	Percentage of labels that referred user to enclosed prescribing information that was absent—detection method 17 (Dill and Generali, 2000)—review of samples
Lack of medication monitoring	Percentage of patients being treated with levothyroxine not receiving minimum monitoring—detection method 44 (Stelfox et al., 2004)—chart review
Documentation errors	Current medications per patient missing from patient record—detection method 0.37 (Wagner and Hogan, 1996)—review of patient record 0.89 (Bedell et al., 2000)—review of patient record
Documentation errors	Percentage of prescription renewals missing from patient record—detection method 15 (Ernst et al., 2001)—review of patient record

Prescription Writing Errors

In a retrospective review of 1,814 prescriptions written by 20 family medicine residents, Shaughnessy and Nickel (1989) found that 21 percent of the prescriptions contained at least one prescription writing error. The errors included omissions (6 percent), prescriptions written for nonprescription products (5 percent), incorrect doses or directions (3 percent), indecipherable quantity to be dispensed (3 percent), unfulfilled legal requirements (1 percent), and incomplete directions (1 percent).

Care Delivery in the Ambulatory Specialty Clinic

Although medication errors occur in ambulatory specialty clinics in association with chemotherapeutic agents, IV infusions, and hemodialysis, there is a lack of data on the incidence of these errors. Only three studies were found—two on hemodialyis and one on chemotherapy.

In one group of 133 ambulatory patients undergoing hemodialysis, the percentage of medication prescribing errors was 97.7 percent; the most frequent errors detected were prescribing medications without indication (30.9 percent), prescribing medications without laboratory-related monitoring (27.6 percent), and not prescribing a medication despite an indication for usage (17.5 percent) (Manley et al., 2003b).

A study carried out in August 2001 through May 2002 reviewed the medications of 133 patients in an ambulatory hemodialysis unit (Manley et al., 2003a). Over a 10-month period, a pharmacist reviewed 5,373 medication orders and identified 354 (6.6 percent) medication-related problems. Most common were medication dosing problems (33.5 percent), adverse drug reactions (20.7 percent), and an indication that was not currently being treated (13.5 percent). At the end of the study period, 0.45 medication-related problems per patient per month had been identified. Extrapolating these finding to the 246,000 U.S. hemodialysis patients would mean that almost 111,000 medication-related problems occur each month.

In a prospective cohort study at three outpatient chemotherapy units, 1,380 adults experienced 203 potential ADEs, none of which caused harm, and 226 children experienced 34 potential ADEs, again none causing harm (Gandhi et al., 2005). Overall, there was a medication error rate of 3 percent (306 out of 10,122 orders).

Potential Drug–Drug and Drug–Disease Interactions

Potential drug–drug interaction rates were found to range from 6.2 to 6.7 percent per year among users of a core group of commonly taken medications. These estimates were derived from health plan administrative data (Solberg et al., 2004). A retrospective analysis of data from the 1995–2000 National Ambulatory Medical Care Survey and National Hospital Ambulatory Medical Care Survey found inappropriate drug–drug combinations in 0.74 percent of visits involving two or more prescriptions and inappropriate drug–disease combinations in 2.58 percent of visits involving at least one prescription (Zhan et al., 2005).

Administering of Samples

Concerns about labeling have been researched for sample medications dispensed from the ambulatory care setting. In one study (Dill and Generali, 2000), involving 35 frequently used sample medications from 16 different manufacturers with nine drug classifications, information on the usual dosage was not present on 12 percent of the labels evaluated; 17 percent gave dosage and frequency; and 9 percent gave dosage, route, frequency, and duration. The remaining 62 percent referred the user to enclosed prescribing information, which in 27 percent of cases was not in fact enclosed.

Lack of Medication Monitoring

The committee identified only one study of medication monitoring in an ambulatory care setting. In a retrospective chart review of 400 outpatients being treated with levothyroxine at a large North American tertiary care hospital, only 56 percent of patients were found to have received minimum monitoring based on criteria derived from the literature and established through expert consensus (Stelfox et al., 2004). Those patients who received the recommended monitoring had fewer levothyroxine-related ADEs than those who did not (1 percent versus 6 percent).

Documentation Errors

Three studies have examined the rate of medication discrepancies in the outpatient medical record. A study in an outpatient geriatric center found that 0.37 of current medications per patient (43 medications/117 patients) were missing from the patient record, and 0.38 of medications per patient (44 medications/117 patients) were included in the record but were not currently being taken by the patient (Wagner and Hogan, 1996). About a third of these errors were judged to have been caused by patients who misreported a medication at a previous visit or changed (stopped, started, or dose-adjusted) a medication between visits. A study carried out in a private practice affiliated with an academic center, involving 312 patients from the practices of five cardiologists and two internists, found that 0.89

of current medications per patient (278 medications/312 patients) were missing from the patient record, and 0.51 of medications per patient (158 medications/312 patients) were included in the record but were not currently being taken by the patient (Bedell et al., 2000). In a family medicine outpatient clinic, pharmacists evaluated 950 prescription-renewal requests for 134 medications and found that 15 percent of prescriptions (147 out of 950) were for medications the patient was taking but were not recorded in the patient's chart (Ernst et al., 2001).

The Community or Mail Order Pharmacy

A medication procurement error led to the inadvertent use of Bicillin C-R to treat syphilis in a Los Angeles clinic (CDC, 2005). In late 1998, the clinic pharmacy received a shipment of Bicillin C-R instead of Bicillin L-A. The pharmacy continued to order Bicillin C-R until March 2004. Other errors in the community pharmacy setting have been associated with telephoned prescriptions and medication dispensing (see Table C-12).

Prescription orders are frequently given by telephone. A study published in 1990 reported that that telephone prescriptions account for over 30 percent of all prescriptions (Spencer and Daugird, 1990). Although telephone prescription errors in the community pharmacy setting have raised concern about patient safety, the committee could only find one study addressing this topic. An observational study conducted in two community pharmacies over 11 days analyzed 813 telephone prescriptions (Camp et al., 2003). The investigators found that 12.4 percent of the telephone prescriptions contained an error. The most common types of errors included prescribing medication for the wrong patient, not providing the patient's telephone number, prescribing the wrong strength, giving the wrong directions for use, and prescribing the wrong medication.

A study conducted in one hospital-based outpatient pharmacy found the rate of dispensing errors to be 12.5 percent (1,229/9,846 prescriptions), and 1.6 percent (155/9,846 prescriptions) of the prescriptions contained

TABLE C-12 Community Pharmacy: Errors

Telephoned prescription errors	**Percentage of telephone prescriptions containing an error— detection method** 12.4 (Camp et al., 2003)—direct observation
Dispensing errors	**Percentage of prescription erroneously dispensed—detection method** 1.7 (Flynn et al., 2003)—direct observation 3.4 (Buchanan et al., 1991)—direct observation 12.5 (Kistner et al., 1994)—audit of filled prescriptions 24 (Allan et al., 1995)—audit of filled prescriptions

errors that had the potential to cause serious harm (Kistner et al., 1994). Another study, conducted in 100 randomly selected community pharmacies, involved the analysis of 100 prescriptions. Allan and colleagues (1995) found 24 dispensing errors, 4 of which were clinically significant. In a cross-sectional, direct observational study at a high-volume outpatient pharmacy, the dispensing error rate was found to be 3.4 percent (Buchanan et al., 1991). In a more recent cross-sectional, direct observational study of 50 community pharmacies (encompassing chain, independent, and health system pharmacies) located in six cities across the United States, the investigators found that the overall dispensing accuracy rate for new and refill prescriptions was 98.3 percent (Flynn et al., 2003). They found 77 errors among the 4,481 prescriptions they analyzed. Of the 77 identified errors, 5 (6.5 percent) were judged to be clinically important. The medication error rate did not differ significantly by pharmacy type or city. This dispensing error rate indicates that there are approximately 4 errors per 250 prescriptions per pharmacy per day, translating to an estimated 51.5 million errors during the filling of 3 billion prescriptions each year.

One study of medication errors involving mail order pharmacy was found (see Table C-13). During September and October 2003, at a highly automated mail order pharmacy practice, the original prescription order was compared with the container contents and label (Teagarden et al., 2005). The overall dispensing error rate was 0.075 percent—16 dispensing errors among 21,252 prescriptions. Of these errors, 14 involved incomplete or incorrect directions on the final label, 1 was due to the entry of an incorrect quantity on the system record, and 1 was due to the omission of the drug on the system record. No errors were associated with the mechanical aspects of the dispensing process.

The Home Care Setting

Two studies have examined prescribing errors in the home care setting (see Table C-14). In an evaluation of 11,689 prescriptions taken by 2,193

TABLE C-13 Mail Order Pharmacy: Errors

Dispensing errors	Percentage of prescription erroneously dispensed—detection method
	0.075 (Teagarden et al., 2005)—audit of filled prescriptions

TABLE C-14 Home Care Setting: Prescribing Errors

Inappropriate prescribing for elderly	Percentage of patients prescribed inappropriate medications
	30 (Meredith et al., 2001)
	40 (Golden et al., 1999)

homebound persons aged 60 and older, investigators found that 10 percent of these prescriptions were inappropriate (according to the Beers criteria) (Golden et al., 1999). Moreover, they found that 40 percent (871 out of 2,193 patients) of the subjects in the study had received at least one inappropriate prescription and that 10.5 percent (230 out of 2,193) had received two or more such prescriptions. A 2001 study analyzed the medication usage of 6,718 elderly home care patients and found that 30 percent had experienced potential medication errors when either the Home Health criteria (Brown et al., 1998) or the Beers criteria (Beers et al., 1992; Beers, 1997) were applied (Meredith et al., 2001).

In another study, self-reports of 101 home health care nurses from 12 agencies in six states showed that 78 percent of 1,467 patients who were in the nurses' care were at increased risk for medication errors because they were taking five or more medications, although such errors actually occurred less frequently (Ellenbecker et al., 2004). The investigators also found that ADEs had occurred in approximately 5 percent of the reported patients.

The Self-Care Setting

Studies on medication errors in the self-care setting have been related largely to medication adherence (see Table C-15). There is a large body of literature on medication adherence, most of which relates to particular disease conditions. In an early study, medication adherence for prescribed medications was estimated at about 50 percent (Sackett and Snow, 1979).

In 2004, a meta-analysis of 569 studies reporting on adherence to medical treatments (328 relating to medications) was published (DiMatteo, 2004). For each study, the adherence rate, as defined by the study author(s), was extracted. The average adherence rate over all studies was 75.2 percent and over all medication studies was 79.4 percent. Adherence rates improved over time: the average rate for pre-1980 studies (80 studies) was 62.6 percent and for 1980–1998 studies (491 studies) was 76.3 percent (p <0.001). However, more recent studies investigating how adherence rates change over time and with frequency of daily dosing have found generally lower rates.

A study in which a medication event monitoring system was used to assess patients' adherence to anticonvulsant medications found the average

TABLE C-15 Self-Care Setting: Adherence Rates

Adherence rates	Percentage medication adherence rate
	80 (Corda et al., 2000)
	76 (Cramer et al., 1989)
	50 (Sackett and Snow, 1979)

adherence rate to be 76 percent during 3,428 patient-days observed (Cramer et al., 1989). The rate decreased, however, when the daily frequency increased: 87 percent for dosing once/day, 81 percent for dosing twice/day, 77 percent for dosing three times/day, and 39 percent for dosing four times/day.

Another study evaluated adherence to medication among health care professionals to estimate the expected upper limit of adherence among the general population. In a self-administered survey, physicians and nurses were asked about their use of prescribed medications for acute and chronic illnesses (Corda et al., 2000). Among the respondents, 301 physicians and nurses had been prescribed medications for acute and/or chronic illnesses within 2 years of the survey. Of 610 prescribed medications, 80 percent were taken as prescribed, with a 77 percent adherence rate for short-term medications and an 84 percent rate for long-term medications.

Sharing of prescription medications appears to be relatively common among children and adolescents (Daniel et al., 2003). In a mail survey of youths aged 9–18 (764 girls and 804 boys), 16 percent of the girls reported borrowing prescription medications from others and 15 percent sharing their prescription medications with someone else; the respective proportions among the boys were 12 and 8 percent. An adolescent obtaining a prescription medication through sharing does not receive the appropriate information about its actions and possible risks. Sharing of potentially teratogenic drugs is of particular concern.

Results similar to the above were obtained in a survey of 963 adult outpatients at a university general internal medicine practice (Shaheen et al., 2004). Of the participants, 16 percent (158/963) reported using someone else's prescription medication. Of those who had been prescribed at least one medication in the past year, 17 percent (147/864) reported sharing their medication with someone else.

The School Setting

The committee found no studies on medication error rates in the school setting. Two studies have addressed this issue. In one study, 649 members of the National Association of School Nurses surveyed reported that 5.6 percent of school children were treated with medications in school; 3.3 percent of these children received medications for attention-deficit hyperactivity disorder (ADHD) (McCarthy et al., 2000). Almost all of the school nurses reported following written guidelines for administering medications, and 75.6 percent reported that they delegated medication administration to assertive unlicensed personnel (66.2 percent secretaries). About half (48.5 percent) reported errors in administering medication. Missing a dose was reported to be the most common error (79.9 percent).

TABLE C-16 Ambulatory Care: ADE Incidence

Study	Events per 100 Patients	ADEs per 100 Patient-Years	Proportion of ADEs Preventable
Gurwitz et al., 2003	Not given	5	28 percent (out of 1,523 ADEs in study)
Gandhi et al., 2000	18 drug complications	Not given	Not reported (394 drug complications in study)
Gandhi et al., 2003	27 ADEs	Not given	20 percent (out of 181 ADEs in study)

Incidence of ADEs During Ambulatory Care

The committee identified three studies on the rate of ADEs in ambulatory clinics (see Table C-16). In one study, using patient surveys and chart review, 394 (18 percent) patients reported a drug complication. Most of these complications were not noted in the medical chart, and it proved impossible to assess what proportion were preventable (Gandhi et al., 2000). A second study found that 162 (25 percent) of the 661 ambulatory care patients studied had experienced an ADE (Gandhi et al., 2003). Of the 181 ADEs found, 13 percent were serious, and 28 percent were ameliorable; 11 percent were attributed to the physician's failure to respond to medication-related symptoms. A third study, involving Medicare patients, found an overall ADE rate of 50.1 per 1,000 patient-years and a preventable ADE rate of 13.8 per 1,000 patient-years (Gurwitz et al., 2003). Of the 38 percent of ADEs that were serious, 42.2 percent were preventable, and of the 62 percent of ADEs that were significant, 18.7 percent were preventable. The preventable ADEs occurred most often at the stages of prescribing (58.4 percent), monitoring (60.8 percent), and administration and patient adherence (21.1 percent).

INCIDENCE OF MEDICATION ERRORS IN PEDIATRIC CARE

It has become clear that the prescribing, dispensing, and administration of medications are associated with a substantial portion of the preventable medical errors that occur with children (Kaushal et al., 2001, 2004). Given the need to tailor all pediatric medication doses to body-size parameters (e.g., weight, body mass index), the fact that children are much less able than adults to double-check their own medications in any setting, and the wide range of appropriate doses for any medication based on the child's size, children are uniquely vulnerable to medication errors. Accurate pediatric medication administration requires accurate weights; proper conversion of pounds to kilograms; the correct choice of appropriate preparations and concentrations; and the ability to measure and administer doses properly, particularly for liquid medications. The ways children differ from adult patients can be summarized by the factors of developmental change, dependency on adults, different disease epidemiology, and demographic characteristics (Forrest et al., 2003). These factors predispose children to patient safety events resulting from, for example, young children needing to rely on adults for dose checking and having to take liquid medications rather than standard-sized pills.

Prescription and Selection of the Drug for the Patient

A number of studies have examined prescription and selection errors associated with medications for pediatric populations (see Table C-17). An inpatient study covering all types of medications carried out at two urban teaching hospitals reported a 4.2 percent error rate (454 physician ordering errors out of 10,778 orders), or 405 prescribing errors per 1,000 patients (Kaushal et al., 2001). Using a broader definition of medication error, a French study reported a higher error rate—24 percent (937 prescribing errors out of 3,943 orders) (Fontan et al., 2003). Also using a broader

TABLE C-17 Hospital Pediatric Care: Prescription and Selection Errors

Medication ordering errors	**Percentage of prescriptions containing an error—detection method** 4.2 (Kaushal et al., 2001)—chart review 24 (Fontan et al., 2003)—chart review
Medication ordering errors in pediatric ICU	**Percentage of prescriptions containing an error—detection method** 30 (Potts et al., 2004)—chart review
Preventable ADEs	**Preventable ADEs per 1,000 admissions** 0.6 (Hardmeier et al., 2004) 1.1 (Bates et al., 1995b) 1.4 (Nebeker et al., 2005)
Gentamicin prescribing in neonatal ICU	**Percentage of prescriptions containing an error—detection method** 13 (14/105) before computerized physician order entry (CPOE) (Cordero et al., 2004)—review of chart and medical record 0 (0/92) post CPOE (Cordero et al., 2004)—review of chart and medical record
Ten-fold prescribing errors intercepted before reaching the patient	**Errors intercepted per 1,000 admissions—detection method** 5.3 (Lesar, 2002b)—incident reports

definition, a still higher rate of 30 percent was observed in a pediatric ICU (2,049 prescribing errors out of 6,803 orders) (Potts et al., 2004).

The French study cited above observed sharply differing error rates for handwritten and computerized prescribing. The study found a handwritten prescribing error rate of 88 percent (518 prescribing errors out of 589 orders) and a computerized prescribing error rate of 11 percent (419 errors out of 3,943 orders) (Fontan et al., 2003).

A more focused study in a neonatal ICU observed 14 Gentamicin prescription dosage errors in 105 very-low-birthweight infants (13 percent error rate) prior to the implementation of computerized physician order entry (CPOE) (Cordero et al., 2004). In 92 post-CPOE infants, no medication errors occurred. In another study in a neonatal ICU, 60 total parenteral nutrition errors were observed out of 557 total parenteral nutrition orders (11 percent error rate) (Lehmann et al., 2004).

Finally, another study evaluated ten-fold prescribing errors that were intercepted before reaching the patient. The occurrence of such errors in a 631-bed tertiary care teaching hospital was 0.53 per 100 pediatric admissions (Lesar, 2002b).

Medication Documentation

Three studies evaluated transcription/documentation errors for medications in hospital pediatric care (see Table C-18). In a study of two academic pediatric units, 85 documentation errors were found in 10,778 orders (0.8 percent) (Kaushal et al., 2001). In another study, 49 pediatric medication cardexes out of 540 (9 percent) were found to disagree in a major way (different dose, wrong medication, wrong frequency or duration, missing route) from the physician's original medication order (Cable and Croft, 2004). In a third study, at the first transcription, 20.7 percent (41 out of 198) of nonchemotherapy prescriptions and 11.8 percent (16 out of 135) of chemotherapy prescriptions were transcribed incorrectly in a pediatric oncohematology unit (Pichon et al., 2002).

TABLE C-18 Hospital Pediatric Care: Documentation Errors

Medication documentation errors	**Percentage of orders containing an error—detection method** 0.8 (Kaushal et al., 2001)—chart review 9 (Cable and Croft, 2004)—chart review
Medication transcription errors in a pediatric oncohematology unit	**Percentage of orders containing an error—detection method** 20.7 nonchemotherapy prescriptions (Pichon et al., 2002)—chart review 11.8 chemotherapy prescriptions (Pichon et al., 2002)—chart review

Preparation and Dispensing of the Drug

The committee identified only four studies addressing errors associated with the preparation and dispensing of medications in hospital pediatric care (see Table C-19). One study was based on chart reviews, which make it difficult to detect dispensing errors, particularly if errors are recognized and corrected before medication is given to the patient (Kaushal et al., 2001). This study estimated the rate of dispensing errors to be 0.05 errors per order written, or 5 dispensing errors per 1,000 patients.

Three other studies examined the proportion of dispensing errors among all reported medication errors. Estimates of this proportion vary widely: 4.5 percent for all types of medication in an inpatient setting (King et al., 2003), 9.3 percent for chemotherapy in an inpatient setting (France et al., 2004), and 58.9 percent for all types of medication in an ICU (Frey et al., 2002).

Administration of the Drug

Rates of drug administration errors have been reported in varying ways (see Table C-20). Administration errors were estimated to be 0.72 errors per 100 orders (or 7 per 100 admissions, or 19.8 per 1,000 patient-days) for all types of medication in an inpatient setting (Kaushal et al., 2001); 23

TABLE C-19 Hospital Pediatric Care: Preparation and Dispensing Errors

Error rates	**Errors per 1,000 patients—detection method** 5 (Kaushal et al., 2001)—chart review
Proportion of dispensing errors among all medication errors	**Percentage of reported errors related to dispensing—detection method** 4.5 percent (inpatient setting) (King et al., 2003)—incident reports 9.3 percent (chemotherapy, inpatient setting) (France et al., 2004)—incident reports 58.9 percent (ICU) (Frey et al., 2002)—incident reports

TABLE C-20 Hospital Pediatric Care: Administration Errors

Error rates, inpatient unit	**Errors per 100 orders—detection method** 0.72 (Kaushal et al., 2001)—chart review
Error rates, inpatient unit	**Errors per 100 admissions—detection method** 7 (Kaushal et al., 2001)—chart review
Error rates, inpatient unit	**Errors per 1,000 patient-days—detection method** 19.8 (Kaushal et al., 2001)—chart review
Error rate, nephrology unit	**Errors as a percentage of opportunities for error—detection method** 23 (Fontan et al., 2003)—chart review

percent of opportunities for administration errors in a pediatric nephrology ward (Fontan et al., 2003); 3.9 errors per 100 charts reviewed for all types of medication in an emergency department (Kozer et al., 2002); and 21.7 acetaminophen dosage errors per 100 patients receiving acetaminophen in an emergency department (Losek, 2004).

Monitoring of the Patient for Effect

Only one study reported on errors involving monitoring of the patient for effects (see Table C-21). Using chart review, this study estimated a rate of 4 errors per 1,000 patients (Kaushal et al., 2001).

Pediatric Care in the Ambulatory and Emergency Department Setting

The majority of pediatric medication error studies identified by the committee were focused on hospitalized patients. Three studies were focused on the ambulatory care setting and two studies on the emergency department setting. Of the three ambulatory care studies, all examined immunizations (see Table C-22). One study, conducted in the United States, defined invalid vaccine doses as doses given before the minimum recommended age, doses not given within the recommended spacing from the previous dose, doses given unnecessarily (defined as 1 year earlier than the required age), and live virus vaccine given too soon after a previous live virus vaccine. This study estimated 4 invalid doses per 100 immunizations given to children, or 36 percent of children being immunized receiving at

TABLE C-21 Hospital Pediatric Care: Monitoring Errors

Monitoring errors	Errors per 1,000 patients—detection method 4 (Kaushal et al., 2001)—chart review

TABLE C-22 Ambulatory Pediatric Care: Immunization Errors

Invalid doses	Invalid doses per every 100 immunizations—detection method 4 (Butte et al., 2001)—chart review
Overimmunized for at least one vaccine	Percentage of children overimmunized—detection method 21 (Feikema et al., 2000)—chart review from National Immunization Screenings
Vaccine doses reported to National Poison Registry	Doses reported per 1 million immunization doses—detection method 11 (Petridou et al., 2004)—incident reports

least 1 invalid dose (Butte et al., 2001). A second study, also conducted in the United States, estimated 21 percent of children being overimmunized for at least one vaccine (Feikema et al., 2000). A third study reported on calls regarding vaccines to the National Poison Control Registry in Greece. The estimate of 11 vaccine errors per 1 million immunization doses likely represents significant underreporting since one would have to consider a vaccine dose to be a poisoning to call this registry (Petridou et al., 2004).

Of the two emergency department studies, one focused on global estimates of prescription and administration errors in this setting, and the other on medication errors with respect to antipyretics (see Table C-23). The first study estimated a rate of 100 prescribing errors per 1,000 patients and 39 administration errors per 1,000 patients (Kozer et al., 2002). The second study found that 22 percent of acetaminophen doses ordered were outside of the recommended 10–15 milligrams/kilogram dose (Losek, 2004).

Incidence of ADEs During Hospitalization

A prospective study analyzed 1,120 patients at two academic pediatric institutions during 1999 using chart, medication order sheet, and medication administration record review, as well as voluntary and solicited reports (Kaushal et al., 2001) (see Table C-24). Twenty-six ADEs were identified—

TABLE C-23 Emergency Department Pediatric Care: Prescription and Administration Errors

Prescribing errors	**Errors per 1,000 patients—detection method** 100 (Kozer et al., 2002)—chart review
Administration errors	**Errors per 1,000 patients—detection method** 39 (Kozer et al., 2002)—chart review
Acetaminophen doses ordered outside recommended range	**Percentage of doses ordered outside recommended range—detection method** 22 (Losek, 2004)—chart review

TABLE C-24 Hospital Care: Pediatric ADE Incidence During Hospitalization

Study	ADEs per 100 Admissions	ADEs per 1,000 Patient-Days	Proportion of ADEs Preventable
Kaushal et al., 2001	2.3	6.6	19 percent (out of 26 ADEs in the study)
Holdsworth et al., 2003	6	7.5	(76 ADEs in the study)

2.3 per 100 admissions or 6.6 per 1,000 patient days; 19 percent of the ADEs were considered preventable.

A later prospective study analyzed 1,197 consecutive admissions (corresponding to 922 patients and 10,164 patient days) at a general pediatric unit and a pediatric ICU in a metropolitan medical center (Holdsworth et al., 2003). Seventy-six ADEs were identified—6 per 100 admissions or 7.5 per 1,000 patient days.

INCIDENCE OF MEDICATION ERRORS IN PSYCHIATRIC CARE

Many studies of medication errors associated with psychotropic medication were conducted as part of either larger general medical–surgical studies or ADE-reporting databases or were limited to geriatric populations in settings not restricted to psychiatric care, such as nursing homes and ambulatory clinics.

General Medical–Surgical Studies

An 18-month study in a tertiary care hospital used computerized monitoring to identify 701 ADEs, including 18 due to psychotropic drugs (2.4 percent) (Classen et al., 1991). A study using several active detection approaches, including daily chart review, among 4,031 medical–surgical inpatients found 247 ADEs (6.5 per 100 admissions) (Bates et al., 1993). Psychotropic medications represented 7 percent of all medication errors. A more recent study of hospitalized patients found that psychotropic drugs accounted for 0.41 percent of serious medication errors (Bates et al., 1998). After CPOE and a team intervention to prevent ADEs were implemented, this rate fell to 0.16 percent. A study using pharmacist detection of prescribing errors with potential for harm in a teaching hospital found that among 11,186 errors, 146 (1.3 percent) were associated with psychotropic medications (Lesar et al., 1997).

Geriatric Populations in Settings Not Restricted to Psychiatric Care

Older patients may be particularly vulnerable to the harmful effects of psychotropic medications (Monette et al., 1995). A 1-year study of 18 nursing homes reported that among 546 ADEs (1.89 per 100 resident-months), 193 (35 percent) were due to psychotropic medications (Gurwitz et al., 2000). A greater proportion of ADEs due to psychotropic medications (63 percent), as compared with all other drug classes (43 percent), was judged to be preventable.

One study found that psychotropic medications represented 23 percent of inappropriate medication orders prescribed in nursing homes (Beers et al., 1992). Two other studies found that older adults in ambulatory settings received even higher proportions of inappropriate psychotropic medications—27 percent (Aparasu and Fliginger, 1997) and 44 percent (Mort and Aparasu, 2000).

Psychiatric Hospitals

The committee identified two studies that examined the incidence of medication errors in a mental health setting (see Table C-25). The more recent of these retrospectively studied 31 state psychiatric inpatients over 2 months of care, for a total of 1,448 patient-days (Grasso et al., 2003). Nine errors were self-reported using the usual incident reporting process, whereas an independent multidisciplinary review team found 2,194 errors for the same 31 patients and episodes of care. There were 1,443 administration errors, accounting for more than half of the total (66 percent); 498 transcription errors (23 percent); 239 prescription errors (11 percent); and 14 dispensing errors (less than 1 percent). Nineteen percent of errors were rated as having a low risk of harm, 23 percent as having a moderate risk, and 58 percent as having a high risk.

The other study of ADEs included both inpatient and outpatient settings and focused on the frequency, severity, causes, and costs of ADEs in an integrated system of care that included medical and psychiatric patients (Senst et al., 2001). In this setting, medication errors were implicated in 13.6 percent of psychiatric readmissions, with medication nonadherence (considered part of the usual lexicon of medication errors) being implicated in 69 percent of hospitalizations. The rate of ADEs during psychiatric hospitalization was 4.2 per 100 admissions.

TABLE C-25 Psychiatric Care: Medication Errors

Prescribing errors	Errors per 1,000 patient-days—detection method 165 (Grasso et al., 2003)—chart review
Transcription errors	Errors per 1,000 patient-days—detection method 334 (Grasso et al., 2003)—chart review
Administration errors	Errors per 1,000 patient-days—detection method 997 (Grasso et al., 2003)—chart review
Dispensing errors	Errors per 1,000 patient-days—detection method 10 (Grasso et al., 2003)—chart review
ADEs	Errors per 100 admissions—detection method 4.2 (Senst et al., 2001)—chart review

The committee's literature review yielded no reports focused specifically on medication errors in outpatient mental health settings, nor have there been medication error incidence studies in settings where psychologists have prescriptive authority. Finally, no studies were found on the incidence and characteristics of medication errors in substance abuse settings, including all settings where medical detoxification of individuals treated for alcohol, sedative hypnotic, or opiate withdrawal occurs. All of these are areas in which data are badly needed.

ERROR RATES: MUCH MORE NEEDS TO BE DONE

Where incidence rates of medication errors have been systematically measured, such errors have been found to be common and at unacceptably high levels. Errors in the administration of IV medications appear to be particularly prevalent. Reasonably well-researched stages of the medication-use process include prescribing, dispensing, and administering in hospitals; prescribing in ambulatory clinics; dispensing in community pharmacies; prescribing in the home care setting; medication adherence in the self-care setting; and inappropriate use of psychotropic drugs.

Where it is possible to compare the results of multiple studies, estimates of error rates vary widely. Much but not all of this variation can be explained by differences in definition and identification methods. Even when the definition of error is standardized and the same identification method is used, however, substantial variation in administration error rates by institution have been found (Barker et al., 2002). Taking account of this variability, the underlying error rates are unacceptably high.

Over the past decade, much scholarly activity and substantial government resources have been directed at determining the extent and scope of medication errors. Yet there are still broad aspects of the medication-use process for which we have little or no understanding of error rates. These include the selection and procurement of medications, monitoring of the effectiveness of medications in all care settings, medication use in schools, medication use in psychiatric care, and the use of over-the-counter and complementary and alternative medications.

The committee concludes that still greater effort is needed in all care settings to identify the incidence of medication errors—both to measure the extent and scope of such errors and to assess the impact of error prevention strategies.

REFERENCES

Ageno W, Squizzato A, Ambrosini F, Dentali F, Marchesi C, Mera V, Steidl L, Venco A. 2002. Thrombosis prophylaxis in medical patients: A retrospective review of clinical practice patterns. *Haematologica* 87(7):746–750.

AGS (American Geriatrics Society). 2002. American Geriatrics Society (AGS) Panel on Persistent Pain in Older Persons. The management of persistent pain in older persons. *Journal of the American Geriatrics Society* 50(Suppl. 6):S205–S224.

Ahmad HA, Geissler A, MacLellan D. 2002. Deep venous thrombosis prophylaxis: Are guidelines being followed? *Australian and New Zealand Journal of Surgery* 72(5):331–334.

Alexander KP, Peterson ED, Granger CB, Casas AC, Van de Werf F, Armstrong PW, Guerci A, Topol EJ, Califf RM. 1998. Potential impact of evidence-based medicine in acute coronary syndromes: Insights from GUSTO-IIb. Global use of strategies to open occluded arteries in acute coronary syndromes trial. *Journal of the American College of Cardiology* 32(7):2023–2030.

Allan EL, Barker KN, Malloy MJ, Heller WM. 1995. Dispensing errors and counseling in community practice. *American Pharmacy* NS35(12):25–33.

Aparasu RR, Fliginger SE. 1997. Inappropriate medication prescribing for the elderly by office-based physicians. *The Annals of Pharmacotherapy* 31(7–8):823–829.

Aujesky D, Guignard E, Pannatier, Cornuz J. 2002. Pharmacological thromboembolic prophylaxis in a medical ward: Room for improvement. *Journal of General Internal Medicine* 17(10):788–791.

Baldwin VR. 1992. *An Analysis of Subjective and Objective Indicators of Quality of Care in North Carolina Homes for the Aged*. PhD diss. University of North Carolina at Chapel Hill.

Barker KN, Mikeal RL, Pearson RE, Illig NA, Morse ML. 1982. Medication errors in nursing homes and small hospitals. *American Journal of Hospital Pharmacy* 39:987–991.

Barker KN, Flynn EA, Pepper GA, Bates DW, Mikeal RL. 2002. Medication errors observed in 36 health care facilities. *Archives of Internal Medicine* 162(16):1897–1903.

Bates DW, Leape LL, Petrycki S. 1993. Incidence and preventability of adverse drug events in hospitalized adults. *Journal of General Internal Medicine* 8(6):289–294.

Bates DW, Boyle DL, Vander Vliet MB, Schneider J, Leape L. 1995a. Relationship between medication errors and adverse drug events. *Journal of General Internal Medicine* 10(4): 100–205.

Bates DW, Cullen DJ, Laird N, Petersen LA, Small SD, Servi D, Laffel G, Sweitzer BJ, Shea BF, Hallisey R, Vander Vliet M, Nemeskal R, Leape LL. 1995b. Incidence of adverse drug events and potential adverse drug events. Implications for prevention. ADE Prevention Study Group. *Journal of the American Medical Association* 274:29–34.

Bates DW, Leape LL, Cullen DJ, Laird N, Petersen LA, Teich JM, Burdick E, Hickey M, Kleefield S, Shea B, Vander Vliet M. 1998. Effect of computerized physician order entry and a team intervention on prevention of serious medication errors. *Journal of the American Medical Association* 80(15):1311–1316.

Bedell SE, Jabbour S, Goldberg R, Glaser H, Gobble S, Young-Xu Y, Graboys TB, Ravid S. 2000. Discrepancies in the use of medications: Their extent and predictors in an outpatient practice. *Archives of Internal Medicine* 160(14):2129–2134.

Bedouch P, Labarere J, Chirpaz E, Allenet B, Lepape A, Fourny M, Pavese P, Girardet P, Merloz P, Saragaglia D, Calop J, Francois P. 2004. Compliance with guidelines on antibiotic prophylaxis in total hip replacement surgery: Results of a retrospective study of 416 patients in a teaching hospital. *Infection Control and Hospital Epidemiology* 25(4):302–307.

Beers MH. 1997. Explicit criteria for determining potentially inappropriate medication use by the elderly. An update. *Archives of Internal Medicine* 157(14):1531–1536.

Beers MH, Ouslander JG, Fingold SF, Morgenstern H, Reuben DB, Rogers W, Zeffren MJ, Beck JC. 1992. Inappropriate medication prescribing in skilled-nursing facilities. *Annals of Internal Medicine* 117(8):684–689.

Bernabei R, Gambassi G, Lapane K. 1998. Management of pain in elderly patients with cancer. SAGE Study Group. Systematic Assessment of Geriatric drug use via Epidemiology. *Journal of the American Medical Association* 279:1877–1882.

Bobb A, Gleason K, Husch M, Feinglass J, Yarnold PR, Noskin GA. 2004. The epidemiology of prescribing errors. *Archives of Internal Medicine* 164(7):785–792.

Boockvar K, Fishman E, Kyriacou CK, Monias A, Gavi S, Cortes T. 2004. Adverse events due to discontinuations in drug use and dose changes in patients transferred between acute and long-term care facilities. *Archives of Internal Medicine* 164(5):545–550.

Brown MN, Lapane KL, Luisi AF. 2002. The management of depression in older nursing home residents. *Journal of the American Geriatrics Society* 50:69–76.

Brown NJ, Griffin MR, Ray WA, Meredith S, Beers MH, Marren J, Robles M, Stergachis A, Wood AJ, Avorn J. 1998. A model for improving medication use in home health care patients. *Journal of the American Pharmaceutical Association* 38(6):696–702.

Buchanan TL, Barker KN, Gibson JT, Jiang BC, Pearson RE. 1991. Illumination and errors in dispensing. *American Journal of Hospital Pharmacy* 48(10):2137–2145.

Butte AJ, Shaw JS, Bernstein H. 2001. Strict interpretation of vaccination guidelines with computerized algorithms and improper timing of administered doses. *The Pediatric Infectious Disease Journal* 20(6):561–565.

Cable G, Croft J. 2004. Agreement between pediatric medication orders and medication cardex. *Journal for Healthcare Quality* 26(2):14–19.

Calabrese AD, Erstad BL, Brandl K, Barletta JF, Kane SL, Sherman DS. 2001. Medication administration errors in adult patients in the ICU. *Intensive Care Medicine* 27(10):1592–1598.

Camp SC, Hailemeskel B, Rogers TL. 2003. Telephone prescription errors in two community pharmacies. *American Journal of Health-System Pharmacy* 60(6):613–614.

Campbell SE, Walke AE, Grimshaw JM, Campbell MK, Lowe GD, Harper D, Fowkes FG, Petrie JC. 2001. The prevalence of prophylaxis for deep vein thrombosis in acute hospital trusts. *International Journal for Quality in Health Care* 13(4):309–316.

CDC (Centers for Disease Control and Prevention). 2005. Inadvertent use of Bicillin C-R to treat syphilis infection—Los Angeles, California, 1999–2004. *Morbidity and Mortality Weekly Report* 54(9):217–219.

Chopard P, Dorffler-Melly J, Hess U, Wuillemin WA, Hayoz D, Gallino A, Bachli EB, Canova CR, Isenegger J, Rubino R, Bounameaux H. 2005. Venous thromboembolism prophylaxis in acutely ill medical patients: Definite need for improvement. *Journal of Internal Medicine* 257(4):352–357.

Classen DC, Pestotnik SL, Evans RS, Burke JP. 1991. Computerized surveillance of adverse drug events in hospital patients. *Journal of the American Medical Association* 266:2847–2851.

Classen DC, Pestotnik SL, Evans RS, Lloyd JF, Burke JP. 1997. Adverse drug events in hospitalized patients. Excess length of stay, extra costs, and attributable mortality. *Journal of the American Medical Association* 277(4):301–306.

Cohen-Mansfield J, Lipson S, Werner P, Billig N, Taylor L, Woosley R. 1999. Withdrawal of haloperidol, thioridazine, and lorazepam in the nursing home: A controlled, double-blind study. *Archives of Internal Medicine* 159(15):1733–1740.

Cooper JW. 1987. Drug-related problems in nursing homes: Medication errors. *Nursing Homes* 36(2):6–13.

Cooper JW. 1999. Adverse drug reaction-related hospitalizations of nursing facility patients: A 4-year study. *Southern Medical Journal* 92(5):485–490.

Cooper S, Zaske D, Hadsall R, Freemont D, Fehr S, Suh D. 1994. Automated medication packaging for long-term care facilities: An evaluation. *The Consultant Pharmacist* 9(1):58–70.

Corda RS, Burke HB, Horowitz HW. 2000. Adherence to prescription medications among medical professionals. *Southern Medical Journal* 93(6):585–589.

Cordero L, Kuehn I, Kumar RR, Mekhjian HS. 2004. Impact of computerized physician order entry on clinical practice in a newborn intensive care unit. *Journal of Perinatology* 24(2):88–93.

Cramer JA, Mattson RH, Prevey ML, Scheyer RD, Ouellette VL. 1989. How often is medication taken as prescribed? A novel assessment technique. *Journal of the American Medical Association* 261(22):3273–3277.

Daniel KL, Honein. MA, Moore CA. 2003. Sharing prescription medication among teenage girls: Potential danger to unplanned/undiagnosed pregnancies. *Pediatrics* 111(5):1167–1170.

Dean B, Schachter M, Vincent C, Barber N. 2002. Prescribing errors in hospital inpatients: Their incidence and clinical significance. *Quality & Safety in Health Care* 11(4):340–344.

Dean BS, Allan EL, Barber ND, Barker KN. 1995. Comparison of medication errors in an American and a British hospital. *American Journal of Health-System Pharmacy* 52(22):2543–2549.

Dill JL, Generali JA. 2000. Medication sample labeling practices. *American Journal of Health-System Pharmacy* 57(22):2087–2090.

DiMatteo MR. 2004. Variations in patients' adherence to medication recommendations: A qualitative review of 50 years of research. *Medical Care* 42(3):200–209.

Ellenbecker CH, Frazier SC, Verney S. 2004. Nurses' observations and experiences of problems and adverse effects of medication management in home care. *Geriatric Nursing* 25(3):164–170.

Ernst ME, Brown GL, Klepser T, Kelly MW. 2001. Medication discrepancies in an outpatient electronic medical record. *American Journal of Health-System Pharmacy* 58(21):2072–2075.

Feikema SM, Klevens RM, Washington ML, Barker L. 2000. Extraimmunization among U.S. children. *Journal of the American Medical Association* 283(10):1311–1317.

Flynn EA, Barker KN, Pepper GA, Bates DW, Mikeal RL. 2002. Comparison of methods for detecting medication errors in 36 hospitals and skilled-nursing facilities. *American Journal of Health-System Pharmacy* 59(5):436–446.

Flynn EA, Barker KN, Carnahan BJ. 2003. National observational study of prescription dispensing accuracy and safety in 50 pharmacies. *Journal of the American Pharmaceutical Association* 43(2):191–200.

Fontan JE, Maneglier V, Nguyen VX, Loirat C, Brion F. 2003. Medication errors in hospitals: Computerized unit dose drug dispensing system versus ward stock distribution system. *Pharmacy World & Science* 25(3):112–117.

Forrest CF, Shipman SA, Dougherty D, Miller MR. 2003. Outcomes research in pediatric settings: Recent trends and future directions. *Pediatrics* 111(1):171–178.

Forster AJ, Murff HJ, Peterson JF, Gandhi TK, Bates DW. 2005. Adverse drug events following hospital discharge. *Journal of General Internal Medicine* 20:317–323.

France DJ, Cartwright J, Jones V, Thompson V, Whitlock JA. 2004. Improving pediatric chemotherapy safety through voluntary incident reporting: Lessons from the field. *Journal of Pediatric Oncology Nursing* 21(4):200–206.

Freeman C, Todd C, Camilleri-Ferrante C, Laxton C, Murrell P, Palmer CR, Parker M, Payne B, Rushton N. 2002. Quality improvement for patients with hip fracture: Experience from a multi-site audit. *Quality & Safety in Health Care* 11(3):239–245.

Frey B, Buettiker V, Hug MI, Waldvogel K, Gessler P, Ghelfi D, Hodler C, Baenziger O. 2002. Does critical incident reporting contribute to medication error prevention? *European Journal of Pediatrics* 161(11):594–599.

Gambassi G, Forman DE, Lapane KL, Mor V, Sgadari A, Lipsitz LA, Bernabei R, on behalf of The SAGE Study Group. 2000. Management of heart failure among very old persons living in long term care: Has the voice of trials spread? *American Heart Journal* 139(1): 85–89.

Gandhi TK, Burstin HR, Cook EF, Puopolo Al, Haas JS, Brennan TA, Bates DW. 2000. Drug complications in outpatients. *Journal of General Internal Medicine* 15:149–154.

Gandhi TK, Weingart SN, Borus J, Seger AC, Peterson J, Burdick E, Seger DL, Shu K, Federico F, Leape LL, Bates DW. 2003. Adverse drug events in ambulatory care. *New England Journal of Medicine* 348(16):1556–1564.

Gandhi TK, Bartel SB, Shulman LN, Verrier D, Burdick E, Cleary A, Rothschild JM, Leape LL, Bates DW. 2005. Medication safety in the ambulatory chemotherapy setting. *Cancer* 104(11):2477–2483.

Gerety MB, Cornell JE, Plichta DT, Eimer M. 1993. Adverse events related to drugs and drug withdrawal in nursing home residents. *Journal of the American Geriatrics Society* 41(12): 1326–1332.

Golden AG, Preston RA, Barnett SD, Llorente M, Hamdan K, Silverman MA. 1999. Inappropriate medication prescribing in homebound older adults. *Journal of the American Geriatrics Society* 47(8):948–953.

Granger CB, Steg PG, Peterson E, Lopez-Sendon J, Van de Werf F, Kline-Rogers E, Allegrone J, Dabbous OH, Klein W, Fox KA, Eagle KA, GRACE Investigators. 2005. Medication performance measures and mortality following acute coronary syndromes. *The American Journal of Medicine* 118(8):858–865.

Grasso BC, Genest R, Jordan CW, Bates DW. 2003. Use of chart and record reviews to detect medication errors in a state psychiatric hospital. *Psychiatric Services* 54(5): 677–681.

Gray SL, Sager M, Lestico MR, Jalaluddin M. 1998. Adverse drug events in hospitalized elderly. *The Journals of Gerontology. Series A, Biological Sciences and Medical Sciences* 53(1):M59–M63.

Gupta N, Kaul-Gupta R, Carstens MM, Franga D, Martindale RG. 2003. Analyzing prophylactic antibiotic administration in procedures lasting more than four hours: Are published guidelines being followed? *The American Surgeon* 69(8):669–673.

Gupta S, Rappaport HM, Bennett LT. 1996a. Inappropriate drug prescribing and related outcomes for elderly Medicaid beneficiaries residing in nursing homes. *Clinical Therapeutics* 18(1):183–196.

Gupta S, Rappaport HM, Bennett LT. 1996b. Polypharmacy among nursing home geriatric Medicaid recipients. *The Annals of Pharmacotherapy* 30(9):946–950.

Gurwitz JH, Noonan JR, Soumerai SB. 1992. Reducing the use of H2 receptor antagonists in the long term setting. *Journal of the American Geriatrics Society* 40:359–364.

Gurwitz JH, Sanchez-Cross MT, Eckler MA, Matulis J. 1994. The epidemiology of adverse and unexpected events in the long-term care setting. *Journal of the American Geriatrics Society* 42(1):33–38.

Gurwitz JH, Field TS, Avorn J, McCormick D, Jain S, Eckler M, Benser M, Edmondson AC, Bates DW. 2000. Incidence and preventability of adverse drug events in nursing homes. *The American Journal of Medicine* 109(2):87–94.

Gurwitz JH, Field TS, Harrold LR, Rothschild J, Debellis K, Seger AC, Cadoret C, Fish LS, Garber L, Kelleher M, Bates DW. 2003. Incidence and preventability of adverse drug events among older persons in the ambulatory setting. *Journal of the American Medical Association* 289(9):1107–1116.

Gurwitz JH, Field TS, Judge J, Rochon P, Harrold LR, Cadoret C, Lee M, White K, LaPrino J, Mainard JF, DeFlorio M, Gavendo L, Auger J, Bates DW. 2005. The incidence of adverse drug events in two large academic long-term care facilities. *The American Journal of Medicine* 118(3):251–258.

Handler SM, Nace DA, Studenski SA, Fridsma DB. 2004. Medication error reporting in long term care. *The American Journal of Geriatric Pharmacotherapy* 2(3):190–196.

Hardmeier B, Braunschweig S, Cavallaro M, Roos M, Pauli-Magnus C, Giger M, Meier PJ, Fattinger K. 2004. Adverse drug events caused by medication errors in medical inpatients. *Swiss Medical Weekly* 134(45–46):664–670.

Heineck I, Ferreira MB, Schenkel EB. 1999. Prescribing practice for antibiotic prophylaxis for 3 commonly performed surgeries in a teaching hospital in Brazil. *American Journal of Infection Control* 27(3):296–300.

Holdsworth MT, Fichtl RE, Behta M, Raisch DW, Mendez-Rico E, Adams A, Greifer M, Bostwick S, Greenwald BM. 2003. Incidence and impact of adverse drug events in pediatric inpatients. *Archives of Pediatrics & Adolescent Medicine* 157(1):60–65.

Hutt E, Pepper GA, Vojir C, Fink R, Jones KR. 2006, in press. Assessing appropriateness of pain medication prescribing practices in nursing homes. *Journal of the American Geriatrics Society*.

Jha AK, Kuperman GJ, Teich JM, Leape L, Shea B, Rittenberg E, Burdick E, Seger DL, Vander Vliet M, Bates DW. 1998. Identifying adverse drug events: Development of a computer-based monitor and comparison with chart review and stimulated voluntary report. *Journal of the American Medical Informatics Association* 5(3):305–314.

Kaushal R, Bates DW, Landrigan C, McKenna KJ, Clapp MD, Federico F, Goldmann DA. 2001. Medication errors and adverse drug events in pediatric inpatients. *Journal of the American Medical Association* 285(16):2114–2120.

Kaushal R, Jaggi T, Walsh K, Fortescue EB, Bates DW. 2004. Pediatric medication errors: What do we know? What gaps remain? *Ambulatory Pediatrics* 4(1):73–81.

King WJ, Paice N, Rangrej J, Forestell GJ, Swartz R. 2003. The effect of computerized physician order entry on medication errors and adverse drug events in pediatric inpatients. *Pediatrics* 112(3 Pt. 1):506–509.

Kistner UA, Keith MR, Sergeant KA, Hokanson JA. 1994. Accuracy of dispensing in a high-volume, hospital-based outpatient pharmacy. *American Journal of Hospital Pharmacy* 51(22):2793–2797.

Kozer E, Scolnik D, Macpherson A, Keays T, Shi K, Luk T, Koren G. 2002. Variables associated with medication errors in pediatric emergency medicine. *Pediatrics* 110(4): 737–742.

Krumholz HM, Chen J, Rathore SS, Wang Y, Radford MJ. 2003. Regional variation in the treatment and outcomes of myocardial infarction: Investigating New England's advantage. *American Heart Journal* 146(2):242–249.

LaPointe NM, Jollis JG. 2003. Medication errors in hospitalized cardiovascular patients. *Archives of Internal Medicine* 163(12):1461–1466.

Learhinan ER, Alderman CP. 2003. Venous thromboembolism prophylaxis in a South Australian teaching hospital. *The Annals of Pharmacotherapy* 37(10):1398–1402.

Lehmann CU, Conner KG, Cox JM. 2004. Preventing provider errors: Online total parenteral nutrition calculator. *Pediatrics* 113(4):748–753.

Lesar TS. 2002a. Prescribing errors involving medication dosage forms. *Journal of General Internal Medicine* 17(8):579–587.

Lesar TS. 2002b. Tenfold medication dose prescribing errors. *The Annals of Pharmacotherapy* 36(12):1833–1839.

Lesar TS, Briceland LL, Delcoure K, Parmalee JC, Masta-Gornic V, Pohl H. 1990. Medication prescribing errors in a teaching hospital. *Journal of the American Medical Association* 263(17):2329–2334.

Lesar TS, Lomaestro BM, Pohl H. 1997. Medication-prescribing errors in a teaching hospital. A 9-year experience. *Archives of Internal Medicine* 157(14):1569–1576.

Lisby M, Nielsen LP, Mainz J. 2005. Errors in the medication process: Frequency, type, and potential clinical consequences. *International Journal for Quality in Health Care* 17(1): 15–22.

Losek JD. 2004. Acetaminophen dose accuracy and pediatric emergency care. *Pediatric Emergency Care* 20(5):285–288.

Manley HJ, Drayer DK, Muther RS. 2003a. Medication-related problem type and appearance rate in ambulatory hemodialysis patients. *BMC Nephrology* 22:4–10.

Manley HJ, McClaran ML, Overbay DK, Wright MA, Reid GM, Bender WL, Neufeld TK, Hebbar S, Muther RS. 2003b. Factors associated with medication-related problems in ambulatory hemodialysis patients. *American Journal of Kidney Disease* 41(2):386–393.

McCarthy AM, Kelly MW, Reed D. 2000. Medication administration practices of school nurses. *The Journal of School Health* 70(9):371–376.

McCormick D, Gurwitz JH, Goldberg RJ, Becker R, Tate JP, Elwell A, Radford AJ. 2001. Prevalence and quality of warfarin use for patients with atrial fibrillation in the long term care setting. *Archives of Internal Medicine* 161:2458–2463.

Meredith S, Feldman PH, Frey D, Hall K, Arnold K, Brown NJ, Ray WA. 2001. Possible medication errors in home healthcare patients. *Journal of the American Geriatrics Society* 49(6):719–724.

Monette J, Gurwitz JH, Avorn J. 1995. Epidemiology of adverse drug events in the nursing home setting. *Drugs Aging* 7(3):203–211.

Moore C, Wisnivesky J, Williams S, McGinn T. 2003. Medical errors related to discontinuity of care from an inpatient to an outpatient setting. *Journal of General Internal Medicine* 18(8):646–651.

Mort JR, Aparasu RR. 2000. Prescribing potentially inappropriate psychotropic medications to the ambulatory elderly. *Archives of Internal Medicine* 160(18):2825–2831.

Nebeker JR, Hoffman JM, Weir CR, Bennett CL, Hurdle JF. 2005. High rates of adverse drug events in a highly computerized hospital. *Archives of Internal Medicine* 165(10):1111–1116.

Petersen LA, Normand SL, Leape L, McNeil BJ. 2001. Comparison of use of medications after acute myocardial infarction in the Veterans Health Administration and Medicare. *Circulation* 104(24):2898–2904.

Petersen LA, Normand SL, Druss BG, Rosenheck RA. 2003. Process of care and outcome after acute myocardial infarction for patients with mental illness in the VA health care system: Are there disparities? *Health Services Research* 38(1 Pt. 1):41–63.

Petridou E, Kouri N, Vadala H, Dalamaga M, Sege R. 2004. Frequency and nature of recorded childhood immunization-related errors in Greece. *Journal of Toxicology. Clinical Toxicology* 42(3):273–276.

Pichon R, Zelger GL, Wacker P, Vodoz AL, Humbert J. 2002. Analysis and quantification of prescribing and transcription errors in a paediatric oncology service. *Pharmacy World & Science* 24(1):12–15.

Potts AL, Barr FE, Gregory DF, Wright L, Patel NR. 2004. Computerized physician order entry and medication errors in a pediatric critical care unit. *Pediatrics* 113(1 Pt. 1): 59–63.

Quenon JL, Eveillard M, Vivien A, Bourderont D, Lepape A, Lathelize M, Jestin C. 2004. Evaluation of current practices in surgical antimicrobial prophylaxis in primary total hip prosthesis—a multicentre survey in private and public French hospitals. *The Journal of Hospital Infection* 56(3):202–207.

Roe MT, Parsons LS, Pollack CV, Canto JG, Barron HV, Every NR, Rogers WJ, Peterson ED. 2005. Quality of care by classification of myocardial infarction: Treatment patterns for ST-segment elevation vs. non-ST-segment elevation myocardial infarction. *Archives of Internal Medicine* 165(14):1630–1636.

Ruths S, Straand J, Nygaard HA. 2003. Multidisciplinary medication review in nursing home residents: What are the most significant drug-related problems? The Bergen District Nursing Home (BEDNURS) study. *Quality & Safety in Health* 12(3):176–180.

Sackett DL, Snow, JC. 1979. *Compliance in Health Care*. Baltimore, MD: Johns Hopkins University Press.

Sanborn TA, Jacobs AK, Frederick PD, Every NR, French WJ. 2004. Comparability of quality-of-care indicators for emergency coronary angioplasty in patients with acute myocardial infarction regardless of on-site cardiac surgery (report from the National Registry of Myocardial Infarction). *The American Journal of Cardiology* 93(11):1335–1339.

Scott-Cawiezell J, Pepper GA, Madsen R, Petroski G, Vogelsmeier A, Zellmer D. 2005. Level of nursing credential and interruptions: What is the impact on nursing home medication administration accuracy? Unpublished manuscript in preparation for project funded by AHRQ 5UC1 HS 14281-02.

Scott IA, Denaro CP, Flores JL, Bennett CJ, Hickey AC, Mudge AM, Atherton J. 2003. Quality of care of patients hospitalized with congestive heart failure. *Internal Medicine Journal* 33(4):140–151.

Senst BL, Achusim LE, Genest RP, Consentino LA, Ford CC, Little JA, Raybon SJ, Bates DW. 2001. Practical approach to determining costs and frequency of adverse drug events in a health care network. *American Journal of Health-System Pharmacy* 58(12):1126–1132.

Shaheen AW, Palker T, Walter EB, Galanko JA, Shaheen NJ, Dolor RJ. 2004. Prescription medication sharing in primary care. In: *Abstracts of Submissions Accepted for Presentation: 27th Annual Meeting, Chicago, IL*. Washington, DC: Society of General Internal Medicine. Pp. 197.

Shaughnessy AF, Nickel RO. 1989. Prescription-writing patterns and errors in a family medicine residency program. *The Journal of Family Practice* 29(3):290–295.

Siple JF, Joseph CL. 1992. Medication discrepancies on admission to a nursing home. *American Journal of Hospital Pharmacy* 49(2):397–400.

Sloane PD, Gruber-Baldini AL, Zimmerman S, Roth M, Watson L, Boustani M, Magaziner J, Hebel JR. 2004. Medication undertreatment in assisted living settings. *Archives of Internal Medicine* 164(18):2031–2037.

Solberg LI, Hurley JS, Roberts MH, Nelson WW, Frost FJ, Crain AL, Gunter MJ, Young LR. 2004. Measuring patient safety in ambulatory care: Potential for identifying medical group drug-drug interaction rates using claims data. *The American Journal of Managed Care* 10(11 Pt. 1):753–759.

Spencer DC, Daugird AJ. 1990. The nature and content of telephone prescribing habits in a community practice. *Family Medicine* 22(3):205–209.

Stelfox HT, Ahmed SB, Fiskio J, Bates DW. 2004. An evaluation of the adequacy of outpatient monitoring of thyroid replacement therapy. *Journal of Evaluation in Clinical Practice* 10(4):525–530.

Tan LH, Tan SC. 2004. Venous thromboembolism prophylaxis for surgical patients in an Asian hospital. *Australian and New Zealand Journal of Surgery* 74(6):455–459.

Taxis K, Barber N. 2003. Ethnographic study of incidence and severity of intravenous drug errors. *British Medical Journal* 326(7391):684.

Taxis K, Dean B, Barber N. 1999. Hospital drug distribution systems in the UK and Germany—a study of medication errors. *Pharmacy World & Science* 21(1):25–31.

Teagarden JR, Nagle B, Aubert RE, Wasdyke C, Courtney P, Epstein RS. 2005. Dispensing error rate in a highly automated mail-service pharmacy practice. *Pharmacotherapy* 25(11):1629–1635.

Tissot E, Cornette C, Demoly P, Jacquet M, Barale F, Capellier G. 1999. Medication errors at the administration stage in an intensive care unit. *Intensive Care Med* 25(4):353–359.

Tissot E, Cornette C, Limat S, Mourand JL, Becker M, Etievent JP, Dupond JL, Jacquet M, Woronoff-Lemsi MC. 2003. Observational study of potential risk factors of medication administration errors. *Pharmacy World & Science* 25(6):264–268.

Vaisbrud V, Raveh D, Schlesinger Y, Yinnon AM. 1999. Surveillance of antimicrobial prophylaxis for surgical procedures. *Infection Control and Hospital Epidemiology* 20(9): 610–613.

van den Bemt PM, Postma MJ, van Roon EN, Chow MC, Fijn R, Brouwers JR. 2002. Cost-benefit analysis of the detection of prescribing errors by hospital pharmacy staff. *Drug Safety* 25(2):135–143.

van Dijk KN, Pont LG, de Vries CS, Franken M, Brouwers JR, de Jong-van den Berg LT. 2003. Prescribing indicators for evaluating drug use in nursing homes. *The Annals of Pharmacotherapy* 37(7):1136–1141.

van Kasteren ME, Kullberg BJ, de Boer AS, Mintjes-de Groot J, Gyssens IC. 2003. Adherence to local hospital guidelines for surgical antimicrobial prophylaxis: A multicentre audit in Dutch hospitals. *The Journal of Antimicrobial Chemotherapy* 51(6):1389–1396.

Vogelsmeier A, Scott-Cawiezell J, Zellmer D. 2005, in press. Barriers to safe medication administration in the nursing home. *Journal of Geriatric Nursing.*

Wagner MM, Hogan WR. 1996. The accuracy of medication data in an outpatient electronic medical record. *Journal of the American Medical Informatics Association* 3(3):234–244.

Winterstein AG, Johns TE, Rosenberg EI, Hatton RC, Gonzalez-Rothi R, Kanjanarat P. 2004. Nature and causes of clinically significant medication errors in a tertiary care hospital. *American Journal of Health-System Pharmacy* 61(18):1908–1916.

Wirtz V, Taxis K, Barber ND. 2003. An observational study of intravenous medication errors in the United Kingdom and in Germany. *Pharmacy World & Science* 25(3):104–111.

Won A, Lapane K, Gambassi G, Bernabei R, Mor V, Lipsitz LA. 1999. Correlates and management of nonmalignant pain in the nursing home. SAGE Study Group. Systematic Assessment of Geriatric drug use via Epidemiology. *Journal of the American Geriatrics Society* 47:936–942.

Won AB, Lapane KL, Vallow S, Schein J, Morris JN, Lipsitz LA. 2004. Persistent nonmalignant pain and analgesic prescribing patterns in elderly nursing home residents. *Journal of the American Geriatrics Society* 52(6):867–874.

Young HM, Sikma SK, Bothell SL, Christlieb C, Trippett LSJ. 2005. Medication observations in assisted living: Methodological issues. *Gerontological Association of America Meeting in Orlando, FL, November 19, 2005.*

Zhan C, Correa-de-Araujo R, Bierman AS, Sangl J, Miller MR, Wickizer SW, Stryer D. 2005. Suboptimal prescribing in elderly outpatients: Potentially harmful drug-drug and drug-disease combinations. *Journal of the American Geriatrics Society* 53(2):262–267.

Zullich SG, Grasela TH, Fiedler-Kelly JB, Gengo FM. 1993. Changes in prescribing patterns in long-term care facilities and impact on incidence of adverse events. *NIDA Research Monograph* 131:294–308.

D

Medication Errors: Prevention Strategies

Many organizations and researchers have recommended specific interventions for preventing medication errors (See Box D-1). This appendix reviews the empirical evidence in support of these interventions in three care settings (hospital, nursing home, and community care), in pediatric and psychiatric care, and in relation to over-the-counter (OTC) and complementary and alternative medications.

PREVENTION STRATEGIES FOR HOSPITAL CARE

The committee reviewed published error reduction strategies of 10 organizations (see Box D-1). The methods used by these organizations for selecting and supporting their recommended interventions varied from those based on expert opinion to more rigorous evaluation of the literature; some organizations did not explicitly state the method used. Most proposed interventions are based on expert opinion.

The most evidence-based summaries were produced by the Agency for Healthcare Research and Quality (AHRQ). These summaries of specific practices were derived from a rigorous review of the published literature using strict article inclusion criteria and a standardized hierarchy for rating the strength of evidence for any particular intervention. These recommendations have been criticized, however, because of issues related to applying the usual evidence criteria to safety interventions (Leape et al., 2002). The National Quality Forum followed a rigorous process of interpreting the AHRQ recommendations to develop standards using an expert panel.

> **BOX D-1**
> **Organizations with Published Prevention**
> **Strategies for Hospital Care**
>
> - Agency for Healthcare Research and Quality (Shojania et al., 2001)
> - American Society of Health-System Pharmacists (American Society of Health-System Pharmacists, 1996)
> - Institute for Healthcare Improvement (IHI, 2005)
> - Institute of Medicine (IOM, 2000)
> - Institute for Safe Medication Practices (ISMP, 2005b),
> - Joint Commission on Accreditation of Healthcare Organizations (JCAHO, 2005a)
> - Massachusetts Coalition for the Prevention of Medical Errors (MCPME, 1999)
> - National Quality Forum (NQF, 2003)
> - National Coordinating Council for Medication Error Reporting and Prevention (NCCMERP, 2005b)
> - Pathways for Medication Safety (Pathways for Medication Safety, 2002)
> - U.S. Pharmacopeia (USP, 2005)

The Joint Commission on Accreditation of Healthcare Organizations (JCAHO) selects its patient safety goals from a pool of recommendations that are first identified by members of the Sentinel Event Advisory Group. These recommendations are selected because they are considered either evidence-based or, much more typically, consensus-based or practical. Similarly, the Institute for Safe Medication Practices generally develops its guidelines based on careful analysis of reported errors. These recommendations are then peer-reviewed prior to their release.

Recommendations for preventing medication errors are made by the National Coordinating Council for Medication Error Reporting and Prevention's committee of experts in the field. The Massachusetts Coalition for the Prevention of Medical Errors developed best-practice recommendations for the prevention of medication errors based on a special consensus panel.

The American Society of Hospital Pharmacists (ASHP) convened a multidisciplinary conference on preventing medication errors. Recommendations from the ASHP derive largely from these expert panels. Along with the ASHP, both the American Medical Association and the American Nurses Association participated in this multidisciplinary conference.

Recommended Approaches

Table D-1 summarizes the error reduction strategies recommended by the organizations listed in Box D-1. In general, most organizations

TABLE D-1 Recommendations for the Prevention of Medication Errors in Hospital Care

Recommended Practice	Recommending Body	Strength of Evidence Supporting Efficacy
Technological Interventions		
Implement computerized provider order entry (CPOE)	IOM, NCCMERP, MCPME, ASHP, IHI, NQF, PMS, AHRQ	Medium strength
Implement bar coding technology at the point of care	NCCMERP, MCPME, ASHP, PMS, AHRQ	Limited evidence
Ensure availability of pharmaceutical decision support	IOM, MCPME, ASHP	Limited evidence
Use pharmaceutical software	IOM, MCPME, ASHP	Lower strength
Use automated medication dispensing devices	AHRQ	Lower strength
Ensure free-flow protection on all general-use and patient-controlled analgesia (PCA) intravenous (IV) infusion pumps	NCCMERP, JCAHO	Limited evidence
Interventions Utilizing Clinical Pharmacists		
Have a central pharmacist supply high-risk IV medications and pharmacy-based admixture systems	IOM, MCPME, PMS	Limited evidence
Include a pharmacist during rounds of patient care units	IOM, MCPME, ASHP, AHRQ	Medium strength
Utilize pharmacist counseling of patients	NCCMERP	Limited evidence
Have a pharmacist available on call after hours of pharmacy operation	MCPME	Medium strength
Have a pharmacist review all medication orders before first doses	ASHP, NQF	Limited evidence
Interventions Related to the Medication-Use Process		
Establish a controlled formulary in which the selected medications are based more on safety than on cost	PMS	Limited evidence
Standardize prescription writing and prescription rules, and eliminate certain abbreviations and dose expressions	IOM, NCCMERP, ASHP, IHI, ISMP, NQF, JCAHO, USP	Limited evidence

continued

TABLE D-1 continued

Recommended Practice	Recommending Body	Strength of Evidence Supporting Efficacy
Limit and formally structure verbal communication of medication prescriptions	NCCMERP, ASHP, NQF, JCAHO	Limited evidence
Implement unit dosing	IOM, MCPME, NQF, AHRQ	Lower strength
Implement standard processes for medication doses, dose timing, and dose scales in a given patient care unit	IOM, IHI, ISMP, USP	Limited evidence
Monitor for look-alike and sound-alike medications	IHI, ISMP, JCAHO, USP	Limited evidence
Limit the number of different kinds of common equipment	IOM	Limited evidence
Do not store concentrated solutions of hazardous medications on patient care units, and limit the number of drug concentrations available in the organization	IOM, MCPME, JCAHO, ISMP	Limited evidence
Employ special procedures and written protocols for the use of high-risk IV and oral medications	OM, MCPME, IHI, INQF, PMS, ISMP, AHRQ, USP	Medium strength
Institute policies and procedures regarding labeling of all medications	NCCMERP, NQF, ISMP, JCAHO, USP	Limited evidence

Miscellaneous Nontechnological Interventions

Adopt a systems-oriented approach to medication error reduction	IOM, NCCMERP, MCPME, ASHP, IHI, PMS, ISMP, USP	Limited evidence
Use improved communication practices, such as always resolving medication discrepancies prior to administration	NCCMERP, ASHP, IHI, JCAHO	Limited evidence
Take steps to reduce workplace fatigue, such as planned naps, careful scheduling, or light therapy	IHI, ISMP, USP	Lower strength
Create a culture of safety	NCCMERP, ASHP, IHI, NQF, PMS, ISMP, USP	Limited evidence
Collect a medication history, and reconcile the list with the patient and other providers during care transitions	ISMP, JCAHO, USP	Limited evidence

TABLE D-1 continued

Recommended Practice	Recommending Body	Strength of Evidence Supporting Efficacy
Improve the work environment for medication preparation, dispensing, and administration	IOM, ASHP, IHI, NQF	Limited evidence
Improve error detection and reporting, and promote a nonpunitive atmosphere	NCCMERP, MCPME, ASHP, NQF, PMS	Limited evidence
Make relevant patient information available at the point of care	IOM, MCPME, IHI	Indirectly supported through evidence on CPOE, electronic medication administration record (MAR), and bar coding
Use failure modes and effects analysis or other strategies for risk management	NCCMERP, PMS, ISMP	Limited evidence
Improve patients' knowledge about their treatment	IOM, MCPME, IHI, PMS	Limited evidence

NOTE: AHRQ = Agency for Healthcare Research and Quality; ASHP = American Society of Hospital Pharmacists; IHI = Institute for Healthcare Improvement; IOM = Institute of Medicine; ISMP = Institute for Safe Medication Practices; JCAHO = Joint Commission on Accreditation of Healthcare Organizations; MCPME = Massachusetts Coalition for the Prevention of Medical Errors; NCCMERP = National Coordinating Council for Medication Error Reporting and Prevention; NQF = National Quality Forum; PMS = Pathways for Medication Safety; USP = U.S. Pharmacopeia.
SOURCE: ASHP, 1993; No Author, 1996; MCPME, 1999; IOM, 2000; Shojania et al., 2001; PMS, 2002; NQF, 2003; IHI, 2005; ISMP, 2005b; JCAHO, 2005a; NCCMERP, 2005b.

recommend implementing computerized provider order entry (CPOE) and bar coding at the bedside, although the evidence supporting bar coding remains weak. Other specific interventions supported by multiple groups include involving clinical pharmacists in patient rounds, implementing and utilizing unit dosing, standardizing prescription writing and prescription rules and eliminating certain abbreviations, utilizing special written protocols for high-risk medications, and limiting as well as standardizing verbal medication orders. Additional general recommendations embraced by most organizations include adopting a systems-oriented approach to medication errors, creating a culture of safety, and improving medication error identification and reporting.

For studies of interventions to reduce medication errors, inclusion criteria derived from AHRQ-sponsored analysis of patient safety practices were used (Shojania et al., 2001). Only studies with the following study design were included: (1) randomized controlled trial; (2) nonrandomized controlled trial; (3) observational studies with controls. The same grading scale was modified to indicate the strength of evidence supporting a particular intervention: greatest, high, medium, lower, limited. This approach results in an overly conservative assessment of the evidence supporting a particular procedure, and these limitations have been well characterized previously (Leape et al., 2002).

Most of the recommendations have limited evidence to support their efficacy. The evidence appears strongest for recommendations to implement CPOE, include pharmacists in medication-intensive areas in the hospital, and use standardized written protocols for high-risk medications.

Evaluation of Recommended Approaches

Interventions to reduce medication errors can be divided into four categories: CPOE and decision-support systems, use of clinical pharmacists, automated medication dispensing systems, and a final category that includes all other proposed strategies.

Computerized Provider Order Entry and Decision-Support Systems

Ten studies evaluated CPOE and decision-support systems for medication error reduction. Two of these studies were randomized controlled trials, and the remaining eight used a before–after design. All ten studies demonstrated a statistically significant reduction in medication errors. Rates of medication errors were reduced by 13–86 percent, and rates of preventable adverse drug events (ADEs) by 17–62 percent.

Two studies at Brigham and Women's Hospital, Boston, Massachusetts, examined the impact of CPOE with clinical decision support on medications errors and ADEs. The first found that nonintercepted serious medication errors decreased by 55 percent, from 10.7 to 4.86 events per 1,000 patient-days (p = 0.01). Preventable ADEs declined by 17 percent, but this was not statistically significant (Bates et al., 1998). The second study, consisting of a baseline period followed by the implementation of CPOE with decision support and then three study periods, demonstrated significant reductions in all medication errors (excluding missed-dose errors) and nonintercepted serious medication errors (Bates et al., 1999). The non-missed-dose medication error rate fell 81 percent, from 142 per 1,000 patient-days in the baseline period to 26.6 per 1,000 patient days in period 3 (p <0.0001). The nonintercepted serious medication error rate declined 86 percent over the same time frame (p = 0.0003). However, the decline in ADEs/1,000 patient days from 14.7 to 9.6 was not statistically significant.

Neither study was sufficiently powered to detect a difference in the preventable ADE rate.

The remaining eight studies examined more focused aspects of the medication-use process. Another study at Brigham and Women's Hospital studied the impact of the implementation of a range of clinical decision-support tools for improving physician prescribing practices. Following the implementation of computerized decision support, use of the recommended histamine$_2$-blocker rose from 15.6 to 81.3 percent of orders (p <0.001); the standard deviation of drug doses decreased by 11 percent (p <0.001); the proportion of doses that exceeded the maximum decreased from 2.1 to 0.6 percent (p <0.001); use of the approved dosing frequency for ondansetron hydrochloride increased from 6 to 75 percent of orders (p <0.001); and use of subcutaneous heparin for thrombosis prophylaxis in patients on bed rest increased from 24 to 46 percent of eligible cases (p <0.001).

At the Regenstrief Institute for Health Care, Indianapolis, Indiana, a study investigated the impact of computerized reminders on physician test-ordering behavior (Overhage et al., 1997). During a 6-month trial, reminders about corollary orders were presented to 48 intervention physicians and withheld from 41 control physicians. Intervention physicians executed the suggested corollary orders in 46.3 percent of instances when they received a reminder, compared with 21.9 percent among control physicians (p <0.0001).

Two studies were carried out at LDS Hospital, Salt Lake City, Utah. The first compared a computerized antibiotic selection consultant with physician antibiotic selection (Evans et al., 1994). The antibiotic consultant suggested an antibiotic regimen to which all isolated pathogens were shown to be susceptible for 453 out of 482 culture results (94 percent), while physicians ordered an antibiotic regimen to which all isolated pathogens were susceptible for 369 out of 482 culture results (77 percent) (p <0.001). The second study found that computer-assisted decision support for ordering antibiotics in an intensive care unit (ICU) resulted in improved quality of care (Evans et al., 1998). During the intervention period, all 545 patients admitted were cared for with the aid of the anti-infectives management program. Measures of processes and outcomes were compared with those for the 1,136 patients admitted to the same unit during the 2 years before the intervention period. Use of the program led to significant reductions in orders for drugs to which the patients had reported allergies (35 versus 146 during the preintervention period, p <0.01), excess drug dosages (87 versus 405, p <0.01), and antibiotic-susceptibility mismatches (12 versus 206, p <0.01). There were also marked reductions in adverse events caused by anti-infective agents (4 versus 28, p <0.02).

A study at Brigham and Women's Hospital, Boston, Massachusetts, examined a computerized decision-support system for prescribing drugs that adjusted drug dose and frequency based on the patient's renal insufficiency. The proportion of prescriptions deemed appropriate by dose increased from 54 to 67 percent after the intervention (p <0.001), and by frequency increased from 35 to 59 percent (p <0.001) (Chertow et al., 2001).

The Section of General Internal Medicine, University of Illinois at Chicago, investigated the impact of computer alerts relating to the appropriate monitoring and use of digoxin (Galanter et al., 2004). Checking for unknown serum values rose after implementation from 6 to 19 percent for digoxin levels, 9 to 57 percent for potassium, and 12 to 40 percent for magnesium (p <0.01 for all comparisons).

A study at the Division of General Internal Medicine, Vanderbilt University Medical Center, Nashville, Tennessee, examined the impact of a CPOE system with clinical decision support designed to adjust medication doses of psychotropic medications in geriatric patients (Peterson et al., 2005). The intervention increased prescription of the recommended daily dose from 19 to 29 percent (p <0.001), reduced the incidence of ten-fold dosing from 5 to 2.8 percent (p <0.001), and reduced the prescription of nonrecommended drugs from 10.8 to 7.6 percent of total orders (p <0.001). Patients in the intervention group had a lower in-hospital fall rate—0.28 falls per 100 patient-days as compared with 0.64 falls per 100 patient-days (p = 0.001).

Researchers at the Mount Sinai Medical Center, New York, New York, investigated the impact of a CPOE system with clinical decision support linked to pharmacist and nurse feedback, designed to adjust medication doses in patients with renal insufficiency (Nash et al., 2005). The baseline rate of excessive dosing was 23.2 percent of administered medications requiring adjustment for renal insufficiency given to patients with renal impairment on the participating units. The rate fell to 17.3 percent with nurse feedback and 16.8 percent with pharmacist feedback in the participating units (p <0.05 for each, relative to baseline). The rates of excessive dosing for the rest of the hospital were largely unchanged over the same time periods.

One recent critique (Berger and Kichak, 2004) of two key studies on the medication-related safety benefits of CPOE (Bates et al., 1998, 1999) suggested that while CPOE (with decision support) has the potential to deliver benefits, there was some question as to whether these benefits had been adequately demonstrated since the 1998 study did not show that the preventable ADE rate had been reduced. The problem with this argument is that the studies that have been conducted were powered to detect a difference not in the preventable ADE rate, but in the serious medication error rate; no adequately powered studies of the preventable ADE rate have been carried out. A number of subsequent studies have also found that CPOE can reduce medication error rates in the inpatient setting.

It is clear as well that computer systems can introduce errors of their own (Ash et al., 2004; McDonald et al., 2004; Koppel et al., 2005), and may even worsen outcomes in some instances. A recent study that raises substantial concern observed an unexpected increase in mortality coincident with CPOE implementation (Han et al., 2005). Although this study had a number of methodological flaws, the increase in mortality was large, and the authors postulated that the increase may have been due to delays in care caused by policies related to the introduction of CPOE and the technology itself. The committee acknowledges that there can be unintended consequences if health care providers do not carefully plan and implement major clinical transformations such as CPOE (Phibbs et al., 2005). Successful implementation requires redesign of health care delivery processes (Levick, 2005) and continuous monitoring for problems during the implementation phase, followed by the rapid introduction of system fixes (Bates, 2005). Finally, high rates of ADEs may continue after the implementation of CPOE in the absence of decision support for drug selection, dosing, and monitoring (Nebeker et al., 2005).

Role of the Clinical Pharmacist

Three hospital-based studies evaluated the role of the clinical pharmacist. In two of these studies, a clinical pharmacist accompanied the medical team during daily rounds and was available throughout the day for consultation. One study, carried out in a medical ICU in a large urban teaching hospital, demonstrated a reduction in the preventable ADE rate of 66 percent, from 10.4 to 3.5 per 1,000 patient-days (p <0.001) (Leape et al., 1999). The pharmacist made 366 recommendations related to drug ordering, 362 of which (99 percent) were accepted by physicians. Another study, carried out in a general medicine unit, demonstrated a reduction of 78 percent in preventable ADEs, from 26.5 to 5.7 per 1,000 patient-days (Kucukarslan et al., 2003). There were 150 documented interventions recommended by the pharmacist during the rounding process, 147 (98 percent) of which were accepted by the team. A third study utilized a clinical pharmacist to review prescriptions for vancomycin to determine the appropriateness of use (Anglim et al., 1997). The proportion of inappropriate prescriptions written was reduced from 61 to 30 percent of orders (p <0.001).

An additional study did not study pharmacists, but evaluated the impact on medication errors of nurses with special medication safety education (Greengold et al., 2003). In this study, the dedicated medication safety nurses had no effect.

Automated Medication-Dispensing Systems

Four studies evaluated automated medication-dispensing devices. In the only randomized trial, now more than 20 years old, a bedside automatic medication-dispensing machine was associated with a statistically significant reduction in medication error rate from 15.9 percent within the control group (a decentralized unit dose system) to 10.6 percent within the intervention group (Barker et al., 1984). In another study, implementation of an automated drug-dispensing system led to a reduction in medication errors, largely those related to time of administration, from 16.9 to 10.4 percent (p <0.001) (Borel and Rascati, 1995). This result is consistent with that of a later study demonstrating that the introduction of an automated medication-dispensing device led to an increase in the number of medications administered as scheduled from 59 to 77 percent of doses (p = 0.02) (Shirley, 1999). The remaining study reported on the introduction of automated medication-dispensing devices into a cardiovascular surgery unit and a cardiovascular ICU. Medication error rates decreased for patients in the surgical unit but increased for patients in the cardiothoracic unit; neither difference was statistically significant (Schwarz and Brodowy, 1995).

The AHRQ-funded review of patient safety practices concluded that the evidence provided by the above studies does not support the use of automated dispensing devices to reduce medication errors (Shojania et al., 2001).

Other Studies

National disease registries have become an important mechanism for correcting both under- and overprescribing of medications in hospitals for certain important groups of patients—those with ST elevation and non–ST elevation acute coronary syndrome and acute heart failure (Ferguson et al., 2003; Peterson et al., 2004; Jha et al., 2005).

A randomized control trial in a cardiac surgical ICU tested the efficacy of smart IV infusion pumps (incorporating an integrated decision-support system)—the intervention period. In the control period, the decision-support software was inactive. Although many errors were found that would not otherwise have been detected, the rates of serious medication errors in the control and intervention periods were not different (Rothschild et al., 2005).

A randomized controlled trial evaluated a continuous quality improvement initiative designed to increase the use of preoperative beta-blockers in patients undergoing coronary artery bypass graft surgery (Ferguson et al., 2003). The intervention included a call to action to a physician leader at the study site; educational products; and periodic longitudinal, site-specific feedback benchmarked on national averages. Over a 2.5-year period, the use of beta-blockers increased by 7.3 percent in the intervention sites compared with 3.6 percent in the control sites (p = 0.04).

Two randomized controlled trials examined the impact of patient educational interventions on medication errors. In one study, geriatric patients either participated in a self-medication program or received standard care (Pereles et al., 1996). Participation in the self-medication program did not increase the proportion of patients who were able to self-medicate on discharge from the hospital. Adherence, however, was improved by the program. The self-medication group had made statistically significant fewer medication errors than the control group at 1-month follow-up. In the other trial, intervention patients received drug safety information and their medication list, and the control group received drug safety information only. There was a nonsignificant difference between intervention patients and controls in the ADE and close-call rates (Weingart et al., 2004).

A final study evaluated whether medical interns exposed to an ICU schedule designed to minimize sleep deprivation might make fewer medication errors (Landrigan et al., 2004). The intervention group schedule was designed to eliminate extended work shifts and reduced the number of hours worked per week. The control group followed the traditional ICU call schedule. The interns allocated to the traditional call schedule made more serious medication errors than the intervention group (99.7 versus 82.5 per 1,000 patient-days, p = 0.03). The interns on the traditional schedule also made more than five times as many serious diagnostic errors (18.6 versus 3.3 per 1,000 patient-days, p <0.001). The results of this study suggest that limiting extended work shifts can reduce the medication error rate.

PREVENTION STRATEGIES FOR NURSING HOME CARE

Interventions to prevent medication errors in nursing home care fall into five categories: regulation, education and academic detailing, profiling and feedback, medication therapy management, and the use of technology.

Regulation

Much of the research relevant to medication safety in nursing homes has focused on documenting the overuse of psychotropic drugs prior to 1990 and evaluating the factors that influenced changes, and in some cases improved use of these drugs. Federal regulation of the use of psychotropic drugs in Medicaid- and Medicare-certified nursing homes became law in 1987 as the Nursing Home Reform Amendments of the Omnibus Budget Reconciliation Act (OBRA) of 1987 (P.L. 100-203), also known as OBRA-

87. Guidelines were implemented for antipsychotic drug use in October 1990 and for anti-anxiety drug use in April 1992. OBRA-87 regulations required that for psychotropic drugs there be an appropriate diagnostic indication, dosages within established limits, documentation of target symptoms, documentation of effect on target symptoms, documentation of presence or absence of side effects, and documentation of behavioral interventions in addition to the use of psychotropic medications (Gurvich and Cunningham, 2000). In 1999, the regulations were expanded to include a modified version of the Beers criteria.

The committee identified several studies of the impact of regulation on the use of psychotropic drugs in nursing homes. These studies used different data sources, including chart reviews, Minimum Data Set (MDS) data, Online Survey Certification and Reporting (OSCAR) data, and pharmacy records.

Antipsychotic Drugs

Earlier research established that the use of psychotropic medications was widespread and excessive, as documented by a review (Kane et al., 1993) of studies conducted prior to OBRA. Studies in 1987 and 1988 using chart review and pharmacy records revealed that antipsychotic medications were received by 14.2 percent of 524 nursing home residents in one facility in New York (Lantz et al., 1996), 23 percent of residents of 372 nursing homes in Minnesota (Garrard et al., 1995), 24 percent of residents in 16 skilled nursing facilities in Wisconsin (Svarstad and Mount, 1991; Svarstad et al., 2001), and 26 percent of residents of 12 nursing homes in Massachusetts (Beers et al., 1988).

After the implementation of OBRA regulations for antipsychotic drugs, Garrard and colleagues (1995) noted an 8 percent decrease in the prevalence of antipsychotic medications. Lantz and colleagues (1996) found a modest 3.8 percent decline in use of antipsychotic drugs over a 10-year period in one nursing home, which was not statistically significant, possibly because of low baseline levels (12.4 percent). A mean reduction of 38 percent of antipsychotic drug use was found in 16 nursing homes post-OBRA, with a range of an 85 percent reduction to a 19 percent increase (Svarstad et al., 2001). A comparable magnitude of change (17.8 to 12.5 percent) was noted within 13 months of OBRA implementation in data collected by a large pharmacy consulting company (Kane et al., 1993). The number of patients requiring antipsyhotic drugs was essentially unchanged in a Veterans Affairs (VA) nursing home in Wisconsin, but the average haloperidol equivalent dose decreased over a 4-month period after OBRA from 12.5 to 7 mg per day (Slater and Glaser, 1995). In another study, in an academic nursing home in Chicago, OBRA was credited with discontinuation or lowered doses in 27.6 percent of residents with dementia diagnoses only, 33.3 percent with psychiatric diagnosis only, and 36 percent with both diagnoses (Semla et al., 1994).

Similar improvements in antipsychotic drug use were found in the medical records of 99 clients in a Wisconsin intermediate care facility for mental retardation, including decreased antipsychotic dosage, decreased number of persons who used antipsychotics, decreased use of as-needed psychotropics, and increased use of other psychotropics (Howland, 1993). These results are significant, since OBRA-87 was initially directed to this population, as well as older institutional residents.

Kidder (1999) used a federal government study from 1974, studies in the literature, and OSCAR data to conclude that antipsychotic drug prescription decreased from a stable level of 33.65 percent pre-OBRA to 16.05 percent post-OBRA (Kidder, 1999). This Health Care Financing Administration (now Centers for Medicare and Medicaid Services [CMS]) official also concluded that fears of deleterious effects from limiting antipsychotic drug use had not been realized, since MDS data and studies identified no decrement, and possible improvement, in behavior and activities of daily living among nursing home residents during the implementation of OBRA.

Anti-Anxiety Drugs

The impact of OBRA on anti-anxiety drug use is confounded by the staggered implementation of the OBRA guidelines for antipsychotic and anti-anxiety drugs, since many studies were conducted in the interval between implementation of the respective policies. Based on data prior to the passage of OBRA, Beers and colleagues (1988) reported that of those residents of 12 Massachusetts nursing homes receiving benzodiazepines, 30 percent were taking a long-acting agent, a category that had been associated with increased sedation, falls, and other adverse events. The typical dosage was relatively high for older patients, at 7.3 mg diazepam equivalent per day, which is nearly 50 percent higher than the geriatric dosage in the OBRA guidelines (Gurvich and Cunningham, 2000).

Kane and colleagues (1993) cited data from a large California pharmacy consulting company to introduce the concern that compensatory prescribing of benzodiazepines might replace antipsychotic use. The baseline routine prescribing rate prior to the OBRA antipsychotic guidelines increased from 5.25 to 7.6 percent in November 1991. Similar results were found in a study of one VA nursing home where prescription of benzodiazepines increased from 42 to 48 percent of residents coincident with the time of implementation of the OBRA antipsychotic guidelines (Slater and Glaser, 1995). Conversely, no change in benzodiazepine use was associated with the implementation of the OBRA antipsychotic guidelines in a follow-up study of 1,650 residents in 16 nursing facilities in Wisconsin published before the implementation of the anti-anxiety guidelines (Svarstad and Mount, 2001a) and in a study of 372 nursing homes in Minnesota (Garrard et al., 1995).

In a 6-year retrospective study in one private, nonprofit nursing home in Georgia conducted in 1994, the rate of anti-anxiety drug use of 22 percent immediately before the implementation of the psychotropic drug regulations (up from 15.5 percent in 1988) decreased significantly to 8.9 percent in 1994, 2 years after the implementation of the anti-anxiety drug regulations (Taylor et al., 2003). A 10-year follow-up study comparing 1984 and 1994 rates of prescription indicated that OBRA implementation coincided with a declined in the prescription of anxiolytic and sedative/hypnotic medications from 12.1 to 6.4 percent (p <0.01) (Lantz et al., 1996). Comparison of the rates of prescription of benzodiazepines during 1986–1989 and those in 1993–1994 using a stratified random sample of 16 skilled nursing facilities in Wisconsin showed an increase from 18.1 to 22.8 percent, which was not statistically significant (Svarstad et al., 2001).

A comparison conducted of chronic benzodiazepine use by Medicaid residents in nursing homes before 1990 and during 1993–1994 to assess the impact of the OBRA guidelines documented a decline of only 3.9 percent, which was not statistically significant (Svarstad and Mount, 2001a). Only the ratio of licensed nurses to residents was associated with improvement in medication appropriateness. Using publications and national datasets, Kidder (1999) determined that following OBRA, national rates of anti-anxiety drug use increased slightly from 10.62 percent (or 13.1 percent if nonrepresentative data were excluded) to 14.29 percent, and hypnotic medication use decreased from 10.62 to 6.83 percent.

Use of Antidepressants

While the use of antipsychotic medication has decreased, the use of antidepressants has increased since the implementation of OBRA (Lantz et al., 1996; Svarstad et al., 2001; Taylor et al., 2003). This may be attributed to increased education about undertreatment of depression, availability of safer medications, and responsiveness of depression in older adults. Lapane and Hughes (2004) found that depression was more likely to be addressed in larger nursing facilities or facilities staffed with a full-time physician, whereas increased antipsychotic drug use was found in facilities that were government-owned, had more licensed nurses, and had more residents reliant on Medicaid funding. Kidder (1999) also noted that antidepressant use had increased from 12.64 to 24.9 percent during the implementation of OBRA, although he observed that the increase began pre-OBRA as safer agents emerged and probably was not due to substitution for drugs covered by the OBRA regulations.

Compliance with Regulations

Llorente and colleagues (1998) examined compliance with the OBRA regulations on psychotropic drugs. They found that none of the eight nursing homes examined were in full compliance with the regulations pertaining to these medications. Only three guidelines had compliance means greater than 70 percent: appropriate diagnosis, drug dosage within limits, and documentation for target symptoms of the psychotropic drug. Documented behavioral intervention had the lowest compliance of 44.5 percent (Llorente et al., 1998). The Office of Inspector General (OIG) found that 85 percent of psychotropic drug use in nursing homes was appropriate. Inappropriate psychotropic drug use was attributed to drug dose too high, drug not justified, lack of documented benefit of drug, wrong type of drug, or duplicated drug (OIG, 2001).

Education and Academic Detailing

Five studies of educational approaches, including academic detailing, were reviewed. One of the studies involved education of nursing staff only, two involved education of physicians only, and two involved education of both. Education of physicians generally included some form of academic detailing involving individual or small-group face-to-face drug therapy education, often in the physician's office.

Education of Nursing Staff

In a single-group pretest–posttest design, 30 licensed nurses (registered and licensed practical nurses) in five nursing homes in North Carolina received a packet of educational materials describing appropriate drug administration techniques, prepared by the consultant pharmacist (Ruffin and Hodge, 1995). The outcome studied was medication administration errors as determined by observation and the clinical significance of errors as determined by guidelines published by the American Society of Consultant Pharmacists. The mean error rate decreased from 10.56 to 2.87 (p = 0.0026) for all routes. Significant differences were noted for the ophthalmic and oral routes, but not for metered dose inhalers or transdermal routes. In addition to the overall weaknesses of the single-group design, the lack of description of the intervention or measurement of the "dose" of the intervention is a major limitation of this study, since it is unknown how many of the nurses read the educational materials. No information was provided about the types of errors, although it appears that most were wrong-technique errors, which would be quite different from the findings of other observational studies.

Academic Detailing of Physicians

In an important randomized controlled trial, 435 physicians (Avorn and Soumerai, 1983; Soumerai and Avorn, 1987) who were Medicaid prescribers (including 208 who practiced in nursing homes) were assigned to one of three groups: control (no education, n = 165), print-only intervention group (received mailings of four-color brochures; n = 132), and face-to-face intervention group (offered two visits from clinical pharmacists trained in academic detailing, plus mailings; n = 141). Education focused on three drug targets: propoxyphene, vasodilators, and cephalexin. Prescribing outcomes consisted of the average number of prescriptions of the targeted drugs over a 9-month period before and after the intervention, extracted from Medicaid prescribing data. In this classic study, physicians who received the face-to-face intervention and mailings showed reduced prescribing of target drugs by 14 percent compared with controls (p <0.0001), and participation in the second visit was the best predictor of improvement. The extent of nursing home practice was not related to reduction of prescribing.

Another quasi-experimental study using a single-group time-series design in one large academic long-term care facility included serial interventions to reduce inappropriate use of H_2-receptor blockers (Gurwitz et al., 1992). Group discussions with all members of the medical staff emphasizing unsubstantiated indications of H_2-receptor blockers and printed educational materials constituted the first intervention. When the frequency of prescriptions reached a predetermined threshold, a booster intervention of additional small-group discussion and a list of patients under the physician's care receiving the drugs was provided. The outcome measures were prevalence of H_2-receptor blocker therapy, estimated cost savings, and estimated resource costs. There was a sudden reduction (maximal 59.1 percent) in prescriptions for H_2-receptor blockers after the first intervention, which persisted for 11 months, and a return to baseline in 19 months. More modest reductions (32.1 percent) occurred with the second intervention, with substantial cost savings from the overall program.

Education of Nurses and Physician Staff

In an intervention aimed at reducing the use of psychotropic medications in nursing homes, six matched pairs of nursing homes were randomly assigned to an educational program in geriatric psychopharmacology for physicians, nurses, and aids or to a no-treatment control group. Experimental homes had significantly better scores on an index of inappropriateness of psychoactive prescribing (–27 versus –6 percent), as well as greater discontinuation of antipsychotics (32 versus 14 percent), benzodiazepines (20 versus 9 percent), and antihistamine hypnotics (45 versus 21 percent).

Residents in experimental homes showed less deterioration in cognitive functioning.

Jones and colleagues (Jones et al., 2004, 2005; Hutt et al., 2006) conducted a quasi-experimental study of six matched pairs of nursing homes (N = 12) randomly assigned to receive a multifaceted intervention or control condition. The intervention focused primarily on the nursing home staff, with educational and behavioral components. The physicians were provided an academic detailing intervention in small groups. Control facilities received only a pain resource binder. The outcome measures were based on knowledge testing of nursing staff and quarterly interviews of a 20 percent sample of the residents regarding pain symptoms, with oversampling of Hispanic residents, supplemented by chart review of medication use and collection of MDS data. There were improvements in staff knowledge in some intervention homes, but attitudes were not changed. A measure of appropriateness of prescribing of pain medication improved among residents not in pain (indicating improved prescribing) and in homes where nursing staff's knowledge improved. Instability in staff and leadership impacted the consistent delivery of the intervention in some intervention homes. Resistance of residents to requesting or taking medication was a significant barrier to improving pain outcomes.

Profiling and Feedback

While profiling and feedback have been used as a component of multifactorial educational interventions (Gurwitz et al., 1992; Jones et al., 2004, 2005; Hutt et al., 2006), use of triplicate prescription programs is an intervention that relies primarily on profiling prescribing patterns and monitoring physician prescribing. One copy of the prescription is forwarded to a regulatory agency for monitoring purposes, while one copy goes to the pharmacist, and one is retained by the prescriber. This intervention originated in New York to reduce the abuse and misuse of Schedule II drugs (medically useful drugs with a high abuse potential) in the state.

Zullich and colleagues (1993) reported that the number of benzodiazepine prescriptions written under the triplicate prescribing policy decreased from 80 to 53 percent, depending on the population, but there was concern that benzodiazepines were being replaced by other psychoactive agents in long-term care settings. This descriptive study of residents in 10 nursing homes in western New York who discontinued use of benzodiazepines included chart review and incident report analysis. The decrease in benzodiazepine use was accompanied by a steady increase in the number of orders for alternative agents, including chloral hydrate, diphenhydramine, and phenobarbital. There was no change in the number of adverse events, although statistical power may have been insufficient to detect such changes.

In addition, it is unclear how the relative use of the different classes of medications was quantified.

Another study using the Systematic Assessment of Geriatric drug use via Epidemiology (SAGE) database compared benzodiazepine prescribing in 1994–1995 in New York under a triplicate prescription policy with prescribing in states without a similar policy (VanHaaren et al., 2001). Residents of New York facilities were less likely to be receiving benzodiazepines (4.9 versus 13 percent; odds ratio = 0.42). This study found no increases in substitute drugs.

Castle (2003) compared the use of restraints and psychotropic drugs in a sample of 120 nursing homes that received mailed reports providing feedback on six quality indicators and in 1,171 facilities that did not receive the reports. Use of physical restraints and psychotropic medications was lower in facilities that received the feedback.

Medication Therapy Management

In a randomized cluster trial, the impact of a clinical pharmacy program involving development of professional relationships, nurse education, and individualized drug review by clinical pharmacists was tested in a sample of 905 residents in 13 intervention nursing homes and 2,325 residents in 39 control homes in Australia (Roberts et al., 2001). Use of several drug groups (nonsteroidal anti-inflammatory drugs [NSAIDs], laxatives, H_2-receptor blockers, and antacids) was decreased. Overall, drug use was decreased by 14.6 percent relative to controls. Lack of significance in resident outcomes was attributed to inadequate power. No rationale was given for the mechanism(s) whereby the intervention was expected to improve the outcomes, nor was the relationship aspect of the intervention adequately described.

Another Australian study (Crotty et al., 2004) was a randomized controlled trial of a multidisciplinary case conference intervention on medication appropriateness and resident behavior, compared with external and internal control groups. The intervention consisted of two case conferences including the geriatrician, the pharmacist, residential care staff, and a representative of the Alzheimer's Association to discuss nonpharmacologic management. The medication appropriateness index for benzodiazepines improved during the study in the intervention versus the external control group, while resident behavior was unchanged. Improved medication appropriateness did not extend to the control group of residents in the same facility. The investigators attributed their success compared with a previous unsuccessful trial to direct participation of the physician and selection of the residents by the staff based on behavior problems.

Use of Technology

Four studies describe or evaluate technology interventions in the nursing home setting. Although some are represented as research, the articles are largely experiential and anecdotal. One covers the key issues involved in implementation of CPOE in a Canadian nursing home (Rochon et al., 2005). In a review of bar coded medication administration in a Veterans Administration (VA) facility, 1 recommendation is unique to nursing homes out of 15 relevant to all settings: development of a reliable method to ensure periodic replacement of wristbands was advised to retain scanability, since nursing home patients have extended stays (Patterson et al., 2004). A survey of nurses' perceptions in a Canadian nursing home found strong resistance to the use of an automated dispensing system (Novek et al., 2000). The fourth study describes the use of Geriatric Risk Assessment MedGuide (GRAM) software, which employs MDS data to help detect ADEs (Feinberg et al., 2004).

PREVENTION STRATEGIES FOR COMMUNITY CARE

Interfaces Between Care Settings

Strategies tested for reducing medication errors at the interfaces between care settings include medication education programs and a medication reconciliation process.

Medication Self-Care Education

Two studies that included strategies such as a self-administered medication program or a medication discharge planning program showed significantly improved medication knowledge among patients, reduced medication errors, and lowered hospital readmission rates. A Canadian study compared the effectiveness of a medication education program in the hospital followed by self-administered medications at home (n = 178) versus nurse-administered medications at home (n = 172) (Jensen, 2003). The self-administered medication group had significantly fewer medication errors and medication-related problems compared with the nurse-administered medication group. There was no statistically significant difference between the groups in medication adherence. In another study employing a medication self-care educational program as an intervention, there was a statistically significant difference in the hospital readmission rate within 31 days after discharge between the intervention group (7.7 percent) and the control group (28.6 percent) (p = 0.05) (Schneider et al., 1993).

Medication Reconciliation

The Institute for Safe Medication Practices suggests the following steps for implementing medication reconciliation, a 2006 JCAHO national patient safety goal (ISMP, 2005a; JCAHO, 2005c), at the interface between care settings: obtain the most accurate list of medications possible, plus information such as the dose, frequency, indication, and time of last dose for each medication; prescribe needed medications, taking into consideration the patient's current medications; reconcile medications and resolve discrepancies; reconcile medications again upon each transfer and at discharge; fully resolve any medication discrepancy; share the list with all health care providers; give the list to patients; and encourage patients to share the list with their providers and pharmacists.

In a study in an adult surgical ICU, a medication reconciliation process was instituted. Medical and anesthesia records were reviewed, allergies and home medications were verified with patient/family, and the findings were compared with orders at the time of discharge from the ICU. In a sample of 33 patients, 31 (94 percent) had their discharge orders changed (Pronovost et al., 2003).

The Ambulatory Clinic Setting

Strategies proposed to reduce medication prescribing errors in the ambulatory clinic setting are varied and include prescription writing aids, electronic prescribing with standardized variable fields that prohibit the use of unsafe abbreviations for medication instructions, medication-related computer signals, clinical practice guidelines, in-service education for physician trainees, a physician–pharmacist collaborative medication therapy management service, patient-specific medication-management reports, and voluntary medication error reporting programs. Only a few of these strategies have been evaluated.

Prescription Writing Aids

An educational program for 12 family practice residents that involved evaluation of and feedback on prescription writing by a clinical pharmacist over a 2-year period helped reduce medication prescribing error rates from 14.4 to 6 percent during the last 6 months of the intervention ($p = 0.0002$) (Shaughnessy and D'Amico, 1994).

Eleven providers in an adult internal medicine clinic participated in a trial of a modified paper prescription form. This form contained prompts for medication name, form, strength, dose, route, frequency, refills, quantity, indication, and additional directions. Use of the modified form reduced clinically important prescribing problems (p = 0.007) and decreased omission errors (p = 0.01) (Kennedy and Littenberg, 2004b).

An intervention in an outpatient clinic included a quality improvement review of prescriptions, the use of a self-inking name stamp, and an educational program that gave examples of poorly written prescriptions and emphasized legal requirements. A follow-up survey showed that 72 percent of local community pharmacies saw the stamps being used. When stamps were not used, illegible signatures continued to be a problem (Meyer, 2000).

Proposed strategies for reducing medication administration errors in the ambulatory clinic setting include failure modes and effects analysis, access to patient records for all health care professionals, use of appropriate abbreviations and formulations, standardized protocols, clearly labeled storage bins for medications, and educational training for staff and health care professionals.

Medication Administration

There are two sets of guidelines for medication administration in the ambulatory clinic—for vaccine administration and chemotherapeutic agent administration—but no studies evaluating these guidelines.

U.S. Pharmacopoeia (USP) has proposed the following guidelines for vaccine administration: (1) conduct a failure modes and effects analysis on the names, packaging, and labeling of the available vaccines in each facility; (2) review appropriate vaccine abbreviations and formulations; (3) establish clear protocols on the prescribing, documenting, dispensing, and administering of vaccinations; (4) use an adequate number of clearly labeled storage bins in the refrigerator; and (5) incorporate training sessions regarding the facility's vaccine protocols into physician, pharmacy, and nursing staff meetings (USP, 2003).

The American Society of Health-System Pharmacists has produced guidelines on how to improve the antineoplastic medication-use system and error prevention programs for all care settings (ASHP, 2002). The American Society of Clinical Oncology has developed some specific guidance for outpatient chemotherapy (ASCO, 2003).

Medication Therapy Management

Pharmacist–physician collaborative medication therapy management services, which involve collaborative practice between physicians and pharmacists, have improved medication safety and achieved therapeutic goals. For example, during the period January 1999 through March 2002, the medication therapy management services in the Fairview Clinics System of Minneapolis–St. Paul resolved 5,780 drug therapy problems for 2,524 patients. During this period, the rate of therapeutic goals achieved increased from 74 percent at the time of patients' initial pharmaceutical care encounters to 89 percent at patients' latest encounters (Isetts et al., 2003).

Another collaborative model involving primary care physicians and clinical pharmacists was tested in a group of 197 hypertensive patients (Borenstein et al., 2003). Patients were randomized to an intervention group (physician–pharmacist comanagement) and a control group (physician-only care). Better blood pressure control was achieved in the comanagement group (60 percent) than in the control group (43 percent) (p = 0.02). Furthermore, the investigators found that the average provider visit costs/patient were higher in the usual-care group ($195) than in the comanagement group ($160) (p = 0.02).

In a population-based cohort study between 1996 and 1997, 19,368 physicians were made aware of 24,266 (56 percent) medication alerts via a computerized drug utilization database linked to a telepharmacy intervention that triggered phone calls to physicians by pharmacists. The result was the change of 2,860 (24 percent) medications to a more appropriate therapeutic agent (Monane et al., 1998).

Successful collaborations between pharmacists and physicians can also be achieved with bidirectional communication, collaborative care of mutual patients, identification of a "win–win" opportunity, attention to physician convenience, and balanced dependence between the pharmacist and the physician (Brock and Doucette, 2004).

Medication Monitoring

Retrospective drug utilization reviews have been promoted as a useful tool for detecting and reducing medication errors (Lyles et al., 1998). However, a recent longitudinal ecologic and cohort study of six Medicaid programs that used the same review software in the mid-1990s did not find a reduction in the rate of exceptions to established medication-use criteria or any reduction in the incidence of hospitalization (Hennessy et al., 2003).

In a 5-month prospective observational study carried out in 2001, 215 drug reviews were conducted with 63 patients being treated at an outpatient hemodialysis center. The reviews found 113 drug discrepancies. Electronic drug records were discrepant by one drug record for 60 percent of patients, two drug records for 26 percent of patients, and more than two drug records for 14 percent of patients. Fifty percent of the 113 drug discrepancies put patients at risk for ADEs (Manley et al., 2003).

The Community Pharmacy Setting

Strategies that have been proposed for reducing dispensing errors in the community pharmacy setting include the following:

- A quality working environment (Buchanan et al., 1991; Flynn et al., 1996, 1999)
- Checking of work by another person (Davis, 1990)
- Quality assurance tools at the point of care, such as bar coding equipment (Davis, 1990) and computer tools to screen for drug interactions (Murphy et al., 2004; Malone et al., 2004)
- Access to patient profiles (Davis, 1990)
- Pharmacist training (Davis, 1990)
- Pharmaceutical case management service (Vivian, 2002; Cranor et al., 2003; Curtiss et al., 2004; Chrischilles et al., 2004)
- Patient counseling (Davis, 1990; Rupp et al., 1992; Rupp, 1992; Kuyper, 1993; Grissinger et al., 2003; Becker et al., 2004)
- A quality assurance program and error reporting system (Davis, 1990; Kennedy and Littenberg, 2004a)
- Assessment of the quality of medication safety of community/ambulatory pharmacies—a tool designed by the Institute for Safe Medication Practices and cosponsored by the American Pharmaceutical Association Foundation and the National Association of Chain Drug Stores (ISMP, 2001)

Some of these strategies have been evaluated empirically.

A Quality Working Environment

Good illumination and limited interruptions help reduce error rates. The relationship between the level of illumination and the prescription-dispensing error rate was investigated in a high-volume U.S. Army outpatient pharmacy. The final sample consisted of 10,888 prescriptions dispensed by five pharmacists. An illumination level of 146 foot-candles was associated with a significantly lower error rate (2.6 percent) than the level of 45 foot-candles (3.8 percent) (Buchanan et al., 1991).

In a study to identify the impact of interruptions and distractions on dispensing error rates, 5,072 prescriptions were analyzed and 164 errors detected, for an overall error rate of 3.23 percent. During the study, a total of 2,022 interruptions (2.99 per half-hour per subject) and 2,457 distractions (3.80 per half-hour per subject) were detected. The error rate for sets of prescriptions with one or more interruptions was 6.65 percent and for sets during which one or more distractions occurred was 6.55 percent (Flynn et al., 1999).

The associations between ambient sounds and the accuracy of pharmacists' prescription-filling performance in a pharmacy have been studied. The results suggest that the quality of pharmacists' performance may not be adversely affected by ambient sound: as sound levels increased, the error rate increased to a point, then decreased. Unpredictable sounds, controllable sounds, and noise had a significant effect on pharmacists' performance, resulting (somewhat surprisingly) in a decreased dispensing error rate (Flynn et al., 1996).

Pharmaceutical Case Management Service

The Iowa Medicaid pharmaceutical case management (PCM) program evaluated the effect of PCM on medication safety and health care utilization (Chrischilles et al., 2004). The participants were 2,211 noninstitutionalized Medicaid patients taking four or more chronic medications. Of these, 524 received PCM services and 1,687 did not. In the PCM group, at least one medication problem occurred with nearly one-half (46.1 percent) of medications and 92.1 percent of patients before the PCM program started. By the end of the program, mean medication appropriateness index scores had improved significantly compared with the starting position among PCM recipients (p <0.001). For those aged 65 and older, the percentage of PCM recipients (n = 175) using high-risk medications decreased significantly (p = 0.032) compared with those who did not receive the service (n = 366). No difference in health care utilization or charges was observed between PCM recipients and PCM eligibles who did not receive PCM services, even after reimbursements for those services were included.

The use of medication therapy management has provided benefits on several levels for two large self-insured employers in North Carolina. These employers compensated pharmacists on a fee-for-service basis for providing advisory services to employees with diabetes mellitus (the Asheville Project). As a result, hemoglobin A1c levels were better controlled, and employer total mean medical costs decreased by $1,622 per patient to $3,356 per patient per year (Cranor et al., 2003). Both employers have permanently added the benefit to their health plans.

Another study examining the impact of pharmacy care services for patients with diabetes also produced good results (Garrett and Bluml, 2005). Eighty community pharmacists in five states were reimbursed for pharmacy care services, including scheduled consultations with patients, clinical goal setting, and referrals to diabetes educators. Over the initial year of the program, the group of 256 patients participating in the study showed significant improvements in clinical indicators and higher rates of self-management. Mean total health costs (including the medication therapy costs) were $918 per patient per year less than employers' expected total costs.

A group of 56 patients in a hypertension clinic at the VA medical center in Philadelphia, Pennsylvania, participated in a trial to see whether the intervention of clinical pharmacists improved blood pressure control. Twenty-one patients out of 27 (81 percent) in the intervention group (monthly meetings with a clinical pharmacist) and 8 patients out of 29 (28 percent) in the control group (standard care from physicians) attained their blood pressure goal (p <0.0001) (Vivian, 2002).

Patient Counseling

Outpatient prescription errors at an Indian Health Service pharmacy were reviewed. Mistakes detected after pharmacists had signed off on prescription accuracy were recorded. The review of errors showed that of 323 reported mistakes, 286 (89 percent) had been detected during patient counseling and subsequently corrected (Kuyper, 1993).

The Home Care Setting

Strategies proposed to reduce medication errors in the home care setting have included an intervention in which a nurse, a clinical pharmacist, and physicians collaborated in monitoring the medications of the studied patients (Ahrens et al., 2002; Ahrens, 2003); home visits by pharmacy staff (No Author, 2000); and the implementation of a medication management model (Meredith et al., 2002).

A randomized controlled trial was used to test the efficacy of a medication-use improvement program developed specifically for home health agencies for patients aged 65 and over (Meredith et al., 2002). The intervention group (n = 130) received the usual care (the patients' home care nurses) supported by a clinical pharmacist, while the control group (n = 129) received the usual care. Medication use improved for 50 percent of intervention patients and 38 percent of control patients, an attributable improvement of 12 patients per 100 (p = 0.051). The intervention effect was greatest for therapeutic duplication, with improvement for 71 percent of intervention patients and 24 percent of control patients, an attributable improvement of 47 patients per 100 (p = 0.003).

The Self-Care Setting

Strategies to reduce medication errors in this setting include educational programs and multisystem interventions (e.g., telecommunications plus educational programs). Some educational programs have been successful in increasing medication knowledge and self-efficacy among patients. In a self-management program, asthmatic patients who were taught the appropriate use of inhalers were able to demonstrate the devices' correct use when tested (van der Loos, 1989). In another program, patients who were taking nonaspirin NSAIDs improved the recall of their medication use after being shown lists and pictures of their medications (Kimmel et al., 2003). A telephone system for monitoring and counseling patients with hypertension helped improve medication adherence for 18 percent of the 133 patients who used the system and for 12 percent of the 134 patients in the control group (p = 0.03), and decreased diastolic blood pressure (5.2 mm Hg in telephone users versus 0.8 mm Hg in controls, p = 0.02) (Friedman et al., 1996).

A systematic review of published randomized controlled trials on interventions to improve patients' adherence to prescribed medications (McDonald et al., 2002) found that 49 percent of the interventions tested (19 of 39 interventions in 33 studies) were associated with increases in adherence, while 17 were associated with reported improvement in outcomes. Two studies found that dosing once a day led to higher adherence than dosing twice a day, but not better clinical outcomes (Baird et al., 1984; Girvin et al., 1999). A third study found that dosing twice a day resulted in higher adherence than dosing four times a day and better clinical outcomes as well (Brown et al., 1997). In general, however, the investigators (McDonald et al., 2002) found that the most effective interventions for long-term care were complex; these interventions included more convenient care, information, counseling, reminders, self-monitoring, reinforcement, family therapy, and other forms of supervision. However, the investigators concluded that even the most effective interventions had modest effects.

The School Setting

The website of the Center for Health and Health Care in Schools provides information on state policies regarding the administration of medications in schools (Health in Schools, 2004). The center has also identified a set of issues that a school medication management policy might include, for example, the responsibility for medication use the school is willing to assume, the responsibilities required of the patient and parents, the rules for self-medication, and feedback mechanisms so that parents can learn about a medication's effect (Robinson, 2004). The American Academy of Pediatrics (Committee on School Health, 2003) has also developed a set of guidelines for the administration of medications in schools. Of more practical help, the Florida Society of Health-Systems Pharmacists has developed a resource manual for medication use in schools (Johnson et al., 2003). The committee is not aware of any study evaluating the procedures included in these documents.

PREVENTION STRATEGIES FOR PEDIATRIC CARE

The committee reviewed published error reduction strategies of 10 organizations: the Pediatric Pharmacy Advocacy Group (Levine, 2001), American Academy of Pediatrics/National Initiative for Children's Healthcare Quality (NICHQ, 2005), Institute for Safe Medication Practices (ISMP, 2005b), American Hospital Association (AHA, 2005), National Quality Forum (NQF, 2003), Massachusetts Hospital Association/Massachusetts Coalition for the Prevention of Medical Errors (MCPME, 1999), National Coordinating Council for Medication Errors Reporting and Prevention (NCCMERP, 2005b), AHRQ (Shojania et al., 2001), JCAHO (JCAHO, 2005a), and Institute of Medicine (IOM, 2000).

The committee identified a total of 26 unique recommendations from these organizations for strategies to reduce medication errors in pediatric care (see Table D-2). These recommendations included equipment/software tools, representation of personnel on groups making decisions on pediatric medications, training and competency of personnel, policies, clear labeling, continuous quality improvement efforts, clear and accurate documentation, standardization, patient education, and teamwork improvement. As Table D-2 indicates, none of these recommendations is based on published evidence of effectiveness in children. The vast majority are based on expert opinion (n = 22), with the remainder being based on studies in adult populations (n = 4). No recommendations have supporting pediatric-specific evidence on efficacy, cost-effectiveness, feasibility, appropriateness in different settings, and institutional barriers or risks.

PREVENTION STRATEGIES FOR PSYCHIATRIC CARE

Within psychiatry, no studies have been carried out to evaluate the efficacy of any error prevention strategies. Examples of strategies likely to be relevant to inpatient psychiatry include short-term approaches (for example, medication ordering protocols, unit-dose distribution systems, and patient education) and computerized interventions (for example, CPOE and automated dispensing devices).

PREVENTION STRATEGIES FOR THE USE OF OTC AND COMPLEMENTARY AND ALTERNATIVE MEDICATIONS

The use of OTC and complementary and alternative medications is largely beyond the health care worker's domain, although many of these

TABLE D-2 Recommendations for the Prevention of Medication Errors in Pediatric Care

Recommended Practice	Recommending Body	Evidence Specific to Children	Source of Supporting Evidence
Computerized provider order entry	PPAG, ISMP, AHA, AHRQ, IOM, NQF, MHA, NCCMERP, AAP/NICHQ	None	Adult data/ expert opinion
Automated medication-dispensing devices	PPAG, ISMP, AHA, AHRQ	None	Adult data/ expert opinion
Pediatric presence with formulary management	PPAG, ISMP, AHA, AAP/NICHQ	None	Expert opinion
Appropriate and competent pharmacy personnel and environment	PPAG, ISMP, AHA, NQF, NCCMERP, AAP/NICHQ	None	Expert opinion
Pharmacist available on call when pharmacy is closed	PPAG, ISMP, AHA, MHA	None	Expert opinion
Policies on verbal orders	PPAG, ISMP, AHA, NQF, NCCMERP, AAP/NICHQ, JCAHO	None	Expert opinion
Clear and accurate labeling of medications	PPAG, ISMP, AHA, NQF, NCCMERP	None	Expert opinion
Quality improvement efforts with drug-use evaluation and medication error reporting and review	PPAG, ISMP, AHA, MHA, NCCMERP, AAP/NICHQ	None	Expert opinion
Access of health care workers to current clinical information and references	PPAG, ISMP, AHA, IOM, MHA, NCCMERP, AAP/NICHQ	None	Expert opinion
Emergency medication dosage calculation tools	PPAG, ISMP	None	Expert opinion
Accurate documentation of medication administration	PPAG, ISMP, MHA, NCCMERP	None	Expert opinion
Medication standardization and appropriate storage	ISMP, AHA, IOM, NCCMERP, JCAHO	None	Expert opinion
Training of all health care providers in appropriate medication prescribing, labeling, dispensing, monitoring, and administration	PPAG, ISMP, IOM, NQF, MHA, NCCMERP, AAP/NICHQ, JCAHO	None	Expert opinion
Patient education on medications	ISMP, AHA, IOM, MHA, NCCMERP, AAP/NICHQ	None	Expert opinion

TABLE D-2 continued

Recommended Practice	Recommending Body	Evidence Specific to Children	Source of Supporting Evidence
Direct participation of pharmacists in clinical care	AHRQ, IOM, NQF	None	Expert opinion
Computer detection/alert systems for adverse drug events (ADEs)	AHRQ	None	Adult studies
Reduction of ADEs related to anticoagulants	AHRQ	None	Adult studies
Unit-dose drug distribution systems	AHA, AHRQ, NQF, MHA	None	Adult studies/ expert opinion
Special procedures and written protocols for high-alert medications	AHA, IOM, NQF, MHA, JCAHO	None	Expert opinion
Use of pharmaceutical software	AHA, IOM	None	Expert opinion
Pharmacy-based intravenous (IV) admixture systems	MHA	None	Expert opinion
Use of bar coding for medication administration	MHA, NCCMERP	None	Expert opinion
Standardized equipment (e.g., pumps, weight scales)	AAP/NICHQ	None	Expert opinion
Standardized measurement systems (kilograms)	AAP/NICHQ	None	Expert opinion
Standardized order sheets including areas for weight and allergies	AAP/NICHQ	None	Expert opinion
Team environment for review of orders among nurses, pharmacists, prescribers	AAP/NICHQ	None	Expert opinion

NOTE: AAP/NICHQ = American Academy of Pediatrics/National Initiative for Children's Healthcare Quality (Berlin et al., 1998; Lannon et al., 2001; Gorman et al., 2003; NICHQ, 2005); AHA = American Hospital Association (AHA, 2002, 2005); AHRQ = Agency for Healthcare Research and Quality, report on *Making Healthcare Safer* (Shojania et al., 2001; AHRQ, 2005); IOM = Institute of Medicine (IOM, 2000); ISMP = Institute for Safe Medication Practices (ISMP, 2005b); JCAHO = Joint Commission on Accreditation of Healthcare Organizations (JCAHO, 2005a,b); MHA = Massachusetts Hospital Association/Massachusetts Coalition for the Prevention of Medical Errors (MCPME, 2005a,b); NCCMERP = National Coordinating Council for Medication Error Reporting and Prevention (NCCMERP, 2005a,b); NQF = National Quality Forum (NQF, 2003, 2005); PPAG = Pediatric Pharmacy Advocacy Group (Levine, 2001; ISMP, 2002, 2005b).

medications are taken on the advice of physicians. It is up to consumers to diagnose their problem properly, select the best medical product if it is necessary, read and understand the instructions for its use, take it properly, and know when it is time to terminate the treatment. Many OTC medication errors are due to misdosing or adverse drug–drug interactions. Patients need to understand that OTCs are drugs and, like prescription medications, have both therapeutic value and potential side effects.

A key approach for reducing OTC medication errors is the Food and Drug Administration's (FDA) labeling requirements, mentioned in Chapter 2, which provide information on active ingredients, what the drug is for, dosing levels, and warnings about use. The information requirements on the packaging of complementary and alternative medications are more limited.

Patient self-education is the other major prevention strategy. Much information to improve patient awareness of OTC and complementary and alternative medications is currently available from the Internet, television, books, magazines, and newspapers.

In addition, there are specialized packaging technologies designed to decrease the chances of misuse, such as tamper-resistant and childproof containers and blister packaging that numbers each pill to help the user remember whether the product was taken. Pillboxes divided by time of day and day of week are another low-technology solution.

Still another approach is for the pharmacist to ask those picking up prescription drugs whether they are using any OTC or vitamin/mineral products and to advise them of any issues involved. For example, people taking blood thinners should be advised to speak to their doctor before taking vitamin E.

The committee could find no study on the efficacy of any of the above strategies for preventing medication errors in the use of OTC and complementary and alternative medications.

REFERENCES

AHA (American Hospital Association). 2002. *Pathways for Medication Safety.* [Online]. Available: http://www.medpathways.info/medpathways/tools/tools.html [accessed December 5, 2005].

AHA. 2005. *American Hospital Association.* [Online]. Available: www.aha.org [accessed June 17, 2005].

Ahrens J. 2003. Combatting medication errors in home health. *Caring* 22(1):56–59.

Ahrens J, Feldman PH, Frey D. 2002. Preventing medication errors in home care. *Center for Home Care Policy and Research Policy Briefs* 12:1–6.

AHRQ (Agency for Healthcare Research and Quality). 2005. *Agency for Healthcare Research and Quality.* [Online]. Available: www.ahrq.gov [accessed June 17, 2005].

American Society of Health-System Pharmacists. 1996. Top-priority actions for preventing adverse drug events in hospitals. Recommendations of an expert panel. *American Journal of Health-System Pharmacy* 53(7):747–751.

Anglim AM, Klym B, Byers KE, Scheld WM, Farr BM. 1997. Effect of a vancomycin restriction policy on ordering practices during an outbreak of vancomycin-resistant Enterococcus faecium. *Archives of Internal Medicine* 157(10):1132–1136.

ASCO (American Society of Clinical Oncology). 2003. American Society of Clinical Oncology statement regarding the use of outside services to prepare and administer chemotherapy drugs. *Journal of Clinical Oncology* 21(9):1882–1883.

Ash JS, Berg M, Coiera E. 2004. Some unintended consequences of information technology in health care: The nature of patient care information system-related errors. *Journal of the American Medical Informatics Association* 11(2):104–112.

ASHP (American Society of Health-System Pharmacists). 1993. ASHP guidelines on preventing medication errors in hospitals. *American Journal of Hospital Pharmacy* 50(2):305–314.

ASHP. 2002. ASHP guidelines on preventing medication errors with antineoplastic agents. *American Journal of Health-System Pharmacy* 59(17):1648–1668.

Avorn J, Soumerai SB. 1983. Improving drug-therapy decisions through educational outreach. A randomized controlled trial of academically-based "detailing." *New England Journal of Medicine* 308(4):1457–1463.

Baird MG, Bentley-Taylor MM, Carruthers SG, Dawson KG, Laplante LE, Larochelle P, MacCannell KL, Marquez-Julio A, Silverberg LR, Talbot P. 1984. A study of efficacy, tolerance and compliance of once-daily versus twice-daily metoprolol (Betaloc) in hypertension. Betaloc Compliance Canadian Cooperative Study Group. *Clinical and Investigative Medicine* 7(2):95–102.

Barker KN, Pearson RE, Hepler CD, Smith WE, Pappas CA. 1984. Effect of an automated bedside dispensing machine on medication errors. *American Journal of Hospital Pharmacy* 41(7):1352–1358.

Bates DW. 2005. Computerized physician order entry and medication errors: Finding a balance. *Journal of Biomedical Informatics* 38(4):259–261.

Bates DW, Leape LL, Cullen DJ, Laird N, Petersen LA, Teich JM, Burdick E, Hickey M, Kleefield S, Shea B, Vander Vliet M. 1998. Effect of computerized physician order entry and a team intervention on prevention of serious medication errors. *Journal of the American Medical Association* 280(15):1311–1316.

Bates DW, Teich JM, Lee J, Seger D, Kuperman GJ, Ma'luf N, Boyle D, Leape L. 1999. The impact of computerized physician order entry on medication error prevention. *Journal of the American Medical Informatics Association* 6:313–321.

Becker C, Bjornson DC, Kuhle JW. 2004. Pharmacist care plans and documentation of follow-up before the Iowa Pharmaceutical Case Management program. *Journal of the American Pharmaceutical Association* 44(3):350–357.

Beers MH, Avorn J, Soumerai SB, Everitt DE, Sherman DS, Salem S. 1988. Psychoactive medication use in intermediate-care facility residents. *Journal of the American Medical Association* 260(20):3016–3020.

Berger RG, Kichak JP. 2004. Computerized physician order entry: Helpful or harmful? *Journal of the American Medical Informatics Association* 11(2):100–103.

Berlin CM, McCarver DG, Notterman DA, Ward RM, Weismann DN, Wilson GS, Wilson JT. 1998. Prevention of medication errors in the pediatric inpatient setting. *Pediatrics* 102(2):428–430.

Borel JM, Rascati KL. 1995. Effect of an automated, nursing unit-based drug-dispensing device on medication errors. *American Journal of Health-System Pharmacy* 52(17):1875–1879.

Borenstein GE, Graber G, Saltiel E, Wallace J, Ryu S, Archi J, Deutsch S, Weingarten SR. 2003. Physician-pharmacist comanagement of hypertension: A randomized, comparative trial. *Pharmacotherapy* 23(2):209–216.

Brock KA, Doucette WR. 2004. An exploratory study of the collaboration between pharmacists and physicans. *Journal of the American Pharmaceutical Association* 44(3): 358–365.

Brown BG, Bardsley J, Poulin D, Hillger LA, Dowdy A, Maher VM, Zhao XO, Albers JJ, Knopp RH. 1997. Moderate dose, three-drug therapy with niacin, lovastatin, and colestipol to reduce low-density lipoprotein cholesterol <100 mg/dl in patients with hyperlipidemia and coronary artery disease. *The American Journal of Cardiology* 80(2):111–115.

Buchanan TL, Barker KN, Gibson JT, Jiang BC, Pearson RE. 1991. Illumination and errors in dispensing. *American Journal of Hospital Pharmacy* 48(10):2137–2145.

Castle NG. 2003. Providing outcomes information to nursing homes: Can it improve quality of care? *Gerontologist* 43(4):483–492.

Chertow GM, Lee J, Kuperman GJ, Burdick E, Horsky J, Seger DL, Lee R, Mekala A, Song J, Komaroff AL, Bates DW. 2001. Guided medication dosing for inpatients with renal insufficiency. *Journal of the American Medical Association* 286(22):2839–2844.

Chrischilles EA, Carter BL, Lund BC, Rubenstein LM, Chen-hardee SS, Voelker MD, Park TR, Kuehl AK. 2004. Evaluation of the Iowa Medicaid pharmaceutical case management program. *Journal of the American Pharmaceutical Association* 44(3):337–349.

Committee on School Health American Academy of Pediatrics. 2003. Guidelines for the administration of medication in school. *Pediatrics* 112(3 Pt. 1):697–699.

Cranor CW, Bunting BA, Christensen DB. 2003. The Asheville Project: Long-term clinical and economic outcomes of a community pharmacy diabetes care program. *Journal of the American Pharmaceutical Association* 43(2):173–184.

Crotty M, Halbert J, Rowett D, Giles L, Birks R, Williams H, Whitehead C. 2004. An outreach geriatric medication advisory service in residential aged care: A randomised controlled trial of case conferencing. *Age Ageing* 33(6):612–617.

Curtiss FR, Fry RN, Avey SG. 2004. Framework for pharmacy services quality improvement—a bridge to cross the quality chasm. Part I. The opportunity and the tool. *Journal of Managed Care Pharmacy* 10(1):60–78.

Davis NM. 1990. Detection and prevention of ambulatory care pharmacy dispensing errors. *Hospital Pharmacy* 25(1):18–22.

Evans RS, Classen DC, Pestotnik SL, Lundsgaarde HP, Burke JP. 1994. Improving empiric antibiotic selection using computer decision support. *Archives of Internal Medicine* 154(8):878–884.

Evans RS, Pestotnik SL, Classen DC, Clemmer TP, Weaver LK, Orme JF, Lloyd JF, Burke JP. 1998. A computer-assisted management program for antibiotics and other antiinfective agents. *New England Journal of Medicine* 338(4):232–238.

Feinberg JL, Cameron KA, Lapane KL, Allsworth JE. 2004. The use of GRAM(TM) software to improve patient safety in nursing facilities. *The Consultant Pharmacist* 5:398–413.

Ferguson TB, Peterson ED, Coombs LP, Eiken MC, Carey ML, Grover FL, DeLong ER, Society of Thoracic Surgeons and the National Cardiac Database. 2003. Use of continuous quality improvement to increase use of process measures in patients undergoing coronary artery bypass graft surgery: A randomized controlled trial. *Journal of the American Medical Association* 290(1):49–56.

Flynn EA, Barker KN, Gibson JT, Pearson RE, Smith. LA, Berger BA. 1996. Relationships between ambient sounds and the accuracy of pharmacists' prescription-filling performance. *Human Factors* 38(4):614–622.

Flynn EA, Barker KN, Gibson JT, Pearson RE, Berger BA, Smith LA. 1999. Impact of interruptions and distractions on dispensing errors in an ambulatory care pharmacy. *American Journal of Health System Pharmacists* 56(13):1319–1325.

Friedman RH, Kazis LE, Jette A, Smith MB, Stollerman J, Torgerson J, Carey K. 1996. A telecommunications system for monitoring and counseling patients with hypertension. Impact on medication adherence and blood pressure control. *American Journal of Hypertension* 9(4 Pt. 1):285–292.

Galanter WL, Polikaitis A, DiDomenico RJ. 2004. A trial of automated safety alerts for inpatient digoxin use with computerized physician order entry. *Journal of the American Medical Informatics Association* 11(4):270–277.

Garrard J, Chen V, Dowd B. 1995. The impact of the 1987 federal regulations on the use of psychotropic drugs in Minnesota nursing homes. *American Journal of Public Health* 85(6):771–776.

Garrett DG, Bluml BM. 2005. Patient self-management program for diabetes: First-year clinical, humanistic, and economic outcomes. *Journal of the American Pharmaceutical Association* 45(2):130–137.

Girvin B, McDermott BJ, Johnston D. 1999. A comparison of enalapril 20 mg once daily versus 10 mg twice daily in terms of blood pressure lowering and patient compliance. *Journal of Hypertension* 17(11):1627–1631.

Gorman RL, Bates BA, Benitz WE, Burchfield DJ, Maxwell L, Ring JC, Walls RP, Walson PD, Neff JM, Eichner JM, Hardy DR, Percelay J, Sigrest T, Stucky E. 2003. Prevention of medication errors in the pediatric inpatient setting. *Pediatrics* 112:431–436.

Greengold NL, Shane R, Schneider P, Flynn E, Elashoff J, Hoying CL, Barker K, Bolton LB. 2003. The impact of dedicated medication nurses on the medication administration error rate. *Archives of Internal Medicine* 163(19):2359–2367.

Grissinger MC, Globus NJ, Fricker MP. 2003. The role of managed care pharmacy in reducing medication errors. *Journal of Managed Care Pharmacy* 9(1):62–65.

Gurvich T, Cunningham JA. 2000. Appropriate use of psychotropic drugs in nursing homes. *American Family Physician* 61:1437–1446.

Gurwitz JH, Noonan JR, Soumerai SB. 1992. Reducing the use of H2 receptor antagonists in the long term setting. *Journal of the American Geriatrics Society* 40:359–364.

Han YY, Carcillo JA, Venkataraman ST, Clark RSB, Watson RS, Nguyen TC, Bayir H, Orr RA. 2005. Unexpected increased mortality after implementation of a commercially sold computerized physician order entry system. *Pediatrics* 116(5):1506–1512.

Health in Schools. 2004. *Center for Health and Health Care in Schools: State Policies on Administration of Medications in Schools.* [Online]. Available: http://www.healthin schools.org/sh/mgmtpolicies.asp [accessed August 30, 2005].

Hennessy S, Bilker WB, Zhou L, Weber AL, Brensinger C, Wang Y, Strom BL. 2003. Retrospective drug utilization review, prescribing errors, and clinical outcomes. *Journal of the American Medical Association* 290(11):1494–1499.

Howland, CW. 1993. *Time-Series Evaluation of Nursing Home Reform (1987): Psychotropic Medications Prescribed in a State Center for Adults with Severe/Profound Developmental Disabilities.* PhD diss. University of Wisconsin at Madison.

Hutt E, Pepper GA, Vojir C, Fink R, Jones KR. 2006. Assessing appropriateness of pain medication prescribing practices in nursing homes. *Journal of the American Geriatrics Society* 254(2):231–239.

IHI (Institute for Healthcare Improvement). 2005. *Institute for Healthcare Improvement.* [Online]. Available: http://www.ihi.org [accessed August 22, 2005].

IOM (Institute of Medicine). 2000. *To Err Is Human: Building a Safer Health System.* Washington, DC: National Academy Press.

Isetts BJ, Brown LM, Schondelmeyer SW, Lenarz LA. 2003 Quality assessment of a collaborative approach for decreasing drug-related morbidity and achieving therapeutic goals. *Archives of Internal Medicine* 163(15):1813–1820.

ISMP (Institute for Safe Medication Practices). 2001. *Medication Safety Self Assessment for Community/Ambulatory Pharmacy.* [Online]. Available: http://www.ismp.org/PDF/Book.pdf [accessed November 20, 2005].

ISMP. 2002. *Pediatric Pharmacy Medication Safety Guidelines.* [Online]. Available: http://www.i smp.org/PR/PediatricPharmacyGuidelines.htm [accessed December 5, 2006].

ISMP. 2005a. *Building a Case for Medication Reconciliation.* [Online]. Available: http://www.ismp.org/MSAarticles/20050421.htm [accessed November 11, 2005].

ISMP. 2005b. *Institute of Safe Medication Practices.* [Online]. Available: http://www.ismp.org [accessed August 22, 2005].

JCAHO (Joint Commission on Accreditation of Healthcare Organizations). 2005a. *2006 Critical Access Hospital and Hospital National Patient Safety Goals.* [Online]. Available: http://www.jcipatientsafety.org/show.asp?durki=10293&site=164&return=10289 [accessed August 22, 2005].

JCAHO. 2005b. *Joint Commission on Accreditation of Healthcare Organizations.* [Online]. Available: http://www.jcaho.org [accessed June 17, 2005].

JCAHO. 2005c. *National Patient Safety Goals for 2006 and 2005.* [Online]. Available: http://www.jcaho.org/accredited+organizations/patient+safety/npsg.htm [accessed November 11, 2005].

Jensen L. 2003. Self-administered cardiac medication program evaluation. *Canadian Journal of Cardiovascular Nursing* 13(2):35–44.

Jha AK, Li Z, Orav EJ, Epstein AM. 2005. Care in U.S. hospitals—the Hospital Quality Alliance program. *New England Journal of Medicine* 353(3):265–274.

Johnson PE, Hayes JM, Reinstein VF, Simmons SM, Benson J. 2003. *Medication Use in Schools.* Tallahassee, FL: Florida Society of Health-System Pharmacists.

Jones KR, Fink R, Pepper GA, Hutt E, Vojir CP, Scott J, Clark L, Mellis K. 2004. Improving nursing home staff knowledge and attitudes about pain. *The Gerontologist* 44(4): 469–478.

Jones KR, Fink RM, Clark L, Hutt E, Vojir CP, Mellis BK. 2005. Nursing home resident barriers to effective pain management: Why nursing home residents may not seek pain medication. *Journal of the American Medical Directors Association* 6(1):10–17.

Kane RL, Williams CC, Williams TF, Kane RA. 1993. Restraining restraints: Changes in a standard of care. *Annual Review of Public Health* 14:545–584.

Kennedy AG, Littenberg B. 2004a. Medication error reporting by community pharmacists in Vermont. *Journal of the American Pharmaceutical Association* 44(4):434–438.

Kennedy AG, Littenberg B. 2004b. A modified outpatient prescription form to reduce prescription errors. *Joint Commission Journal on Quality and Safety* 30(9):480–487.

Kidder SW. 1999. Regulation of inappropriate psychopharmacologic medication use in U.S. nursing homes from 1954 to 1997: Part II. *Annals of Long Term Care* 7:56–62.

Kimmel SE, Lewis JD, Jaskowiak J, Kishel L, Hennessy S. 2003. Enhancement of medication recall using medication pictures and lists in telephone interviews. *Pharmacoepidemiol Drug Safety* 12(1):1–8.

Koppel R, Metlay JP, Cohen A, Abaluck B, Localio AR, Kimmel SE, Strom BL. 2005. Role of computerized physician order entry systems in facilitating medication errors. *Journal of the American Medical Association* 293(10):1197–1203.

Kucukarslan SN, Peters M, Mlynarek M, Nafziger DA. 2003. Pharmacists on rounding teams reduce preventable adverse drug events in hospital general medicine units. *Archives of Internal Medicine* 163(17):2014–2018.

Kuyper AR. 1993. Patient counseling detects prescription errors. *Hospital Pharmacy* 28(12): 1180–1181, 1184–1189.

Landrigan CP, Rothschild JM, Cronin JW, Kaushal R. 2004. Effect of reducing interns' work hours on serious medical errors in intensive care units. *New England Journal of Medicine* 351(18):1838–1848.

Lannon CM, Coven BJ, France FL, Hickson GB, Miles PV, Swanson JT, Takayama JI, Wood DL, Yamamoto L. 2001. Principles of patient safety in pediatrics. *Pediatrics* 107(6): 1473–1475.

Lantz MS, Giambanco V, Buchalter EN. 1996. A ten-year review of the effect of OBRA-87 on psychotropic prescribing practices in an academic nursing home. *Psychatric Services* 47(9):951–955.

Lapane KL, Hughes CM. 2004. Which organizational characteristics are associated with increased management of depression using antidepressants in US nursing homes? *Medical Care* 42(10):992–1000.

Leape LL, Cullen DJ, Clapp MD, Burdick E, Demonaco HJ, Erickson JI, Bates DW. 1999. Pharmacists participation on physician rounds and adverse drug events in the intensive care unit. *Journal of the American Medical Association* 282(3):267–270.

Leape LL, Berwick DM, Bates DW. 2002. What practices will most improve safety? Evidence-based medicine meets patient safety. *Journal of the American Medical Association* 288(4): 501–507.

Levick DL. 2005. Response to article. *Pediatrics*: letter, December 23, 2005.

Levine SR. 2001. For the Institute for Safe Medication Practices and the Pediatric Pharmacy Advocacy Group: Guidelines for preventing medication errors in pediatrics. *Journal of Pediatric Pharmacology and Therapeutics* 6:426–442.

Llorente MD, Olsen EJ, Leyva O, Silverman MA, Lewis JE, Rivero J. 1998. Use of antipsychotic drugs in nursing homes: Current compliance with OBRA regulations. *Journal of the American Geriatrics Society* 46(2):198–201.

Lyles A, Zuckerman IH, DeSipio SM, Fulda T. 1998. When warnings are not enough: Primary prevention through drug use review. *Health Affairs* 17(5):175–183.

Malone DC, Abarca J, Hansten PD, Grizzle AJ, Amstrong EP, Van Bergen RC, Duncan-Edgar BS, Solomon SL, Lipton RB. 2004. Identification of serious drug-drug interactions: Results of the partnership to prevent drug-drug interactions. *Journal of the American Pharmaceutical Association* 44(2):142–151.

Manley HJ, Drayer DK, McClaran M, Bender W, Muther RS. 2003. Drug record discrepancies in an outpatient electronic medical record: Frequency, type, and potential impact on patient care at a hemodialysis center. *Pharmacotherapy* 23(2):231–239.

McDonald CJ, Overhage JM, Mamlin BW, Dexter PD, Tierney WM. 2004. Physicians, information technology, and health care systems: A journey, not a destination. *Journal of the American Medical Informatics Association* 11(2):121–124.

McDonald HP, Garg AX, Haynes RB. 2002. Interventions to enhance patient adherence to medication prescriptions: Scientific review. *Journal of the American Medical Association* 288(22):2868–2879.

MCPME (Massachusetts Coalition for the Prevention of Medical Errors). 1999. *Massachusetts Hospital Association: Principles and Best Practices Recommendations to Reduce Medication Errors*. Burlington, MA: Massachusetts Hospital Association.

MCPME. 2005a. *Massachusetts Coalition for the Prevention of Medication Errors*. [Online]. Available: http://www.macoalition.org/publications.shtml [accessed June 17, 2005].

MCPME. 2005b. *MHA Best Practice Recommendations to Reduce Medication Errors*. [Online]. Available: http://www.macoalition.org/documents/Best_Practice_Medication_Errors.pdf [accessed June 17, 2005].

Meredith S, Feldman P, Frey D, Giamarco L, Hall K, Arnold K, Brown NJ, Ray WA. 2002. Improving medication use in newly admitted home healthcare patients: A randomized controlled trial. *Journal of the American Geriatrics Society* 50(9):1484–1491.

Meyer TA. 2000. Improving the quality of the order-writing process for inpatient orders and outpatient prescriptions. *American Journal of Health-System Pharmacy* 57(Suppl. 4): S18–S22.

Monane M, Matthias DM, Nagle BA, Kelly MA. 1998. Improving prescribing patterns for the elderly through an online drug utilization review intervention: A system linking the physician, pharmacist, and computer. *Journal of the American Medical Association* 280(14):1249–1252.

Murphy JE, Forrey RR, Desiraju U. 2004. Community pharmacists' responses to drug-drug interaction alerts. *American Journal of Health-System Pharmacy* 61(14):1484–1487.

Nash IS, Rojas M, Hebert P, Marrone SR, Colgan C, Fisher LA, Caliendo G, Chassin MR. 2005. Reducing excessive medication administration in hospitalized adults with renal dysfunction. *American Journal of Medical Quality* 20(2):64–69.

NCCMERP (National Coordinating Council for Medication Error Reporting and Prevention). 2005a. *National Coordinating Council on Medical Error Reduction and Prevention.* [Online]. Available: http://www.nccmerp.org [accessed June 17, 2005].

NCCMERP. 2005b. *National Coordinating Council on Medical Error Reduction and Prevention: Council Recommendations.* [Online]. Available: http://www.nccmerp.org/councilRecs.html [accessed May 25, 2005].

Nebeker JR, Hoffman JM, Weir CR, Bennett CL, Hurdle JF. 2005. High rates of adverse drug events in a highly computerized hospital. *Archives of Internal Medicine* 165(10):1111–1116.

NICHQ (National Initiative for Children's Healthcare Quality). 2005. *National Initiative for Children's Healthcare Quality.* [Online]. Available: http://www.nichq.org [accessed June 17, 2005].

Novek J, Bettess S, Burke K, Johnston P. 2000. Nurses' perceptions of the reliability of an automated medication dispensing system. *Journal of Nurse Care Quality* 14(2):1–13.

NQF (National Quality Forum). 2003. *Safe Practices for Better Healthcare: A Consensus Report.* Washington, DC: NQF.

NQF. 2005. *National Quality Forum.* [Online]. Available: http://www.qualityforum.org [accessed June 17, 2005].

OIG (Office of the Inspector General). 2001. *Psychotropic Drug Use in Nursing Homes (OEI-02-00-00490).* Washington, DC: Department of Health and Human Services.

Overhage JM, Tierney WM, Zhou XH, McDonald CJ. 1997. A randomized trial of "corollary orders" to prevent errors of omission. *Journal of the American Medical Informatics Association* 4(5):364–375.

Pathways for Medication Safety. 2002. *Tools Developed by the American Hospital Association, Health Research and Educational Trust, the Institute for Safe Medication Practices and the Commonwealth Fund.* [Online]. Available: http://www.medpathways.info/medpathways/index.jsp [accessed Aug 22, 2005].

Patterson ES, Rogers ML, Render ML. 2004. Fifteen best practice recommendations for bar code medication administration in the Veterans Health Administration. *Joint Commission Journal of Quality and Safety* 30(7):355–365.

Pereles L, Romonko L, Murzyn T, Hogan D, Silvius J, Stokes E, Long S, Fung T. 1996. Evaluation of a self-medication program. *Journal of the American Geriatrics Society* 44(2):161–165.

Peterson ED, Chen AY, Kontos MC, Smith SC, Pollack CV, Ohman EM, Roe MT. 2004. Associating changes in hospital non-ST-segment elevation acute coronary syndromes guideline adherence with changes in patient outcomes: Results from CRUSADE. *AHA Circulation* 110(Suppl. III):785.

Peterson JF, Kuperman GJ, Shek C, Patel M, Avorn J, Bates DW. 2005. Guided prescription of psychotropic medications for geriatric inpatients. *Archives of Internal Medicine* 165(7): 802–807.

Phibbs CS, Milstein AS, Delbanco SD, Bates DW. 2005. No proven link between CPOE and mortality. *Pediatrics*. Letter, December 19, 2005.

PMS (Pathways for Medication Safety). 2002. *Pathways for Medication Safety. American Hospital Association, Health Research and Educational Trust, and the Institute for Safe Medication Practices*. [Online]. Available: http://www.hret.org/hret/programs/medpath ways.html [accessed December 5, 2005].

Pronovost P, Weast B, Schwarz M, Wyskiel RM, Prow D, Milanovich SN, Berenholtz S, Dorman T, Lipsett P. 2003. Medication reconciliation: A practical tool to reduce the risk of medication errors. *Journal of Critical Care* 18(4):201–205.

Roberts MS, Stokes JA, King MA, Lynne TA, Purdie DM, Glasziou PP, Wilson DA, McCarthy ST, Brooks GE, de Looze EJ. 2001. Outcomes of a randomized controlled trial of a clinical pharmacy intervention in 52 nursing homes. *British Journal of Clinical Pharmacology* 51(3):257–265.

Robinson V. 2004. *Medication Management in Schools: A Systems Approach to Reducing Risk and Strengthening Quality in School Medication Management*. [Online]. Available: http://www.healthinschools.org/sh/introduction.asp [accessed August 30, 2005].

Rochon PA, Field TS, Bates DW, Lee M, Gavendo L, Erramuspe-Mainard J, Judge J, Gurwitz JH. 2005. Computerized physician order entry with clinical decision support in the long-term care setting: Insights from the baycrest centre for geriatric care. *Journal of the American Geriatrics Society* 53(10):1780–1789.

Rothschild JM, Keohane CA, Cook EF, Orav EJ, Burdick E, Thompson S, Hayes J, Bates DW. 2005. A controlled trial of smart infusion pumps to improve medication safety in critically ill patients. *Critical Care Medicine* 33(3):533–540.

Ruffin DM, Hodge FJ. 1995. Pharmacists' impact on medication administration errors in long-term care facilities. *The Consultant Pharmacist* 10(10):1025–1032.

Rupp MT. 1992. Value of community pharmacists' interventions to correct prescribing errors. *The Annals of Pharmacotherapy* 26(12):1580–1584.

Rupp MT, DeYoung M, Schondelmeyer SW. 1992. Prescribing problems and pharmacist interventions in community practice. *Medical Care* 30(10):926–940.

Schneider JK, Hornberger S, Booker J, Davis A, Kralicek R. 1993. A medication discharge planning program: Measuring the effect on readmissions. *Clinical Nursing Research* 2(1):41–53.

Schwarz HO, Brodowy BA. 1995. Implementation and evaluation of an automated dispensing system. *American Journal of Health-System Pharmacy* 52(8):823–828.

Semla TP, Palla K, Poddig B, Brauner DJ. 1994. Effect of the Omnibus Reconciliation Act 1987 on antipsychotic prescribing in nursing home residents. *Journal of the American Geriatrics Society* 42:648–652.

Sending PharmD candidates to patients' homes can avert potential medication problems. 2000. *Clinical Resource Management* 1(12):186–188.

Shaughnessy AF, D'Amico F. 1994. Long-term experience with a program to improve prescription-writing skills. *Family Medicine* 26(3):168–171.

Shirley KL. 1999. Effect of an automated dispensing system on medication administration time. *American Journal of Health-System Pharmacy* 56(15):1542–1545.

Shojania K, Duncan B, McDonald K, Wachter RM. 2001. *Making Health Care Safer: A Critical Analysis of Patient Safety Practices*. Rockville, MD: Agency for Healthcare Research and Quality; publication 01-E058.

Slater EJ, Glaser W. 1995. Use of OBRA-87 guidelines for prescribing neuroleptics in a VA nursing home. *Psychiatric Services* 46(2):119–121.

Soumerai S, Avorn J. 1987. Predictors of physician prescribing change in an educational experiment to improve medications use. *Medical Care* 25:210–222.

Svarstad BI, Mount JK. 1991. Nursing home resources and tranquilizer use among institutionalized elderly. *Journal of the American Geriatrics Society* 38:769–775.

Svarstad BI, Mount JK. 2001a. Chronic benzodiazepine use in nursing homes: Effects of federal guidelines, resident mix, and nurse staffing. *Journal of the American Geriatrics Society* 49(12):1673–1678.

Svarstad BL, Mount JK. 2001b. *Evaluation of Written Prescription Information Provided in Community Pharmacies, 2001.* Rockville, MD: U.S. Food and Drug Administration.

Svarstad BL, Mount JK, Bigelow W. 2001. Variations in the treatment culture of nursing homes and responses to regulations to reduce drug use. *Pyschiatric Services* 52(5): 666–672.

Taylor LF, Strasser DC, Miller SW, Hennessy CH, Archea C. 2003. Psychotropic drug use in a nursing home: A 6-year retrospective. *The Journal of Applied Gerontology* 22(4): 474–489.

Top-priority actions for preventing adverse drug events in hospitals. 1996. Recommendations of an expert panel. *American Journal of Health-System Pharmacy* 53(7):747–751.

USP (U.S. Pharmacopeia). 2003. *Centre for the Advancement of Patient Safety: CAPSLink, October 2003, Errors Involving Vaccines.* [Online]. Available: http://www.usp.org/patientSafety/newsletters/capsLink [accessed November 17, 2005].

USP. 2005. *U.S. Pharmacopeia.* [Online]. Available: http://www.usp.org [accessed August 22, 2005].

van der Loos TL. 1989. [Control of diabetes mellitus with the insulin pen. Adequately managed?]. *Nederlands Tijdschrift Voor Geneeskunde* 133(23):1183–1184.

VanHaaren AM, Lapane KL, Hughes CM. 2001. Effect of triplicate prescription policy on benzodiazepine administration in nursing home residents. *Pharmacotherapy* 21(10): 1159–1166.

Vivian EM. 2002. Improving blood pressure control in a pharmacist-managed hypertension clinic. *Pharmacotherapy* 22(12):1533–1540.

Weingart SN, Toth M, Eneman J, Aronson MD, Sands DZ, Ship AN, Davis RB, Phillips RS. 2004. Lessons from a patient partnership intervention to prevent adverse drug events. *International Journal for Quality in Health Care* 16(6):499–507.

Zullich SG, Grasela TH, Fiedler-Kelly JB, Gengo FM. 1993. Changes in prescribing patterns in long-term care facilities and impact on incidence of adverse events. *NIDA Research Monograph* 131:294–308.

Index

A

Accountability
  performance measurement for, 330
  state reporting systems for, 92
Accreditation
  curricula recommendations, 344
  recommendations for, 22, 329, 335
  See also Joint Commission on
      Accreditation of Healthcare
      Organizations
Acetaminophen, 31, 83, 115
Acute care
  patient monitoring, 84–85
  technologies for improving, 14
  See also Emergency departments
Acute coronary syndromes, 125, 126, 373,
    375
ADEs. *See* Adverse drug events
Adherence. *See* Nonadherence
Administration of medications
  bar coding technology in, 81
  causes of errors in, 81–83
  error detection by observation, 243–244
  error incidence, 4, 28, 110–112, 114–
      115, 369–371, 376–378, 395–396
  error prevention in ambulatory care, 429
  methods, 80
  overrides of automated warnings, 252

patient self-administration, 83–84
in pediatric care, 114–115, 395–396
prevention of errors in, 80–81, 83, 250–
    251
procedure, 79–80
research needs, 21
responsibility, 79
Adverse drug events (ADEs)
  costs, 130–133, 202
  definition, 3, 4–5, 36, 37, 38, 311–312
  detection methods, 237–239, 241–245
  incidence. *See* Incidence of medication
      errors and ADEs
  monitoring for, 238
  mortality, 28
  patient right to know, 7
  as percentage of adverse events, 28, 67
  potential, 37, 109–110
  preventability, 6, 122, 317
  preventable. *See* Preventable adverse
      drug events
  reporting. *See* Surveillance and reporting
  strategies for preventing, 6, 317
  See also Medication errors
Adverse drug reaction, 38
Agency for Healthcare Research and
    Quality, 240, 245, 247, 409
  Center for Quality Improvement and
      Patient Safety, 25